Between Feast and Famine

Between Feast and Famine

Food, health, and the history of Ghana's long twentieth century

John Nott

UCLPRESS

First published in 2025 by
UCL Press
University College London
Gower Street
London WC1E 6BT

Available to download free: www.uclpress.co.uk

A CIP catalogue record for this book is available from The British Library.

ISBN: 978-1-80008-790-3 (Hbk)
ISBN: 978-1-80008-791-0 (Pbk)
ISBN: 978-1-80008-792-7 (PDF)
ISBN: 978-1-80008-794-1 (epub)
DOI: https://doi.org/10.14324/111.9781800087927

Contents

List of figures

List of tables

List of abbreviations

ADAR	*Agricultural Department Annual Report*
ADB	Agricultural Development Bank, Ghana
BMI	body mass index
CI	confidence interval
CMAM	Community-based Management of Acute Malnutrition
CPP	Convention People's Party, Ghana
CRS	Catholic Relief Services
EDAR	*Education Department Annual Report*
ERP	Economic Recovery Programme, Ghana
FAO	Food and Agriculture Organization, UN
FDC	Food Distribution Corporation, Ghana
FPC	Food Production Corporation, Ghana
(G)DHS	(Ghana) Demographic and Health Survey
GDP	gross domestic product
GLSS	Ghana Living Standards Survey
GNTC	Ghana National Trading Corporation
HMSO	Her/His Majesty's Stationery Office, UK
IMF	International Monetary Fund, UN
IPPF	International Planned Parenthood Federation
LSHTM	London School of Hygiene and Tropical Medicine, UK
MDAR	*Medical Department Annual Report*
MGRS	WHO Multicentre Growth Reference Study
MRC	Medical Research Council, UK
MUAC	mid-upper arm circumference
NCHS	National Centre for Health Statistics, US
NGO	non-governmental organisation
NLC	National Liberation Council, Ghana
NRC	National Redemption Council, Ghana
OFY	Operation Feed Yourself, Ghana
PAMSCAD	Programme of Action to Mitigate the Social Costs of Adjustment, Ghana
PEM	protein-energy malnutrition
PNDC	Provisional National Defence Council, Ghana
PP	Progress Party, Ghana

PRAAD/A/K/T	Public Records and Archives Administration Department, Accra/Kumasi/Tamale, Ghana
RH	Rhodes House Library, Oxford, UK
RUTF	Ready to Use Therapeutic Food
SAP	Structural Adjustment Programme
SD	standard deviation
SFC	State Farms Corporation, Ghana
SMC	Supreme Military Council, Ghana
TNA	The National Archives, London, UK
UGFCC	United Ghana Farming Cooperative Council
UN	United Nations
UNICEF	United Nations International Children's Emergency Fund
USAID	United States Agency for International Development
WHO	World Health Organization, UN
WL	Wellcome Library, London

Acknowledgements

This book has been a long time in the making – so long that I am struggling to remember everyone that helped me at the start. I do remember, though, that Shane Doyle was a constant source of advice and quiet reassurance throughout the PhD project on which this book is based. The other academic and support staff at the University of Leeds, and especially the postgraduate community, also made the School of History a happy home for many years. I was lucky to be working on my PhD with a cohort of inspiring, entertaining Africanist PhD students. Rosie Thornley and Lucy Taylor were invaluable sounding boards and even better company; likewise Nicola Ginsburgh and Josh Doble, whose enduring friendship is a gift of many hours spent together in the Katrina Honeyman Room. Vincent Hirribarren sparked my interest in GIS and the possibilities of digital humanities in African history. Alexander Moradi offered invaluable advice regarding historical anthropometry and generously shared his Gold Coast Regiment data. Parts or all of this book have been read and improved by Gareth Austin, Emma-Louise Anderson, Carina Truyts, Eline Schmeets, Megan Vaughan, and three anonymous readers; conversations with Tom Scott-Smith, Alice Wiemers, Mahama Saaka, and Victor Mogre have also been extremely helpful.

Various grants from the Economic and Research Council (ESRC), the Arts and Humanities Research Council (AHRC), the Worldwide Universities Network, the Royal Historical Society, and the US National Institute of Child Health and Human Development enabled me to live, travel, and train in pursuit of my PhD research. I am hugely grateful for the faith these organisations have shown in me.

The staff at the Library of Congress and the other Kluge Fellows resident at the Library provided a collegial and intellectually stimulating environment in Washington. In fact, library and archival staff in the UK, the USA, and in Ghana have always been helpful and patient in spite of endless requests. I am particularly grateful for the staff at the Public Records and Archives Administration (PRAAD) in Tamale, Kumasi, and especially in Accra – the most fun archive I've had the pleasure of visiting. During a short fellowship in Pennsylvania State University's Population Research Institute, Stephen Matthews and other staff and students cultivated my interest in the possibilities and limitations of modern demography. Courses provided by the University of Michigan and the Max Planck Institute for Demographic Research in Rostock helped further these interests. The last chapter of this book was written while a fellow at the Merian Institute for Advanced Studies in Africa (MIASA) at the University of Ghana. This was a blissful period to reflect on and revise the contents of the book while in the company of a remarkable group of scholars.

At the University of Ghana, alongside colleagues at MIASA, Frank Nyame, Matilda Steiner-Asiedu, Stephen Addae, Samuel Agyei-Mensah, Selasi Woanyah, and Obed Harrison all gave me their time and their attention, for which I am extremely grateful. Elsewhere in Accra, Molly Keogh and Maryanne Mathias have always been willing to open their home/office whenever I was passing through, and I have nothing but fond memories of life in Kanda. In Tamale, my deepest thanks are to Salifu and Mary Mahama for sharing their home with me; I was very happy there. Stephen Ali provided a great deal of help and friendship in Tamale, as did Mohammed Attiah and Selina Aboyinga. In Kumasi, Rudolf Steiner, Ekow Mankatah, and Abena Oteng all provided valuable advice and assistance.

In conducting this research, it has been a great privilege to speak with some of the most important figures in the history of nutrition and public health, both in and outside of Ghana. With Fred Sai, Joseph Oliver-Commey, and Rosanna Agble in Accra; with Sam Bugri in Tamale; and with Hebe Welbourn, Roger Whitehead, and Harold Alderman elsewhere. Their dedication to improving the health and wellbeing of people around the world has been a great source of inspiration.

Although this book was on pause for much of my time there, working at Maastricht University's Faculty of Arts and Social Sciences (FASoS) – alongside Anna Harris, Sally Wyatt, Harro van Lente, Bernike Pasveer and other wonderful colleagues – introduced me to the utility of science and technology studies for the history of medicine. These ideas became an essential part of the book as it later developed. Time well spent with colleagues and friends at FASoS, often at De Poort, was both intellectually rewarding and an indispensable source of comfort during years complicated by Covid lockdowns. For this, and for many other kindnesses, I am eternally grateful to Dani Shanley, Ilias Alami, Shiro Inoue, Ricky Janssen, Andrea Wojcik, and, especially, Rachel Vaden Allison.

More recently, at the University of Edinburgh, I had the time and space to complete some of the outstanding work on this book, and was gifted with a project which complemented its focus. Whilst at Edinburgh

I have been grateful for generative conversations on and around the history of epidemiology with Lukas Engelmann, Carolina Mayes, Cristina Moreno-Lozano, Gladys Kostyrka, Karissa Patton, Rob Smith, Christos Lynteris, Jana Lohrova, Marlee Tichenor, and Kit Lieutaud. The work conducted at Edinburgh has been supported by funding from the European Research Council (ERC) under the European Union's Horizon 2020 Research and Innovation Programme (Grant Agreement No. 947872).

At UCL Press, Pat Gordon Smith believed in this project straight away, while Matthew Browne helped it find its home here. Thanks also to the entire UCL Press production team for turning this manuscript into a reality. Any errors are, of course, entirely my own.

I am always grateful for my family and friends – for the companionship, disinterest, and perspective of old friends outside of academia, and for everyone that put me up and put up with me while I was working on this project. In particular, and years ago, while writing the bulk of this book, my life was anchored to and enriched by the communities of friends living in and passing through our homes at Tordorff Terrace, Harefield Road, and De Lacey Mount. In more recent years I have been blessed with the love, care, and unwavering partnership of Kat Hunfeld, whose team I am endlessly proud to be on. Finally, for my parents. My dad, Terry, encouraged my bookishness and sparked my interest in history when I was very young. My mum, Carol, made me go to school when I would rather have been doing anything else. I may not have even considered university without the encouragement, support, and kindness of my parents.

1
Nutrition in African history, the history of nutrition in Africa

In 1938, Dr F.M. Purcell, an Anglo-Irish physician then in the employ of the Colonial Medical Service, was tasked with surveying the relationship between food and health across what was then the Gold Coast, and what is now Ghana. Purcell's work here was demanded because of two *relatively* recent developments: the formal extension of British-colonial government across huge swathes of the African continent, and the crystallisation of nutrition as a fundamental determinant of health. After several years' study, Purcell's final report divided the Gold Coast into three, applying this new science to the primary ecologies which made up this new polity: the fishing villages along the Atlantic coast; the wealthy central rainforest belt; and the dry Northern savannah. Dividing the colony in this way offered a means to consider 'the diet and nutrition of three contrasting peoples in the Gold Coast ... in relation to their environment and occupation'.[1] In this respect, Purcell's research built out of the then common knowledge that the Gold Coast – as with most of the colonies which made up the British Empire – was a place of remarkable diversity in terms of food economics, food culture, family construction, and the many other socioeconomic determinants of good and bad nutrition. In the decades which have passed since Purcell submitted his report, this salient point has been somewhat forgotten. Instead, with both academic analyses and popular portrayals tending to focus on periods of particular hardship, or on places which are particularly prone to hunger, Africa is habitually cast as a place of famine, food insecurity, and poor nutrition. But this is only part of the story.

The relationship between food and health has changed dramatically since the start of the twentieth century, when nutritional science emerged as a coherent scientific discipline. At the same time, foodways, food economies, and the domestic economies by which people are fed have changed in response to the dramatic shifts of the long twentieth century. Stretching from the late 1800s and into the present, these years are unmatched in terms of political, economic, scientific, social, demographic, and environmental upheaval. In few parts of the world have these changes been more dramatic than in Africa south of the Sahara. Although there are now many histories which speak to this change, a tendency to focus on times of crisis and places of precarity allows for the endurance of what the Nigerian novelist Chimamanda Ngozi Adichie has described as the 'single stories' which tend to define the African past. These include the histories of disease, hunger, and malnutrition which, even if not entirely untrue, are always incomplete.[2]

Take, for instance, John Iliffe's seminal 1987 history of poverty in Africa, which suggested that the continent's primary food-health concern shifted from famine to malnutrition part-way through the colonial period.[3] If sub-Saharan Africa was indeed caught in this process, it was never uniform. Severe famines have affected Ethiopia, Nigeria, the Sahel, the Sudan, and the horn of Africa since the middle of the twentieth century. Less severe, more isolated periods of want have occurred in many other parts of the continent.[4] In other areas, however, there is scant recorded history of hunger. Micro-level histories which exist outside of these time-spaces have already begun to trouble these ideas. In Ghana's rainforest, as in fertile rainforest economies elsewhere, famine was conspicuously absent from the historical record, although other forms of food-related disease may have been widespread, if not necessarily severe.[5]

Concentration on foodways in crisis environments has, however, tended to overlook these spaces, contributing to narratives which naturalise African food insecurity while also erasing histories of food security elsewhere. Focusing on flashpoints of food crisis also fails to countenance the processes which contribute to malnutrition in times and places less affected by dramatic manifestations of dearth. By extending the history of the hungry beyond periods of particular hunger, this book provides the framework for a broader history of nutrition in the twentieth century.[6] By broadening the geographic focus, it offers a means to properly integrate these changes across a more representative range of environments. As epidemics of diet-related chronic disease spread rapidly throughout contemporary Ghana – as elsewhere in the world – these histories provide critical context for the future of public health.

Towards a historical geography of food and health

The lines drawn during the 1884–5 Berlin Conference divided the African continent between the then major European powers, with little thought to the social coherence of these new spaces. The comparison which formed the basis of Purcell's nutrition survey was a direct result of this process. Purcell's survey, and to some extent this book, are directed by the political geography of the Gold Coast as it was administered from the start of the twentieth century (see Figures 1.1 to 1.4). By this time, the Gold Coast Colony, a narrow strip along the Atlantic seaboard, had been a primary entrepôt for the Atlantic trade in gold, ivory, and enslaved people for several centuries.[7] Dotted with European fortifications from the fifteenth century, the Colony came under the formal control of the British Government in 1821. In the fertile rainforests a little way inland, the Asante Kingdom arbitrated the Atlantic trade, straddling the coast and the interior as the region's principal political, economic, and military power during the immediate precolonial period.[8] Asante was brought violently into the British Empire at the end of the 1800s, and only following a drawn-out series of wars which had spanned most of the nineteenth century. The Northern Territories, the last area to come under formal colonial control, grouped together a loose conglomeration of ethnic groups and rival precolonial kingdoms which stretched across the savannah. The unification of these three spaces as the Gold Coast, and their endurance as independent Ghana, offers the ready comparison of markedly different nutrition environments which are, nonetheless, bound together as an ostensibly unified polity. For our purposes, the comparison is starkest between Asante and the North.[9]

Though distinct in many respects, communities in the North of Ghana are united by a depth of shared history which is illustrated by a degree of linguistic commonality. The North's grain-crop economies are fed by a single rainy season which is supplemented by animal wealth, while patrilineal social structures and the greater influence of Islam speak to a trans-Saharan cultural orientation. Denied human capital investment during the colonial period – primarily to encourage labour migration to the more economically productive areas in the south of the colony – Northern history consolidates further into the twentieth century.[10]

Asante, on the other hand, was a global centre of gold production between the eleventh and seventeenth centuries. Gold wealth combined with the kingdom's fertile forest ecology to allow for a remarkable level of economic security; a centralised and expansionist political system;

more varied modes of production; and a degree of cultural homogeneity, defined by Akan languages and matrilineal inheritance.[11] Until the second half of the twentieth century, urbanisation occurred largely in the south. Tied as they were to forest industry and, later, to the Atlantic orientation of the colonial economy, cities required a degree of economic security and political centralisation which was largely absent from this part of the West African savannah. Adjacent to forts, ports, and the

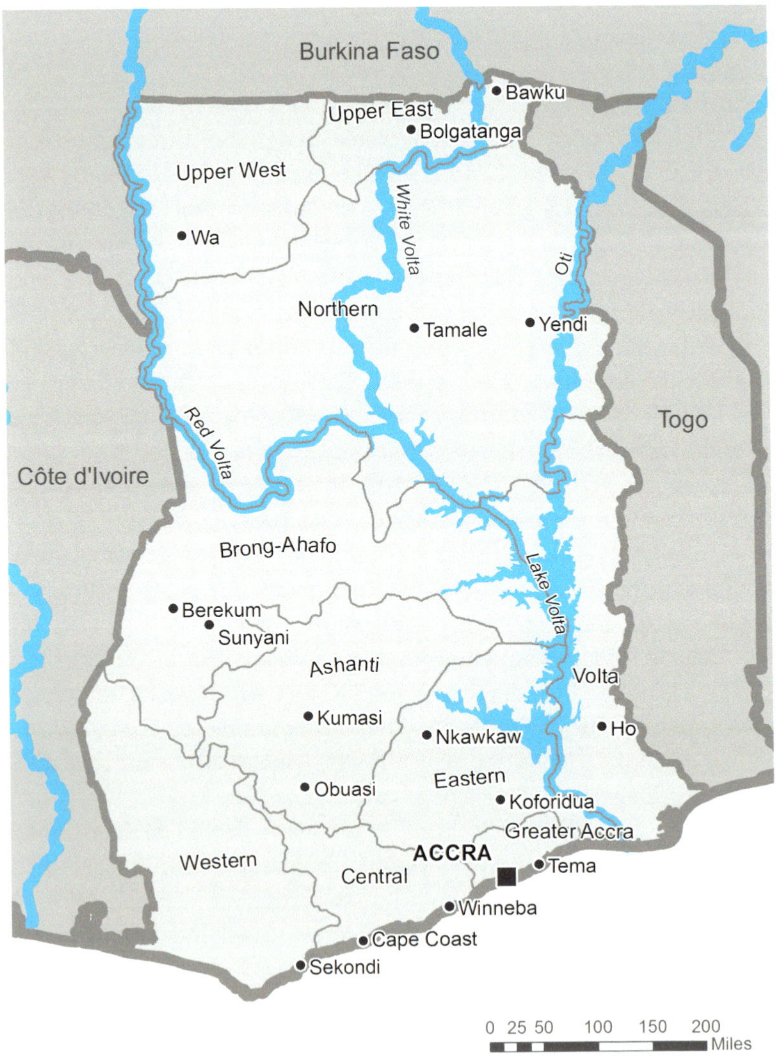

Figure 1.1 Towns and regions in Ghana as administered between 1983 and 2018.[12]

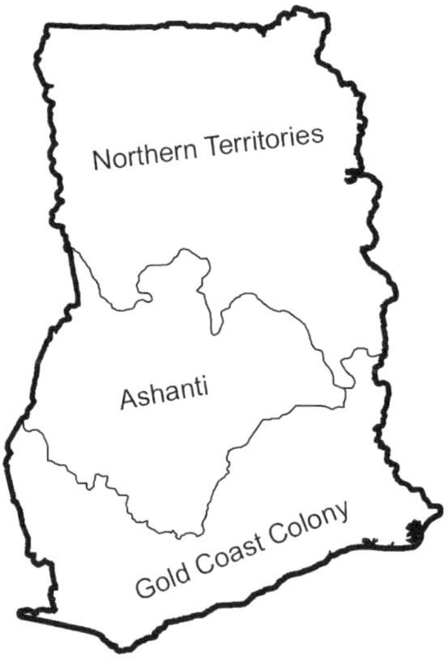

Figure 1.2 The Gold Coast as administered in 1931.[13]

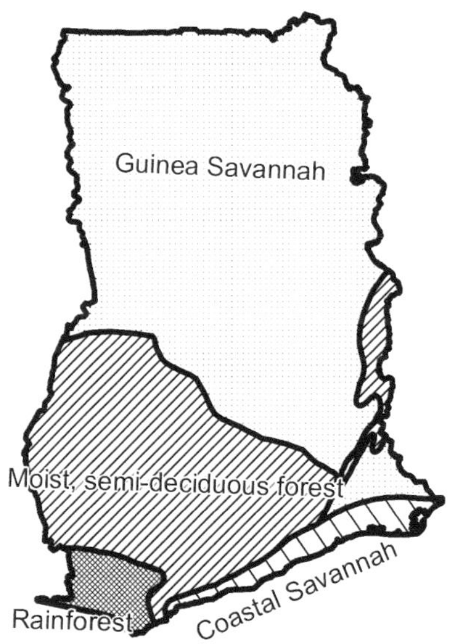

Figure 1.3 Ghana's main agroecological areas.[14]

centres of colonial administration – and with high population densities and increasingly marketised food economies – nutrition in urban areas was often an exaggeration of similar trends apparent in the surrounding forests.[15]

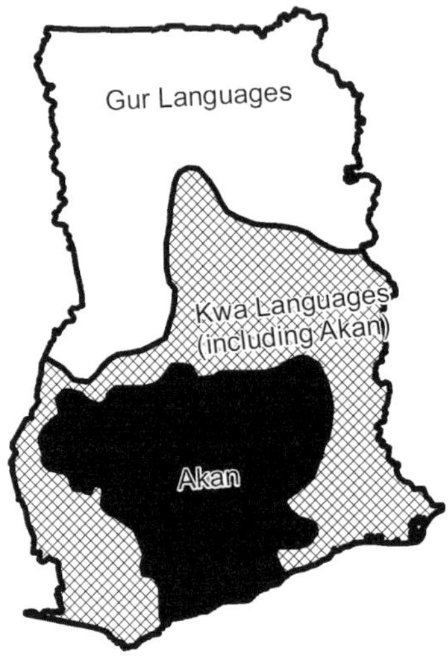

Figure 1.4 Ghana's main ethnolinguistic divisions.[16]

Although recognising the influence of ecology on nutrition, we should be hesitant of often ahistorical ideas around environmental determinism. Instead, critical insights into how these spaces have come into being are drawn from broadly Marxian analyses of economic development.[17] To this end, and alongside Ghana's clear spatial divisions, extreme fluctuations in the Ghanaian macroeconomy also provide readily contrasted historical environments, offering a means to consider the relationship between nutrition and the broad economic shifts which have defined Africa's long twentieth century. As the wealthiest dependency in British-colonial Africa, an independent state which experienced significant post-colonial decline, and the recent posterchild of International Monetary Fund (IMF)-led 'neoliberal' development, Ghana also permits an unusually sharp framework for longitudinal study. From the trade in commodities and, more profitably, people in the precolonial nineteenth century, to the neoliberal turn of the 1980s and 1990s, Ghana's economic trajectory has had various effects on the domestic and food economies which underwrite nutritional health in the distinct geographies which make up the country.

None of the changes of the twentieth century were more dramatic than colonisation and the ascendency of colonial capitalism. Although indigenous forms of profit-producing private industry were common throughout the region prior to the nineteenth century, greater integration of African and imperial commodity and capital markets further induced the buying and selling of land and labour, while also stimulating the slow subsidence of subsistence agriculture and the gradual growth of market-dependency.[18] Yet imperial involvement in Africa's emerging market economies – through interference with land tenure or monopolies on marketing, for instance – has also been said to have stymied the development of a more extensive and efficient cash-crop market, or the expansion of an indigenous capitalist class.[19] Unlike in settler colonies, the majority of land in the Gold Coast remained under African ownership. Colonial promotion of small-scale indigenous producers underlined the environmental advantage and efficiency of the forest economy.[20] Agricultural and economic growth emanated primarily from Asante, which grew to quickly become the centre of global cocoa production. Much of the labour required for economic expansion was derived from the Northern Territories, an area seen by the colonial government as an unproductive and unprofitable backwater. Although Asante was the economic driver of this new polity, the infrastructural investments which act as a boon to good health were concentrated to the south of the cocoa belt, in the expanding towns and cities along the Atlantic coast.

How the ascendency of colonial capitalism variously affected mothers and children is at the heart of this story. Although nutrition influences health throughout our lives, the most dramatic manifestations of deficiency occur in infancy. Since young children have little ability to feed themselves and growing, undeveloped bodies demand more careful feeding than adults – as well as more food and more nutritious food as a percentage of body weight – malnutrition is often not a failure of food but of feeding. This might mean that feeding is insubstantial, imperfect, or unhygienic, especially during breastfeeding or while weaning. Indeed, malnutrition remains a primary cause of child mortality worldwide; a 2013 review suggested that inadequate or inappropriate feeding was responsible for 3.1 million, or 45 per cent, of child deaths internationally.[21] Many of these tragedies can be understood as a failure of 'social reproduction' or 'domestic reproduction'. As contrasted with production for betterment or profit, social reproduction is the basal labour necessary to ensure biological survival across generations. Although the provision of food, shelter, and warmth actively drives the productive labour force, the value granted to social reproduction is historically and spatially transient, and is ultimately dependent on the nature of local modes of production, something which changed radically over the course of the twentieth century.[22] Histories of famine and childhood malnutrition in Africa have emphasised how family relations and social contracts adapted to the new forms and various failures of capitalist production.[23] In this respect, nutritional health is shaped by the intimate and gendered demands of distinct economies, and the relative social value of domestic reproduction in these time-spaces; clinical deficiencies, when they occur, are often the result of domestic constraint and domestic compromise.[24]

The social and spatial orientation of colonial economic development cast a long shadow over independent Ghana. Although it was the first sub-Saharan colony to win independence from Britain, in 1957, the decades which followed highlighted the fragility of Ghana's export economy. The statist, socialist agenda pursued by Kwame Nkrumah, Ghana's first president, provided widespread social reforms – improving access to medicine, education, and other drivers of good health – yet struggled to right macroeconomic concerns. Into the 1970s and early 1980s, economic contraction translated into political turmoil, which, in turn, precipitated a period of widespread food insecurity. As in the nineteenth and early twentieth centuries, these hardships were not suffered evenly across the country. In 1983, Jerry John Rawlings' military government embraced an early IMF/World Bank-led Structural Adjustment Programme (SAP) as a means to both economic and political stability. It was, by and large, successful, and the 2000 general election saw the nation's first transfer of power from one democratically elected regime to another. Four more free and fair elections have since passed. Today a stalwart African democracy, recently exploited oil reserves have helped move Ghana into the World Bank's classification of 'Lower Middle-Income Country'. However, and although democratic process has been forwarded as a necessary insurance against hunger, childhood malnutrition has endured. In what has been described as a 'double burden' of disease, malnutrition today combines with emergent epidemics of diet-related non-communicable disease.[25]

Clearly, the relationship between food and health has changed significantly over the course of the long twentieth century, but change has not been uniform across the country. Any epidemiology of nutrition is a reflection on the historical geography of the foodways and domestic economies which shape dietary and feeding regimens, even if such studies rarely engage with the historical determinants of health. Indeed, this is the basis of a long tradition of nutrition surveying, of which Purcell's report forms an early example. Subsequent national-level nutrition surveys took place in Ghana in 1961–2 and 1986.[26] Since the 1980s, nutrition indices in the form of anthropometric measurements (height, weight, body mass index [BMI], child growth indictors, and so on) have been routinely recorded within the glut of cross-sectional surveys of population health or living standards. These metrics have become political actors in their own right, with improvements in average anthropometry indicating national progress against first the Millennium Development Goals (2000–15) and then the Sustainable Development Goals (2016–30).[27] Although this book is necessarily reliant on such data, it takes that the science of nutrition – just as the nutrition environment itself – must be understood as historically contingent.

Science and its subjects

The social and economic instability of Ghana's long twentieth century was matched only by the instability of nutritional science during this same period. Hugh Trowell, one of the physicians most intimately involved in British-colonial research on nutrition in Africa, summed up the capricious nature of the field in a 1975 article, complaining that 'experts now tell me that I must call it Protein-Energy-Malnutrition, but never mind; probably they will change it again'.[28] His frustration is not entirely surprising; Trowell had spent much of the 1940s and 1950s conflicted over what to call the confounding manifestation of childhood malnutrition which he had been seeing with some regularity in hospitals across Kenya and Uganda. At first he wrote about 'infantile pellagra' and then 'malignant malnutrition'.[29] Eventually he came to settle on 'kwashiorkor', a word taken from the Ga language and from earlier observations of infant illness in the area around Accra, today the capital city of Ghana.[30] After having literally written the book on kwashiorkor in 1954, Trowell clearly thought that the name, at least, had been put to bed.[31] The problem, however, was apparently the experts:

> Experts should never be consulted about the status of a new idea in medicine. They are almost always wrong; they have climbed on the steps of their own research to a pinnacle of great eminence; they are hostile to a new idea which may challenge their pre-conceived notions.[32]

Unhappy with the pedants directing subsequent science (and apparently unaware of the irony of this statement), Trowell also goes on to describe his 1935 visit to a Harley Street 'palace of the expert', a trip which ended up misdirecting his own research into malnutrition.[33] The experts that could be trusted, as detailed in Trowell's intellectual genealogy of kwashiorkor, were the colonial service physicians practising and publishing from all over a colonised continent. Curiously, Trowell fails to consider that colonisation might have played a role, either in the incidence of nutritional disease or in the development of his own expertise.

This is another book which is often about kwashiorkor. As with Trowell's history, it takes that it is impossible to disentangle expert opinion from the competition and egoism inherent within narratives of scientific discovery.[34] Unlike Trowell's accounting, however, this history suggests that the incidence of childhood malnutrition in twentieth-century Africa and scientific analyses of such deficiencies are impossible to divorce from the political economy of colonial government.

The history of health is, then, as much a history of medicine as a history of disease. Unpicking the relationship between European imperial government and the development of nutritional science has proved a fertile site for research into the history of medicine over the past several decades. Under empire, nutrition research was often an appendage of 'tropical medicine', a geographically specific form of medical science which often involved contrasting the apparent ill-health of colonised peripheries with the apparent vigour of metropolitan centres.[35] The orientation of this research encouraged a particular focus on clinical manifestations of deficiency. Indeed, the very concept of malnutrition was 'discovered' in British-colonial India in the interwar years.[36] Later, in African colonies, research shifted in order to focus on epidemics of malnutrition in childhood.[37] In these spaces, physicians were confronted by dramatic manifestations of deficiency, kwashiorkor in particular, which was rarely seen in British hospitals at the time.[38] However, couched as it was in the imperial logic of the 'civilising mission', much of the scientific analysis struggled to align the epidemiology of deficiency diseases with relatively recent changes to foodways and domestic economies. Instead, conclusions tended to emphasise hierarchical assumptions regarding diets and childrearing norms in Africa, and their distance from those commonly found in Europe.[39]

Loosely defined, difficult to measure, and poorly understood by both policymakers and consumers, nutritional science has always been remarkably subjective. According to Gyorgy Scrinis, this is because the 'nutritionist' paradigm – the dominant form of dietetics throughout the twentieth century – involves the reductive concentration on individual nutrients at the expense of the social interactions between food and health.[40] Concentration on the chemical makeup of food ignores the relevance of feeding in the aetiology of deficiency while also facilitating the appropriation and vulgarisation of nutritional science. Even the word 'malnutrition' is suitably vague. The opacity of the nutritionist paradigm, and the instability of nutritional science, has contributed to the enduring trend of marketised solutions to nutritional deficiency. This often-ignominious history takes in the assent of fortified foods, dietary supplements, 'nutraceuticals', and 'superfoods'.[41] The celebration of specific foods or food groups often derives from insidious ties to the prevailing political economy. As Sidney Mintz explained in his classic study of sugar, for instance, by 'provisioning, sating – and, indeed, drugging – farm and factory workers, [sugar] sharply reduced the overall cost of creating and sustaining the metropolitan proletariat'.[42] Later, as we will see, the colonial-era promotion of baby formula as a means to assuage the growing weight of childrearing ultimately led to an epidemic of what would come to be described as 'commerciogenic malnutrition'.[43] The nature of nutrition epidemiology means that it is usually only much later that the unintended effects of dietary interventions come to be understood.

Recognising the instability and mutability of scientific fact is essential for a more critical form of historical epidemiology, one which takes that both disease and the scientific study of disease are products of a given time and place. Or, in the words of Hannah Landecker, and taken from her history of metabolic disease, 'knowledge is a product of its times. However, times are also a product of knowledge.'[44] In this sense, it is impossible to delineate changes in disease incidence without also considering the technoscientific changes which make illnesses delineable and explain their incidence. Likewise, it is impossible to delineate changes in medical science without also considering the disease environment which it develops in response to. Disease and medicine are, then, co-produced and reflective of the time-spaces which culture their co-production. In our specific case, epidemiological shifts in nutritional health have resulted from the conceptual history of what foods are good and bad for us, as much as from empirical changes to food supply and domestic reproduction.[45]

Detail and definition

The slippery science of nutrition, and the tangled spatial histories of twentieth-century Ghana, leave us with many points of detail which deserve definition, as well as plenty of unstable definitions. Although wary of prescriptive statements about the dietetic or social determinants of good and bad nutrition, detailing nutritional change requires some discussion of nutritional science, as well as some consideration of how nutritional science has been interpreted (or ignored) by historians of Africa.

For reasons related to epidemiological import as well as scientific preoccupation, childhood deficiencies have dominated both the science and history of nutrition in twentieth-century Africa. Initially understood as a severe manifestation of protein deficiency, kwashiorkor would, in later years, come to sit at one extreme of a spectrum of childhood malnutrition described as protein-energy or protein-calorie malnutrition (PEM or PCM). At the other extreme is 'marasmus', which, deriving from the Greek 'to wither', describes the physiological process of starvation. Marasmus generally occurs in infants and is characterised by the progressive wasting of subcutaneous tissue because of inadequate calories and proteins. Marasmus may result from an acute gastric infection or from a simple lack of food. Marasmus is sometimes described as synonymous with 'wasting' or 'undernutrition', itself often taken as a distinct form of malnutrition, one which 'is primarily due to inadequate intake of calories whereas malnutrition is caused by inadequacy of particular, or several, essential nutrients, thus a person who is undernourished is also malnourished, though the converse may not hold'.[46] Kwashiorkor is most often observed in older children, usually during or after weaning and before the age of five or six. The 'classical' theory of kwashiorkor causation argues that kwashiorkor results from a diet moderately adequate in calories but grossly deficient in protein.[47] Alongside the retarded growth common across the spectrum of PEM, symptoms of kwashiorkor include oedema, changes in skin and hair pigmentation, diarrhoea, loss of appetite, irritability, lethargy, anaemia, and the fatty degeneration of the liver. A visually dramatic disease with a complicated pathology that is still not fully understood, as well as a much poorer prognosis than marasmus, kwashiorkor offered a worthy problem for mid-century science – a 'riddle' which, even into the 2000s, required protracted inpatient treatment.[48] Yet, even as early as the 1960s, nutritionists working primarily in Uganda explained that cases of pure kwashiorkor or pure marasmus were very rare, as 'most children have mixed deficiencies ... which defy short precise nomenclature'.[49] As such, the dualistic approach to PEM is not often used today. Moderate or severe acute malnutrition (MAM or SAM) is instead defined according to deviation away from growth standards. However, the telltale oedema associated with kwashiorkor still suggests a 'severe' or 'complicated' form of malnutrition.

Many histories of twentieth-century Africa make some note of childhood malnutrition, but few engage with the various and complex aetiologies of deficiency. Often claims are made as part of important debates regarding changes to food systems and food security during this period. However, as both an empirical health concern intimately related to food supply and a socio-medical construct shaped by the political economy of medical consensus, nutrition is a peripheral aspect of famine and food insecurity as well as something entirely disconnected from hunger. Here nutritionist dietetics – already a historically determined influence on the epidemiology of nutritional illness – is often employed in rhetorical arguments regarding the African past.[50] For instance, and again returning to his pioneering history of African poverty, John Iliffe has argued that 'nutrition was not only the most important food problem of late-colonial Africa but also a sensitive indicator of poverty'.[51] While the first point is likely true for the continent writ large, we should be wary of the linear relationship drawn between poverty and poor nutrition. This ready conflation of poverty and malnutrition is, however, prominent in many histories of Africa. Paul Harrison, for instance, has explained how 'malnutrition is the most acute physical expression of absolute poverty: it is poverty imprinted on human flesh and bone'.[52] This is clearly an over-simplification. Where hunger is a conscious acknowledgement of want, malnutrition is a subconscious, physiological response to dietary inadequacy often couched in culturally and socially subjective understandings of dietary adequacy. Where food may be considered a largely inelastic commodity, 'nutritious' food is much less so, due in part to the pull of food culture. This is not to say that malnutrition and poverty are not interconnected, but to instead emphasise that they are not interdependent.

Many of these arguments are used to colour the history of famine in Africa. Over the past several decades, a broad consensus has formed around the conclusion that population pressure, epidemic disease, and increased demands for labour accompanied increased food insecurity in the decades immediately following the colonial invasion.[53] Yet the precise nature of the early-colonial food crisis is a point of debate. Iliffe has, for instance, argued that colonial famine relief assuaged the threat of epidemic starvation but that the structural impact of colonial rule meant that 'food was regularly available to those who could afford it and regularly scarce for those who could not'.[54] Michael Watts, by contrast, has suggested that famine became more common but less severe under colonialism, that increased competition under colonial capitalism undermined the social contracts and agricultural diversity which had contributed to food security in earlier years.[55] Although commonly taken to be a fundamental juncture in the historiography, it might be argued that Iliffe's endemic hunger as a result of new forms of poverty and Watt's definition of mild famine resulting from falling patronage entitlements are not entirely separate issues. In support of this, and as a history which argues for a more holistic approach to the relationship between food and health, this book assumes a loose but extreme definition of famine as an atypical increase in mortality resulting from epidemic hunger.[56] Such a definition is loose because increased famine mortality is largely the result of infectious disease, and the synergistic relationship between infection and poor nutrition, rather than starvation itself. It is extreme because, as food crises occurring over the past several decades have shown, epidemic hunger does not necessarily lead to increased mortality.[57] By the later decades of the twentieth century, more efficient transport and communications improved state-wide famine relief systems and lessened the severity of famine across the continent.[58] Histories of these later famines have generally focused on the political economy of hunger; on how powerful actors have created or exploited famine in the absence of accountability.[59] Most of these histories have benefited from the malleability of Amartya Sen's 'entitlement approach' to famine.[60] Here, famine can occur even without any aggregate decline in food production. Instead, the victims of famine are those individuals or groups that are unable to acquire food, and have therefore lost their entitlement to food, in any given context. By directing the discourse away from supply-side analyses focusing on food availability, the entitlement approach allows famine to be understood as a group-specific demand failure influenced by disparities in social capital and socioeconomic status. Entitlement is also a useful way to think about malnutrition, at least in the extent to which nutrition relates to crises of food acquisition, dietetic sacrifices, and other dietary responses to worsening economic conditions.[61]

Although detailing the relationship between nutrition and famine over the course of the twentieth century, this is not a history of famine in and of itself. Instead, the indices routinely engaged in the analysis of nutrition are 'nutritional status' and 'nutrition security'. While these are interrelated concepts, it is important to recognise that they are not the same. As a measure of an individual's nutritional health, nutritional status is extrapolated from anthropometry, as well as from the presentation of clinical nutritional disease. Although an individual measure, nutritional status is often averaged out across communities, regions, or nations. Using adult height as a proxy for nutritional status during infancy, the recent emergence of anthropometric history has lent a degree of empiricism to the history of nutritional status, with the average adult height achieved by a given population taken to be an indicator for the nutrition environment during childhood.[62] Indeed, small-scale studies readily illuminate the relationship between height and standard of living; a 1979 Ghanaian study, for instance, found that a 12-year-old in an expensive Accra private school would, on average, tower over their compatriots in deprived parts of the city by a remarkable 12 centimetres.[63] Borrowing these conclusions, longitudinal height data have been compiled from military enlistees, for births in the nineteenth century, as well as from cross-sectional surveys conducted routinely from the 1980s on.[64] Data on infant growth rates, often also taken from these same cross-sectional surveys, can also be used to detail nutritional status in a given time and place. Likewise, hospital data can suggest the community incidence of clinical deficiency but – as with all these datasets – has limitations in the form of inconsistent diagnoses, diagnostic preoccupation, and other questions relating to standardisation and comparability. The use of adult height can also be misleading, as it more properly reflects nutritional status throughout childhood *and* adolescence. Adults born in the Ghanaian savannah are consistently taller than those born in the forest, even though limited health and education infrastructure, a harsher disease environment, and less secure food economies leave children in the North with considerably worse nutrition indices during infancy. Yet widespread 'nutrition insecurity' during these formative years is apparently offset at other points in the life course.[65] In contrast with nutritional status, nutrition security is much harder to measure. More closely related to systemic factors which influence nutritional health, nutrition security reflects the adequacy of food markets, the negative effects of disease environments, and the nature of diet and childrearing practices. Nutrition insecurity suggests a degree of vulnerability which is not necessarily realised and so is less apparent over the short and medium term. What the concept of nutrition security offers, however, is a tool to explain longitudinal, spatial, and social disparities in nutritional status, as well as insight into the epidemiology of clinical deficiency.

Chapter outlines

While the aims of the book and its approach to the history of health are diverse at times, its focus is straightforward, considering the historical epidemiology of nutrition from period to period and place to place. However, and in order to put this narrative history into proper context, the next chapter, Chapter 2, examines the medicine of nutrition as practised in Africa during the first half of the twentieth century. By focusing on the specific history of kwashiorkor, this chapter highlights how the politically informed othering of African nutrition dictated the medicine of malnutrition for much of the century. Chapter 3 gives further context to twentieth-century changes by detailing the social reproduction of health and nutrition in the immediate precolonial period, using demography and anthropology to speak to the nature of nutrition on the eve of colonisation. The various food environments and ecologies of nineteenth-century West Africa shaped understandings of wealth and poverty across discrete spaces, influencing family construction and providing continuing context for the social epidemiology of malnutrition.

Chapters 4 and 5 approach the most important aspects of malnutrition in the Southern and Northern Gold Coast under colonial rule. Focusing primarily on Asante, Chapter 4 concerns the ways in which childrearing and social reproduction changed in response to the new demands of colonial capitalism. In Asante, as elsewhere, average nutritional status improved in conjunction with economic growth. Despite this, the incidence of clinical deficiency saw limited improvement and may have even worsened with the devaluation of Asante motherhood. Here, the nutrition security of dependent children was negatively affected by constraints on social reproduction which were particularly evident across the cocoa belt. These gendered economic shifts pre-empted the rise of 'commerciogenic' malnutrition and precipitated the later epidemic of infant malnutrition which occurred following the market contraction of the 1970s and 1980s. In contrast with the forests, the initial trend of almost exclusively male migration allowed urban women in Southern cities a particularly advantageous position in a period when the value of domestic chores was heavily inflated, underpinning the nutritional advantage of urban childhood into the 1950s. In Chapter 5, the interaction between malnutrition, food insecurity, and migration in the North is addressed in view of established discourses regarding colonial coercion and Northern underdevelopment. Governmental neglect undoubtedly sidelined Northern health and coercion surely damaged Northern food security in these years. However, the development of the colony-wide labour market also provided new avenues for economic self-determination and new forms of wealth and security for those able to secure them, alongside new sources of gendered and generational conflict.

Following on from these colonial histories, Chapter 6 charts the tumultuous history of Ghana's early independent statehood, as well as the distribution of what were, on a national scale, unprecedented levels of malnutrition, peaking in the early 1980s. Political and economic instability in these years exposed the unevenness of Ghanaian development. That widespread want and epidemic malnutrition followed the collapse of the food market revealed the fundamental fragility of Ghana's twentieth-century economy. Acting as a companion to Chapter 2, Chapter 7 details concurrent developments in nutritional science after independence and during the nadir of Africa's twentieth-century crisis, the Malthusian explanations for this crisis and the nature of subsequent, 'neoliberal' approaches to nutrition care. Although nutritional science had moved on from its overtly imperialist construction, change was extremely slow and developments, when they occurred, still tended to reflect a Western political economy of nutrition. In view of the 'neoliberal' turn in both politics and medicine, Chapter 8 considers the epidemiology of malnutrition since Structural Adjustment fundamentally reshaped the Ghanaian economy in the early 1980s. This questions the relationship between malnutrition and market-led development, as well as the extent to which malnutrition can be addressed under the cultural hegemony of neoliberalism and with the tools thus provided. The last chapter, Chapter 9, works as an epilogue to this long history of food and health, initially framing the rise of metabolic disorder as another epidemiological inheritance of the neoliberal political economy. However, as non-communicable diseases which have nonetheless been spreading rapidly, nascent epidemics of diet-related chronic disease echo the outbreaks of kwashiorkor which emerged in the middle of the twentieth century, further illustrating the necessity of historical reflection in the analysis and amelioration of illness in the present.

Notes

1 Public Records and Archives Administration Department, Accra (PRAAD)/ADM/11/1/1294, F.M. Purcell, 'Report of the standing committee to study the important question of human nutrition, 1937–41', p. 138.

2 How these stories seep into analyses of health in the present is explored in Nolwazi Mkhwanazi, 'Medical Anthropology in Africa: The Trouble with a Single Story', *Medical Anthropology*, 35.2 (2016), 193–202.

3 John Iliffe, *The African Poor: A History* (Cambridge: Cambridge University Press, 1987), p. 160.

4 For a survey history of famine, see Cormac Ó Gráda, *Famine: A Short History* (Princeton, NJ: Princeton University Press, 2009).

5 See, for instance, Amanda L. Logan, *The Scarcity Slot: Excavating Histories of Food Security in Ghana* (Berkeley, CA: University of California Press, 2020); John Nott, 'Malnutrition in a Modernising Economy: The Changing Aetiology and Epidemiology of Malnutrition in an African Kingdom, Buganda c.1940–73', *Medical History*, 60.2 (2016), 229–49.

6 In this respect, this book also builds on Elias Mandala's 2005 challenge to African history, which had always discussed 'food or hunger but never the two together'. See Elias C. Mandala, *The End of Chidyerano: A History of Food and Everyday Life in Malawi, 1860–2004* (Portsmouth, NH: Heinemann, 2005), p. 240.

7 I was once told that 'colonial Ghana' is a misnomer, since Ghana was never colonised. The Gold Coast is therefore used to refer to the territory when under colonial rule. To avoid confusion, the administrative area comprising the southernmost stretch of the Gold Coast between the Atlantic and Asante, the Gold Coast Colony, is rarely referred to. Where it is, 'Colony' refers to the administrative area, while 'colony' refers to the entirety of the Gold Coast (see Figure 1.2).

8 'Asante' refers to the historical Asante Kingdom or, less precisely, to those areas which share a cultural, ecological, and economic homogeneity defined by Akan culture, forest agriculture, and matrilineal inheritance. This is an area similar in scope to that of the Crown Colony of Ashanti, as administered by the British from 1901–57 (see Figure 1.2). When discussing the Crown Colony or the much smaller administrative region in postcolonial Ghana (see Figure 1.1), 'Ashanti' or 'Ashanti Region' are used, as per the anglicisation of the word.

9 When discussing what were, between 1983 and 2018, the three northernmost regions of Ghana (Northern, Upper East, and Upper West), the North or Northern are used, capitalised, and employed in contrast with the South or Southern. The administrative 'Northern Region' is distinct and specified wherever used (see Figure 1.1).

10 There are, in comparison with Asante, far fewer histories of the North. Important works include Ivor Wilks, Nehemia Levtzion, and Bruce M. Haight, *Chronicles from Gonja: A Tradition of West African Muslim Historiography* (Cambridge: Cambridge University Press, 1986); Sean Hawkins, *Writing and Colonialism in Northern Ghana: The Encounter Between the LoDagaa and 'the World on Paper'* (Toronto: University of Toronto Press, 2002); Carola Lentz, *Ethnicity and the Making of History in Northern Ghana* (Edinburgh: Edinburgh University Press, 2006). However, due in part to its economic insecurity, at least relative to the forest, the North of Ghana has been an important site for the history of food and food-related research. See, for instance, Jack Goody, *Cooking, Cuisine and Class: A Study in Comparative Sociology* (Cambridge: Cambridge University Press, 1982).

11 Asante's importance in the nineteenth century has also translated into a wealth of historical analysis. See, for instance, Kwame Arhin, 'The Structure of Greater Ashanti (1700–1824)', *Journal of African History*, 8.1 (1967), 65–85; Ivor Wilks, *Asante in the Nineteenth Century: The Structure and Evolution of a Political Order* (Cambridge: Cambridge University Press, 1975); T.C. McCaskie, *Asante Identities: History and Modernity in an African Village, 1850–1950* (Edinburgh: Edinburgh University Press, 2001); Gareth Austin, *Labour, Land, and Capital in Ghana: From Slavery to Free Labour in Asante, 1807–1956* (Rochester, NY: University of Rochester Press, 2005).

12 This map, and other maps throughout this book, have been made with public-domain data from Natural Earth <http://www.naturalearthdata.com> [accessed 3 December 2015].

13 Administrative areas derived from Gold Coast Government, *The Gold Coast Appendices, Containing Comparative Returns and General Statistics of the 1931 Census* (Accra: Government Printer, 1932); for the history of Ghana's spatial administration, see R. Bagulo Bening, *Ghana: Administrative Areas and Boundaries, 1874–2009* (Accra: Ghana Universities Press, 2010).

14 Agroecological areas are based on E.A. Boateng, *A Geography of Ghana* (Cambridge: Cambridge University Press, 1966).

15 Claire Robertson and Gracia Clark's respective accounts of market systems in Accra and Kumasi have provided detailed analysis of the gendered nature of urban food economies. See Claire Robertson, *Sharing the Same Bowl? A Socioeconomic History of Women and Class in Accra, Ghana* (Bloomington, IN: Indiana University Press, 1984); Gracia Clark, *Onions Are My Husband: Survival and Accumulation by West African Market Women* (Chicago, IL: University of Chicago Press, 1994).

16 Ethnolinguistic divisions are based on M. Paul Lewis, Charles D. Fennig, and Gary F. Simons, *Ethnologue: Languages of the World* (Dallas, TX: SIL International, 2016).

17 These ideas, defined largely by dependency theorists in the 1970s, have gone somewhat out of vogue, but it is difficult to conduct a comparative spatial history of Ghanaian development without them. See, for a general elucidation of such ideas, Samir Amin, *Unequal Development: An Essay on the Social Formations of Peripheral Capitalism* (Hassocks, Sussex: Harvester Press, 1976); for Ghana specifically, see R. Bagulo Bening, *Ghana: Regional Boundaries and National Integration* (Accra: Ghana Universities Press, 1999); Jacob Songsore, *Regional Development in Ghana: The Theory and the Reality* (Accra: Woeli, 2003).

18 See, for the nineteenth century, Gareth Austin, '"No Elders Were Present": Commoners and Private Ownership in Asante, 1807–96', *The Journal of African History*, 37.1 (1996), 1–30.

19 See, for Ghana, Geoffrey Barry Kay, *The Political Economy of Colonialism in Ghana: A Collection of Documents and Statistics, 1900–1960* (Cambridge: Cambridge University Press, 1972); Kathryn Firmin-Sellers, *The Transformation of Property Rights in the Gold Coast: An Empirical Analysis Applying Rational Choice Theory* (Cambridge: Cambridge University Press, 1996).

20 Gareth Austin, 'African Economic Development and Colonial Legacies', *International Development Policy*, 1 (2010), 11–32.

21 Robert E. Black et al., 'Maternal and Child Undernutrition and Overweight in Low-Income and Middle-Income Countries', *The Lancet*, 382.9890 (2013), 427–51.

22 See, for instance, Cindi Katz, 'Vagabond Capitalism and the Necessity of Social Reproduction', *Antipode*, 33 (2001), 709–28.

23 See, for instance, Mandala, *The End of Chidyerano*; Megan Vaughan, *The Story of an African Famine: Gender and Famine in Twentieth-Century Malawi* (Cambridge: Cambridge University Press, 1987); Henrietta L. Moore and Megan Vaughan, *Cutting down Trees: Gender, Nutrition, and Agricultural Change in the Northern Province of Zambia, 1890–1990*, Social History of Africa (London: James Currey, 1994); Mary Howard and Ann V. Millard, *Hunger and Shame: Poverty and Child Malnutrition on Mount Kilimanjaro* (London: Routledge, 1997).

24 Although not dealing with these questions explicitly, the most valuable gender history for this book is Jean Allman and Victoria Tashjian, *'I Will Not Eat Stone': A Women's History of Colonial Asante* (Oxford: James Currey, 2000).

25 Amartya Sen, *Development as Freedom* (Oxford: Oxford University Press, 1999); Samuel Agyei-Mensah and Ama de-Graft Aikins, 'Epidemiological Transition and the Double Burden of Disease in Accra, Ghana', *Journal of Urban Health*, 87 (2010), 879–97.

26 Aside from snatches of published material, both of these national surveys seem to have been lost to time. However, hospital records and smaller-scale local surveys offer valuable additional data throughout.

27 Vincanne Adams (ed.), *Metrics: What Counts in Global Health* (Durham, NC: Duke University Press, 2016); Justyna Bandola-Gill, Sotiria Grek, and Marlee Tichenor, *Governing the Sustainable Development Goals: Quantification in Global Public Policy* (Cham: Springer International Publishing, 2022).

28 H.C. Trowell, 'The Beginning of the Kwashiorkor Story in Africa', *Central African Journal of Medicine*, 21.1 (1975), 1–5 (p. 1).

29 H.C. Trowell, 'Infantile Pellagra', *Transactions of the Royal Society of Tropical Medicine and Hygiene*, 33 (1940), 389–404; H.C. Trowell, 'Malignant Malnutrition (Kwashiorkor)', *Transactions of the Royal Society of Tropical Medicine and Hygiene*, 42.5 (1949), 417–42.

30 Cicely D. Williams, 'Kwashiorkor: A Nutritional Disease of Children Associated with a Maize Diet', *The Lancet*, 226 (1935), 1151.

31 H.C. Trowell, J.N.P. Davies, and R.F.A. Dean, *Kwashiorkor* (London: Edward Arnold, 1954).

32 Trowell, 'The Beginning', p. 2.

33 Trowell, 'The Beginning', p. 2.

34 The unintended effects of earlier expertise are vividly detailed in Timothy Mitchell, *Rule of Experts: Egypt, Techno-Politics, Modernity* (Berkeley, CA: University of California Press, 2002); this builds on a wealth of science studies research into the social construction of scientific fact. See, for a classic example, Bruno Latour and Steve Woolgar, *Laboratory Life: The Construction of Scientific Facts* (London: Sage Publications, 1979).

35 Megan Vaughan, *Curing Their Ills: Colonial Power and African Illness* (Stanford, CA: Stanford University Press, 1991); Warwick Anderson, *Colonial Pathologies: American Tropical Medicine, Race, and Hygiene in the Philippines* (Durham, NC: Duke University Press, 2006).

36 Michael Worboys, 'The Discovery of Colonial Malnutrition Between the Wars', in *Imperial Medicine and Indigenous Societies*, ed. by David Arnold (Manchester: Manchester University Press, 1988), pp. 208–25; David Arnold, 'The "Discovery" of Malnutrition and Diet in Colonial India', *The Indian Economic & Social History Review*, 31.1 (1994), 1–26.

37 Jennifer Tappan, *The Riddle of Malnutrition: The Long Arc of Biomedical and Public Health Interventions in Uganda* (Athens, OH: Ohio University Press, 2017).

38 Sjoerd Rijpma, *David Livingstone and the Myth of African Poverty and Disease: A Close Examination of His Writing on the Pre-Colonial Era* (Leiden: Brill, 2015), pp. 436–7.

39 Diana Wylie, *Starving on a Full Stomach: Hunger and the Triumph of Cultural Racism in Modern South Africa* (Charlottesville, VA: University Press of Virginia, 2001); Cynthia Brantley, *Feeding Families: African Realities and British Ideas of Nutrition and Development in Early Colonial Africa* (Portsmouth, NH: Heinemann, 2002).

40 Gyorgy Scrinis, *Nutritionism: The Science and Politics of Dietary Advice* (New York: Columbia University Press, 2013).

41 Lisa Haushofer, *Wonder Foods: The Science and Commerce of Nutrition* (Berkeley, CA: University of California Press, 2022).

42 Sidney W. Mintz, *Sweetness and Power: The Place of Sugar in Modern History* (New York: Penguin, 1986), p. 180.

43 D.B. Jelliffe, 'Commerciogenic Malnutrition?', *Nutrition Reviews*, 30.9 (1972), 199–205.

44 Hannah Landecker, 'Postindustrial Metabolism: Fat Knowledge', *Public Culture*, 25.3 (2013), 495–522 (p. 497).

45 In an attempt to do just this, this book follows calls from economic history for more methodologically pluralist approaches to the causal analysis of health throughout history. See Morten Jerven, 'A Clash of Disciplines? Economists and Historians Approaching the African Past', *Economic History of Developing Regions*, 26.2 (2011), 111–24.

46 N. Kakwani, *On Measuring Undernutrition* (Helsinki: WIDER, 1986), p. 1.

47 It should be recognised that the 'classical' approach to kwashiorkor is not universally accepted. See, for instance, M.H. Golden, 'The Development of Concepts of Malnutrition', *The Journal of Nutrition*, 132.7 (2002), 2117S–2122S.

48 'Riddle' is Jennifer Tappan's apt description of this history: Tappan, *Riddle*; on the contested pathology of kwashiorkor, see, for instance, Golden, 'Development of Concepts'; for a textbook discussion of PEM as understood today, see Truswell, 'Protein-Energy Malnutrition'; for current approaches to the management of malnutrition, see Steve Collins et al., 'Management of Severe Acute Malnutrition in Children', *The Lancet*, 368.9551 (2006), 1992–2000.

49 D.B. Jelliffe and J.P. Stanfield, 'Protein Deficiencies and Calorie Deficiencies', *The Lancet*, 288.7469 (1966), 207–8.

50 Amanda Logan's recent history of Banda, on the edge of the Asante forest, has methodically addressed the endurance of similar tropes in academic writing on food in Africa; see Logan, *The Scarcity Slot*.

51 Iliffe, *African Poor*, p. 161.

52 Paul Harrison, *The Greening of Africa: Breaking through in the Battle for Land and Food* (London: Paladin, 1987), p. 21.

53 Sjoerd Rijpma, 'Malnutrition in the History of Tropical Africa', *Civilisations*, 43.2 (1996), 45–63; Shane Doyle, 'Population Decline and Delayed Recovery in Bunyoro, 1860–1960', *Journal of African History*, 41.3 (2000), 429–58; Jan Kuhanen, *Poverty, Health, and Reproduction in Early Colonial Uganda* (Joensuu, Finland: University of Joensuu, 2005).

54 John Iliffe, *Famine in Zimbabwe, 1890–1960* (Gweru, Zimbabwe: Mambo Press, 1990), p. 79.

55 Michael Watts, *Silent Violence: Food, Famine & Peasantry in Northern Nigeria* (Berkeley, CA: University of California Press, 1983).

56 This 'classic' definition is probably the most common conceptualisation of famine. See, for instance, Ó Gráda, *Famine*, pp. 6–7.

57 Cormac Ó Gráda, *Eating People Is Wrong, and Other Essays on Famine, Its Past, and Its Future* (Princeton, NJ: Princeton University Press, 2015), pp. 174–208; Alex de Waal, 'Famine Mortality: A Case Study of Darfur, Sudan 1984–5', *Population Studies*, 43 (1989), 5–24; Amrita Rangasami, '"Failure of Exchange Entitlements" Theory of Famine: A Response', *Economic and Political Weekly*, 20.4 (1985), 1797–801; for more on this debate, see Paul Howe and Stephen Devereux, 'Famine Intensity and Magnitude Scales: A Proposal for an Instrumental Definition of Famine', *Disasters*, 28 (2004), 353–72.

58 Ó Gráda, *Famine*, pp. 96–7.

59 Alex de Waal, *Famine Crimes: Politics and the Disaster Relief Industry in Africa* (Oxford: James Currey, 1997); David Keen, *The Benefits of Famine: A Political Economy of Famine and Relief in Southwestern Sudan, 1983–1989* (Oxford: James Currey, 1994).

60 Amartya Sen, *Poverty and Famines: An Essay on Entitlement and Deprivation* (Oxford: Oxford University Press, 1981).

61 Nott, 'Malnutrition in a Modernising Economy'.

62 See, for instance, John Komlos (ed.), *Stature, Living Standards, and Economic Development: Essays in Anthropometric History* (Chicago, IL: University of Chicago Press, 1994); Richard H. Steckel, 'Stature and the Standard of Living', *Journal of Economic Literature*, 33.4 (1995), 1903–40.

63 D.K. Fiawoo, 'Physical Growth and the School Environment: A West African Example', in *Physiological and Morphological Adaptation and Evolution*, ed. by William A. Stini (The Hague: Mouton, 1979), pp. 301–14.

64 See, for instance, Alexander Moradi, Gareth Austin, and Joerg Baten, *Heights and Development in a Cash-Crop Colony: Living Standards in Ghana, 1870–1980* (Cape Town: ERSA, 2013).

65 Alexander Moradi and Joerg Baten, 'Inequality in Sub-Saharan Africa: New Data and New Insights from Anthropometric Estimates', *World Development*, 33 (2005), 1233–65.

2
African foodways, British government, and the new science of nutrition

In 1953, with the Gold Coast well on its way to independence, the British-colonial government decided to release a cookbook. Intended to educate its citizens on the relationship between good food and good health, *Gold Coast Nutrition and Cookery* epitomises the farce, tragedy, and hubris which defined European attempts to manipulate African domesticity.[1] Chapter 39 is, for instance, exclusively concerned with the minutiae of that mainstay of British culture, the serving and drinking of tea.[2] While reminding the reader that 'many doctors agree that this is an unnecessary meal', the author goes on to describe one which is 'dainty but light', one in which 'a small table and embroidered cloth is used'. Cups and saucers and teaspoons 'should be grouped round the teapot so that the hostess may fill and hand them to each guest'. Sandwiches are a suitable food for teatime, but bread should be thinly cut, and crusts removed. In its defence, *Gold Coast Nutrition and Cookery* does cover *kenkey*, *fufu*, *tuo zaafi*, and the other starchy paps and vegetable-heavy soups commonly enjoyed throughout West Africa. However, as with the more complex cultural incongruities – such as pies, tarts, soufflés, and groundnut macaroons – many of the authors' suggested sandwiches contain meat or fish or cheese. Naturally, a proper cup of tea also requires milk.

Assumptions around the need for animal milks were also extended to infant feeding and the intimacies of African reproduction. Explaining that 'breastmilk, even during the first six months of a baby's life, does not completely supply his needs, and must be supplemented by other foods', the authors explicitly promote breastmilk substitutes and artificial feeding regimens for infant children.[3] Today, medical advice encourages exclusive breastfeeding for the first six months of life, not only because breastmilk is optimal for child development but also because bottle-feeding increases the risk of gastric infection, impeded nutrient absorption, and acute malnutrition. During the early twentieth century, however, bottle-feeding boomed across the colonial world, the promotion of supplementary foods combining with increased demands on maternal time and the general devaluation of domestic *reproduction* vis-à-vis capitalist *production*.[4] As we will see in later chapters, these pressures were most acute in centres of colonial commerce.[5] By the middle of the twentieth century, the intersection of economic pressures and medical cues combined to foster 'bottle-feeding-diarrhoea syndrome' and new epidemics of malnutrition.[6]

These developments did not go unchallenged. As early as 1939, the paediatrician Cicely Williams had publicly derided the promotion of breastmilk substitutes as 'murder' and 'the most criminal form of sedition'.[7] In 1972, Dick Jelliffe would term this phenomenon 'commerciogenic malnutrition'.[8] The aggressive marketing of breastmilk by foreign multinationals – including by Nestlé, which was then accused of dressing employees as nurses and operating from maternity wards – led to increased public scrutiny, the beginnings of the Nestlé boycott in the early 1970s, and the World Health Organization's 1981 adoption of the International Code of Marketing of Breast-Milk Substitutes. Since childhood malnutrition remains a pressing problem, similar critiques remain relevant – repeated and updated in view of changes to food science, food economics, and medical preoccupation.[9]

Protein, and its apparent absence, lies at the heart of this enduring history. As does the prescience of Cicely Williams. During the early 1930s, and prior to her rallying against the baby food industry, Williams had worked as a paediatrician in the Gold Coast Medical Service. While in Accra, she published two papers on a curious infantile illness, one 'in which some amino acid or protein deficiency cannot be excluded' as its primary cause.[10] Taking 'kwashiorkor', the name used by Accra's indigenous Ga for this set of symptoms, Williams added an acute form of protein malnutrition to the pantheon of single-nutrient deficiencies which had emerged alongside the discovery of nutrients in the nineteenth century.[11]

Nutritional science came of age during the transition to colonial capitalism, as new needs were met by new foods, new foods generated new tastes, and new forms of food insecurity wracked much of the African continent.[12] During these years, Britain's African colonies were among the most important sites for the science of nutrition. Williams's early contributions mean that the Gold Coast is central to this more general scientific history, but this chapter necessarily traces the broader networks of nutritional science, flitting between the Gold Coast and other primary sites of knowledge production. A great deal of the later colonial research into human nutrition took place in Buganda, a kingdom in the south of Uganda. Encompassing Kampala and the fertile areas north of Lake Victoria, Buganda was the epicentre of global nutrition research into the 1970s, hosting the UK's Medical Research Council (MRC) nutrition unit until the political upheaval of the Idi Amin years.[13] Much like Asante, Buganda parlayed the economic security offered by its lush rainforest ecology into political dominance in the decades prior to the formal onset of British-imperial government. Mild manifestations of kwashiorkor were, however, apparently endemic, at least by the late nineteenth century.[14] Here nutrition research concentrated not on shifting continental patterns of hunger or *undernutrition* but on kwashiorkor, defined as protein *malnutrition*, and enveloped in the scientific and political opacity of nutritionist discourse; while 'malnutrition' acknowledges some problem of nutrients, it fails to explain precisely what is wrong with them.[15] Instead, malnutrition suggests a nutritional dichotomy and the capacity for improvement. As a fundamental lack of nutrients, 'undernutrition' is a more substantive failure, one which exists beyond the nutritionist paradigm. Despite this, many histories of malnutrition have conflated these issues or failed to grapple with such distinctions.[16] This chapter takes the view that such distinctions were, however, recognised by imperial administrations, that kwashiorkor was useful in the construction of African alterity, and that its usefulness shaped the later development of nutritional medicine. The history of kwashiorkor, therefore, has just as much to do with an absence of food as it does with an absence of high-protein foods.

Despite the ostensibly universal nature of good and bad nutrition, the construction of kwashiorkor as an endemic and uniquely African form of malnutrition reflected the delicate politics of food in imperial Africa. Defined as a simple deficiency of protein, research into kwashiorkor found favour both because it was scientifically exciting and because it fitted with political expedient ideas of 'African exceptionalism'. Drawing on assumptions regarding the pervasion of poverty and disease in base civilisations and primeval ecologies, African exceptionalism was an important element of the 'civilising mission' and a valuable justification for the continent's colonisation.[17] Such ideas endure in the singular narratives of need which continue to dominate academic writing on African health.[18] As with most traditional understandings of illness in Africa, infantile deficiencies had been conceptualised and prevented within social frameworks.[19] However, science and scientism – as well as the more specific correlates of nutrition and nutritionism – fundamentally undermined any such construction of kwashiorkor. The medicalisation of malnutrition would go on to mar the prevention of malnutrition at the same time as promoting commercial salves and technical treatments for a disease perhaps better understood as a symptom of social dislocation.

Detailing how the conceptual history of malnutrition moved from Europe to non-representative parts of colonial Africa, this chapter works towards a global history of protein deficiency. Southern Uganda features prominently, and the earlier history of kwashiorkor derives from similarly food-secure environments in the Gold Coast forest. Neither area fits comfortably into grand narrative histories of continental hunger, yet it was these environments which shaped the science of nutrition for much of the twentieth century. Although these were important loci for the history of kwashiorkor, the 'discovery' and definition of malnutrition was also intractable from an earlier British experience, a metropolitan image of Africa, and the administration of an economically diverse and often fragile sub-Saharan empire. This trans-imperial history features political and scientific dissonance at all levels of administration – from individual scientists through to colony administrations and Whitehall mandarins.[20] Despite this, nutritional science would still come to reflect, justify, and reinforce the wider imperial mission. Here, active metropolitan involvement in the steering of research and the construction of consensus was complemented by the more passive weight of European history. Although individual scientists subverted the government line in pursuit of a more critical approach, the narrative which won through – that protein deficiency was a heavy and timeless burden of African civilisation, or the lack thereof – reflected both the subconscious politics of contemporary dietetics and the more conscious political misdirection of imperial administration.

The politics of nutrition across the British Empire

In order to understand nutrition in colonial Africa, we first need to consider the development and politicisation of food and nutrition in Europe. Eating has always been political, and dietetics, or the implementation of a certain dietary regimen, has long reflected the ideals of a given political economy.[21] Failure to live up to such ideals helped naturalise deficiency. At the end of the seventeenth century, for instance, Ireland's 'hung'ring for the lazy root' would be used to explain and explain away the Great Hunger 50 years later; potatoes being 'food for a contented slave, not for the hardy and the brave'.[22] Made politically relevant by the metaphor of the body politic, health and virtue were bound together and promoted through a moderate but considered diet.[23]

In the humoral tradition of Hippocrates and then Galen, dominant from the fifth century BCE, food was taken to be the primary recourse against illness.[24] With the rise of nutritionist dietetics during the nineteenth century, humoral understandings of diet were slowly replaced by the scientific analysis of individual nutrients.[25] Experimental nutrition began by investigating the requisite amount of energy necessary for sustenance, while the discovery of protein and the chemical revolution in the eighteenth century broadened understandings of human need.[26] Unprecedented social and economic change during the nineteenth century meant that nutrition was slowly incorporated into the nascent science of epidemiology. The Industrial Revolution promoted the diversification of employment, the industrialisation and globalisation of food production, and widespread movements away from the land. Patterns of consumption changed rapidly in response to huge structural changes in European food economies, while the incidence of nutritional illness changed in turn.[27] Although the economy grew rapidly during the nineteenth century, the sporadic decline of average heights suggests that malnutrition was pervasive among the emergent working class.[28] Scurvy, beriberi, rickets, and pellagra were all linked to diet during these years. The discovery of vitamins during the first decades of the twentieth century granted a satisfying chemical explanation for these correlations and imbued nutritional science with considerable momentum in the medical world.[29]

It was in this context that nutritional medicine became an overtly political concern. 'Physical deterioration' during the later nineteenth century was so marked that height requirements for British military recruits had to be dropped by six inches between 1845 and 1901; the failure rate for turn-of-the-century recruits was estimated to be as high as 60 per cent.[30] Physical disparities between British and Boer infantrymen were assumed to result from the meat-heavy diets of the South African veld and, following the British army's inauspicious display during the South African War (1899–1902), investments in the wellbeing of the poor were increasingly understood as an indirect investment in Britain's status as a global power.[31] In response to fears regarding Britain's declining 'national efficiency', in 1904 the government established an Inter-Departmental Committee on Physical Deterioration.[32] The committee's final report recommended greater state involvement in nutrition, including, among other things, the provision of school meals.[33] In Foucaultian terms, nutritional science contributed to the emergence of 'biopolitics', or the paternalistic extension of state authority over the body of the individual and the collective bodies of the wider populace.[34] By the First World War, elemental nutrients had been elevated to biopolitical objects, tools by which the government might solve problems of wartime food supply and population health.[35] Funding followed nutrition's newfound status and, in the interwar years, nutrition-related research won around one-sixth of all MRC grants.[36]

Extending a politicised concept of nutrition beyond British borders was readily accepted in the context of empire. Investigations into nutrition in European possessions overseas found favour among Whitehall politicians already primed to understand the physical capital of the colonised as an extension of colonial power. Stimulated by the military mechanisms behind European expansion, nutrition research in the colonies initially consisted of debates over what rations were necessary for the good health of White soldiers stationed in the tropics.[37] However, in the mid-1920s, John Boyd Orr, later the first head of the Food and Agriculture Organization of the United Nations (FAO), and John Gilks, then head of the Kenyan Medical Service, undertook a pioneering survey of African nutrition.[38] Comparing the largely vegan diets of the Kikuyu with the meat, blood, and milk-based diets of their Maasai neighbours, Orr and Gilks hoped 'to hasten the improvement of the physical condition of the native and to increase his importance as an economic factor'.[39] During a 1926 visit to the Gold Coast, William Ormsby-Gore, Under-Secretary of State for the Colonies, explained that 'the capacity of labour ... is bound up with the question of food. There are few parts of the world where the study of dietetics is more important than in Africa.'[40] Social engineering by means of nutrition became an increasingly pertinent consideration for civil engineers; the Volta River Project, for instance, employed dieticians from its inception in the 1940s in order to assess the 'human element' necessary for the construction of the Volta Dam.[41] As in Europe, high-protein foods had the greatest biopolitical value. Research in the Gold Coast found that, while adults in the forest belt were not necessarily unhealthy, they were weaker than their counterparts on the coast, where fish was a more consistent element of diet.[42] The government's conclusion was that 'an increased consumption of meat is desirable, especially for those engaged in hard physical labour'.[43]

As an extension of state authority over a given population, biopolitics is practised differently depending upon the specific priorities of a given state. So, although the nutritionist discourse emphasised ostensibly universal, scientific understandings of nutrition, nutrition in the Empire was inextricable from the politics of empire. Central to the practice of imperial rule was the distancing of the colonised 'other' from the metropolitan norm.[44] Differences in diet provided valuable distance between Europeans and their colonial subjects. As part of an imperialised form of 'tropical medicine', nutrition helped establish a stark contrast between the peripheral 'White man's grave' and the vigour and wellbeing of the metropole. The Colonial Office's endorsement of the London School of Hygiene and Tropical Medicine (LSHTM) in the 1890s monopolised healthcare in the tropics, establishing medicine as a formal element of imperial government.[45] The spread of nutritionist dietetics and imperial biopower created an intellectual environment which attracted anthropologists and doctors working in the colonies to the 'otherness' of food and nutrition in the areas to which they had been posted.[46] Such research also helped explain and naturalise the relative economic value of colonised peoples. In India, the wheat and dairy diets of the Sikhs and Pathans were seen as closer to European dietaries and provided scientific credence for their eugenicist designation as 'martial races'. David McCay, Professor of Physiology at Calcutta's Medical College, explained in 1912 that differences in diet 'appear to be the determining factor of the several causes that go to relegate, fix and maintain the position of a people, tribe or race in the category of men'.[47]

In 1933 the League of Nations Health Organisation implored member states to investigate the nutritional status of their colonial subjects, arguing that 'the fact that the greater part of the population of Africa and Asia ... suffers from insufficient or faulty feeding is no longer a secret, and there is more honour to be gained in attempting to improve the situation than in concealing it'.[48] The British response began in 1936, when Colonial Secretary J.H. Thomas sent a circular memo to all British possessions requesting information on the nutritional status of their populations, the state of nutritional research, and possible ways to improve the diets of their subjects. The resulting two-volume report, *Nutrition in the Colonial Empire*, was widely publicised and distributed, its 1939 release promoted by Lord Dufferin on the BBC and Lord Hailey in *The Times*.[49] In *The Times*, Hailey proudly announced that the report covers 'an area of well over two million square miles and with a population ... divided into countless groups having the most different food habits and customs that it is possible to imagine'.[50] In spite of this enormous breadth, *Nutrition in the Colonial Empire* explained that 'Diseases resulting from malnutrition ... prevail almost everywhere among tribal races ... excess of carbohydrate, deficient of fat and first class protein and uncertain or negligible supplies of milk and green vegetable are the outstanding features'.[51] Not only was this description grossly inaccurate, even in the context of contemporary knowledge, but it understated the worth of vegetable matter, overstated the value of animal produce, and created a simple dichotomy between colonial and European diets.[52] This othering of non-European diets was the crux of colonial dietetics, providing scientific justification for the colonisation of consumption as part of the colonial project.

Defining kwashiorkor: the European roots of an African disease

Kwashiorkor is particularly interesting in the context of tropical otherness. Analogous symptoms are rarely described in European histories of health, yet kwashiorkor has assumed such prominence in the wider aetiology of African illness. It is, therefore, worth thinking about why kwashiorkor was so prevalent in Africa yet was apparently absent from the history of European disease. While this certainly resulted from historical and spatial variations in food and domestic economy, it also relates to the political history of food and nutrition in earlier centuries. In this respect, the discovery of kwashiorkor in the 1920s and Brock and Autret's World Health Organization (WHO)-sponsored 1952 conclusion – that kwashiorkor is 'the most serious and widespread nutritional disorder known to medical and nutritional science' – were derived as much from the predispositions of European physicians as they were from the African disease environment.[53]

In biomedical literature, the incidence of kwashiorkor in the Global South is usually taken to be determined by weaning practices, and only then influenced by the food environment. It is likely that the same can also be said for European manifestations of the disease. The 'danger period during weaning' that was described by Hebe Welbourn with regard to kwashiorkor in Uganda was certainly well known in Europe – recorded since at least pre-Christian Greece.[54] In seventeenth-century England, stunted growth, rickets, gastroenteritis, and teething were all associated with weaning. 'Teething' was often cited as a cause of death, and the 'weaning illness' – diarrheal infections as a result of sudden dietary change and increased susceptibility to infection – was common enough to be regarded as 'normal and inevitable'.[55] In the distinct socio-medical environment of proto-industrial London, the

London Bills of Mortality began to record rickets in 1634, as well as its marked increase in subsequent years. Such diagnoses likely combined a number of bone-deforming illnesses of infancy, including wasting, scurvy, and kwashiorkor. This would perhaps account for the emphasis laid by other writers on the occurrence of hepatomegaly – or the enlarged liver later seen as typical in kwashiorkor patients – in cases categorised as rickets. John Graunt's pioneering work of epidemiology, the 1662 *Observations on the Bills of Mortality*, includes discussion of rickets and its relationship with, or confusion for, 'livergrown', another disease recorded in the Bills.[56] It seems likely that kwashiorkor was present in the children of pre- and early-modern Europe, but that contemporary medical discourse could not explain its incidence or speak to its symptoms.

Under similar social and economic pressures to those seen in colonial Africa a century later, localised food economies and the domestic economy of childrearing changed enormously during the Industrial Revolution.[57] As a result, the symptoms that would later be associated with kwashiorkor are more plainly visible in European medical literature. By the 1700s, accounts of oedematous malnutrition in infant children were commonly listed in popular paediatric textbooks and, from the nineteenth century, medical attention began to explicitly address food, feeding, and deficiency in the modernising economy.[58] Symptoms now usually associated with kwashiorkor – such as wasting; oedema in the legs, arms, and stomach; fatty livers; skin disorders; loose stools; and other intestinal problems – were regularly described in irritable and apathetic children that had been weaned too early or onto insubstantial diets.[59] In the early twentieth century, diagnoses of such disorders emphasised the overconsumption of starch, rather than a deficiency of protein. In 1906 Czerny and Keller described Mehlnährschaden, or 'damage by starch'.[60] In subsequent years, reports came from Europe and the United States further detailing 'injuries produced by starch' and 'diseases of infants due to prolonged feeding with excess carbohydrates'.[61]

By this time, however, low-protein diets were becoming less common, at least in Western Europe. Although not often consumed by the majority of the population, animal produce was central to European perceptions of dietary value, something at least in part related to the history of class stratification. In his elucidation of this point, Jack Goody referenced Walter Scott's *Ivanhoe*: '"Swine is good Saxon" said the Jester "but … pork, I think, is good Norman-French; and so when the brute lives, and is in charge of a Saxon slave, she goes by her Saxon name, but becomes a Norman … when she is carried to the Castel-hall."'[62]

The same being true for sheep and mutton, cows and beef, calves and veal, meat had long been an aspirational expenditure. As average income increased, the consumption of animal produce grew in tandem. The 'democratisation' of meat consumption over the course of the nineteenth century has been said to constitute a 'food revolution' which greatly increased the relative protein content of European diets and more firmly aligned meat and health in European medicine.[63] By the mid-1800s, the medical consensus was that meat 'exceed[s] all other foods in nutritional power' and access to meat became thought of as a fundamental right.[64] Products such as Liebig's Extract of Meat (now Oxo) and Johnston's Fluid Beef (now Bovril), emerged from the 1840s in order to provide the poor with affordable animal protein, sparking the long-standing trend of marketing manufactured food-like supplements to the poor, rather than addressing shortcomings in the supply of real food.[65]

In the years following the First World War, protein deficiencies became increasingly interesting to a medical community recently exposed to the destitution of the poor in the ghettos of Europe and the dust bowls of North America.[66] Primed to ascribe particular importance to protein, research suggested that 'hunger oedema' or 'war dropsy' was the result of inadequate protein intake.[67] The question of protein in the presentation of oedema appeared to be confirmed in the later 1920s, when low-protein diets produced an analogous form of kwashiorkor in white rats.[68] It was only in the later 1940s, in the unique clinical environments of the wartime Minnesota Starvation Study and in postwar German orphanages, that oedema was seen in undernourished patients with relatively high-protein diets.[69] Prior to this, researchers were naturally drawn to these curious, oedematous presentations of want and, in the European cultural environment, diets deficient in protein were seen to be particularly flawed.

These developments accompanied the expansion of European involvement in Africa and served to highlight the differences between the democratised European dietetic and latterly constructed ideas of the 'average' African diet. Even the earliest physicians exploring Africa highlighted the lack of meat as a chief cause of European ill-health on the continent. In the Gold Coast, Joseph Dupuis was of the opinion that 'many fall victim to the climate from the adoption of a course of training improperly termed prudential; viz. a *sudden* change of diet, from *ship's fare* to a scanty sustenance of vegetable matter'.[70] The relative disinterest in meat as a staple in Africa was also considered particularly curious. In Sierra Leone in the early 1800s, the physician Thomas Winterbottom, for instance, noted that:

> An African, who has been feasted with every delicacy which an European table can afford, yet if rice has not constituted a part of his entertainment, will say, he has had *no meat* for so long a time, and on his return home will recur to his beloved food with redoubled ardour.[71]

Linguistics offers some insight into the culturally specific value of food. In French, 'meat', *viande*, derives from the Latin, 'to live'. For the Tallensi of north-eastern Ghana, meat is delicious, certainly, but it is not 'food' in the same way as porridge. Instead, meat is *valeg*, or 'gluttony'. In the fragile Tallensi food economy, and unlike a generalised European pattern, meat was shared widely, while arable produce is more commonly secreted away.[72] By the 1920s, vegetable-based diets in the Akan forest were taken to be actively 'dangerous'.[73]

The advent of tropical medicine facilitated the spread of nutrition research into fertile ground outside of Europe, where oedematous malnutrition was found to be particularly prevalent. In Latin America, symptoms later defined as kwashiorkor were described in a number of articles from 1908.[74] In literature emanating from the French Empire, doctors described the 'Swelling [disease] of Vietnam' as early as 1913.[75] Similar groups of symptoms were also being described in the British Empire by at least the 1920s.[76] Yet it was the work of Cicely Williams which cemented kwashiorkor as an illness undocumented in Western medical literature. Despite its global incidence, her conclusions would spark decades of debate and research into primarily African presentations of the illness.

In earlier years, however, European doctors in Africa had been relatively dismissive of such conditions, even though they were readily apparent. In the 1870s, a German doctor travelling in the Loango Kingdom (now part of the Democratic Republic of Congo) found children with protruding abdomens, 'just as white children, who had consumed large quantities of carbohydrate-rich food in early youth'.[77] Early doctor-explorers like David Livingstone and Thomas Winterbottom had received their medical training in the particular nutrition environment of the Industrial Revolution. However, as Sjoerd Rijpma explains, by the 1920s it was 'not surprising that [Williams] called it a "new disease": the symptoms were hardly seen in Europe then'.[78]

In the absence of effective medical communication, it was not until later in the twentieth century that the numerous descriptions of kwashiorkor began to be brought together.[79] Williams's work was particularly attractive largely because it emphasised an absence of dietary protein, rather than an excess of starch. Dermatological signs – sometimes described as 'crazy-pavement dermatitis' – were also made more dramatic by their presentation on Black skin, as well as by the White-colonial obsession with Blackness.[80] In later accounts, dyspigmentation was central to the differential diagnosis of kwashiorkor, and was the only significant distinction between kwashiorkor and Mehlnährschaden, 'an infantile syndrome of nutritional oedema with little or no alteration in skin and hair pigment [which] has been described in European infants'.[81] Instead, 'the degree to which dyspigmentation can be taken as evidence of kwashiorkor' was forwarded as a potential indicator 'in studying the frequency and importance of the syndrome' at the population level.[82] In general, Williams's lengthy descriptions of kwashiorkor stood out because, through the prism of British tropical medicine, this definition fitted with the established otherness of African life, something which was only exacerbated by Williams's use of, and, subsequently, the global adoption of, Ga nomenclature.

Williams's apparently punitive 1936 transfer to Malaya restricted her ability to work on kwashiorkor. Research, however, intensified under the industry of Hugh Trowell and the cohort collected around Kampala's Mengo Hospital. Trowell's progress was slow and frustrated by the complicated pathology of kwashiorkor. In 1937, after feeding patients with cow's milk, liver, and all known vitamins and continuing to lose around 40 per cent of them, Trowell was convinced that kwashiorkor was not a simple single-nutrient deficiency.[83] The mysterious aetiology of the disease only began to unfold in 1942 after Jack Davies, Mengo's new pathologist, showed up degenerated pancreases in post-mortem examinations. This, Trowell and Davies would go on to explain, suggested that patients were unable to digest their food due to a shortage of pancreatic secretions; it also explained why supplements failed to relieve patients in advanced cases. By 1946, it was suggested that a lack of protein could severely harm the tissues and organs of the body because it restricted the ability to create new tissue. The functioning of the liver and the pancreas were gradually undermined, leading to a decline in enzyme production and the restriction of nutrient absorption. The subsequent failure to digest led to diarrhoea and, because of excessive fat, an enlarged liver.[84]

Trowell's research was, however, hindered by the reservations of colonial administrators. In Uganda, R.S.F. Hennessey, a politically minded pathologist who would later become Principal Medical Officer of the Uganda Protectorate, took little interest in kwashiorkor. Prior to his promotion, Hennessey would perform a number of autopsies in the space of an hour, mainly on vital organs extracted by students and medical assistants. Jack Davies, taking 50 sections of one cadaver, found the critical pancreatic degenerations on his first attempt.[85] It is difficult to say whether Hennessey's failure to do more to investigate the pathology of kwashiorkor was due to incompetence or wilful ignorance. In any case, he was certainly resistant to Trowell's investigations. Trowell describes Hennessey as saying 'Oh, there's nothing in Kwashiorkor. It's just that they're not very well fed, then they pick up malaria, hookworms, and all the rest of it. What's the mystery? There is no new complaint here.'[86] Both Hennessey and John Hall, the Governor of Uganda, tried to privately dissuade Trowell from keeping on with his kwashiorkor work, Hall once asking 'where will all this racket end?'[87] Citing Roger Whitehead, a long-time director of the MRC nutrition unit in Uganda and then The Gambia, the historian Jennifer Tappan suggests that, unlike previously unknown vitamin and mineral deficiencies which provided opportunities for science to improve the lives of colonial subjects, 'protein malnutrition pointed to the poverty of colonial populations'.[88]

It is, however, important to realise that the concerns of the administration inside individual colonies were not necessarily the same as those in Whitehall. While in-country administrators were understandably reluctant to draw attention to a high incidence of kwashiorkor, protein deficiencies were still more palatable than a fundamental lack of food, especially if they could be presented as an endemic problem of the African environment. Emphasising that 'the native food problem is not so much one of quantity as one of quality', Whitehall promoted a narrative in which the presence of kwashiorkor could actively alleviate metropolitan responsibility for malnutrition in the colonies.[89] Since subsequent research concentrated on areas with highly visible burdens of kwashiorkor and a relative lack of undernutrition, much of the resultant literature emphasised a cultural proximity to malnutrition. Accounts such as Welbourn's late 1950s survey of Ugandan kwashiorkor patients found that no families appeared poor, while some seemed comparatively well-to-do.[90] Earlier, in the mid-1940s, the Ugandan administration had stated that 'the majority of children in Buganda show signs of malnutrition'. This was not necessarily a problem. Malnutrition, the same report would explain, 'is not due so much to absolute poverty as to ignorance, conservatism and superstition'.[91] These were enduring and malleable conclusions. In 1962, under Apartheid, the South African minister of health spoke in parliament in order to explain that there was no famine or undernutrition in the country but, because of custom, ignorance, and immorality, kwashiorkor was still present.[92]

There was a year between the receipt of replies to the 1936 Thomas circular and the final publication of *Nutrition in the Colonial Empire*. Over the course of that year, representative preliminary reports were 'depoliticised' by the Colonial Office to remove any suggestion that low wages, inadequate returns from cash-crops, and declines in food production were complicit in the pervasive pattern of malnutrition.[93] In the Gold Coast, as elsewhere, reports circulated after the Colonial Office's initial request for information suggested that, contrary to the conclusions that were published later, the colony's greatest nutritional problem was not a deficiency of quality foods (although that was a concern) but endemic undernutrition and the recurrent threat of famine in particular areas.[94]

In response to Whitehall's request for information on colonial nutrition, the Gold Coast government seconded F.M. Purcell to undertake a detailed investigation into nutrition across the colony's three main agroeconomic regions – the dry Northern savannah, the rainforest, and the coastal plain. Inaction and official indifference marred Purcell's investigation. Audrey Richards, the pioneering anthropologist and sometime colonial officer, later explained that, 'in spite of our circulars, the Heads of the technical services (medicine, agriculture and education), do not seem to have cooperated very closely'.[95] After two years and some 200 pages, Purcell's foremost concern was that, throughout the savannah, 'there is a severe shortage of every kind of food during several months yearly'.[96] On the completion of his report, 'a senior officer' had told him that '"this report will not be sent home … as it reveals neglect on the part of the local administration in the Northern Territories" … unofficially it was explained to me that "no one may starve in the British Empire"'.[97]

It was, in fact, sent to London, although nearly two years after its completion. On receipt of the report, S. Culwick, the Nutrition Officer to the Colonial Office, noted that 'two and a half years ago the [Gold Coast] Nutrition Committee agreed to … immediate measures to meet these local shortages … it would appear that has not been followed up'.[98] Disappointed by the official response to his work, Purcell had already resigned his position and gone to the press, 'venting his grievances' in a 1943 letter to the editor of *West Africa*.[99] Purcell's revelations were reprinted a number of times between 1943 and 1946, and were notable because they jarred with official representations of nutritional health in the colonies. In 1946, the *West African Review* took it upon itself to remind readers that 'we must avoid the error of supposing that shortage of vital foods, present and pending, is something affecting Germans alone'.[100] In its response, the Colonial Office explained that 'short term, local relief measures operate for the periodical acute hunger in the villages of the territories, but the solution of the problem is a matter for long-term development'.[101] At the behest of Oliver Stanley, the Secretary of State for the Colonies, Governor Alan Burns was asked to explain the state of nutrition in the north. Assuring Stanley that 'I am by no means complacent about the situation which the Purcell Report reveals', Burns stressed that 'the problems of nutrition can only be tackled effectively on a long term basis and in conjunction with the many other problems with which we are faced'.[102]

Starvation was a difficult problem for governments to contend with. Humanitarianism had come of age and absolute failures of subsistence were widely seen as a governmental responsibility, if not a direct failure of imperial government.[103] In his unpublished reply to the 1936 Thomas circular, the Director of the Gold Coast's Medical Department suggested as much, since 'so much attention has been devoted to the cocoa and mining industries ... food produced on their farms is apt to be overlooked'.[104] Similar critiques were common throughout the 1930s.[105] In 1939, Audrey Richards summed up the opinion of many scholars and some administrators, writing that the diet and health of the colonised 'has deteriorated in contact with white civilisation rather than the reverse'.[106] However, as Michael Worboys has explained, through publications like *Nutrition in the Colonial Empire* Whitehall sought to reframe malnutrition from an epidemic, structural problem resulting from colonialism 'to an endemic one for which colonialism had little responsibility and over which it could exercise little control'.[107]

The promotion of protein malnutrition as Africa's greatest nutritional concern complemented this more general process. Constructed as a problem of ignorance and backwardness, the high incidence of kwashiorkor in Uganda never earned much consternation from London. Despite reservations from Hennessey and Hall inside the Protectorate, the research undertaken in Uganda came to be considered a boon to the British Empire. At the end of his speech inaugurating Kampala's new Makerere Medical School in 1951, then Colonial Secretary James Griffith announced that 'the medical school is known throughout the whole of Africa ... for the magnificent research work of Dr. Hugh Trowell'.[108] As Tappan has explained, Makerere was taken by the MRC's chief executive, Sir Harold Himsworth, to be a 'model for medical research in the tropics'.[109] Although Himsworth expected Makerere to be built on universalistic understandings of health, kwashiorkor research found political favour because it also fitted with exceptionalist ideas of African primitivism, African diet, and the African disease environment.

This is a distinction which deserves to be stressed. Although we should be hesitant to speak of a coherent 'imperial science', the delicate politics of famine and the emotive politics of food did shape medical discourse.[110] The influence of systemic pressures – not only the contemporary politics of empire but also the weight of the European past and of past scientific consensus – were borne out in the medicine of malnutrition. In the Gold Coast, Purcell's gravest concerns were reserved for the hungry in the Northern savannah. Although oedematous infant malnutrition was apparently endemic in the rainforest, his tone is much lighter when the focus shifts to Akim: 'then to consider fruits; the ignorance and indifference to fruits is astonishing. There are oranges, bananas, pineapples, pawpaw, mango, guava &c – yet no Akan housewife would think of making a banana fritter; and they have never even heard of a pineapple soufflé!'[111] The relative abundance of food meant that there was nothing sombre to be said about nutrition here and, as in *Gold Coast Nutrition and Cookery*, the soufflé again appears as a touchstone of civility. As a problem of ignorance and indifference, malnutrition here was to be remedied with the slow march of European civilisation and the slow spread of scientific knowledge.

Colonising kwashiorkor: tropical medicine and indigenous knowledge

Cicely Williams was remarkable in part because she listened to her patients and her Ga colleagues, responding to the cultures she encountered with a degree of sensitivity uncommon in colonial doctors.[112] In her second paper on kwashiorkor, she began by explaining that such symptoms were understood by the Ga as 'the disease the deposed baby gets when the next one is born'.[113] In her Doctor of Medicine thesis, she saw 'the most uncomprehending indignation, rage and bitterness in a child of three years old who found that his place on his mother's back was suddenly usurped by a new baby'.[114] As part of his broader disregard for Williams's work, Hugh Stannus, then the Empire's leading authority on nutrition, brushed such observations aside, stating that the transliteration of kwashiorkor was irrelevant and a 'common superstition', since, even 'among the Wa-yao of Central Africa the disease, whatever it may be, is called *litango lya kututa* – each successive child is said to push (*kututa*) the previous one into its grave'.[115] Operating within the nutritionist dietetic, and in view of exceptionalist ideas of African health, scientific consensus narrowly framed kwashiorkor as a simple deficiency of protein. Clearly, however, the aetiology of kwashiorkor was understood by the colonised in a very different way. In 1954, Trowell et al. listed some 32 names for kwashiorkor taken from a handful of African and Asian countries, most of which suggest the same social aetiology of the disease – short birth spacing and short breastfeeding durations.[116] For those prone to the disease, kwashiorkor did not necessarily relate to diet but was instead tied to household makeup, conjugal responsibility, and the highly personal intricacies of childrearing.

If protein deficiency was indeed endemic during the early twentieth century, it may more accurately be seen as a reaction to the gendered pressures of the colonial economy (see Chapters 3 and 4). Protracted breastfeeding and sexual abstinence were increasingly untenable throughout the twentieth century, with birth spacing durations declining almost universally across the continent.[117] This was, in part, a result of colonial biopolitics. In the Belgian Congo, perhaps the most extreme example of engineered pronatalism, 'birth bonuses' worth five days' pay were given to contracted labourers working on plantations and in mines across the colony.[118] In less invasive regimes, such as the Gold Coast, state-sponsored baby shows formed a mechanism of 'social regulation, if not social control' as early as the 1920s. Mothers were encouraged to bring up children according to Western ideals and rewarded with sugar, soap, and children's clothes when these conditions were met.[119] The systemic influence of capitalist development compounded such policies. Again in the Gold Coast, male ownership of extra-subsistence produce severely undermined the value of childbearing, childrearing, and food production, the biologically and socially ascribed outputs of female labour.[120] Accompanying the pervasive devaluation of such labour was a similarly pervasive pattern of gendered conflict.[121] While domestic pressures reflected the various ideals of colonial governments and the shifting and spatially bounded demands of capital formation, domestic compromise was a fairly universal phenomenon across imperial Africa.

Endemic kwashiorkor could be utilised as a tool for colonial governance partly because the medicalisation of the disease stripped it of its social and economic context.[122] Reducing kwashiorkor to a deficiency of protein allowed for its presentation as a failure on the part of African mothers, communities, and cultures. In this respect, kwashiorkor helped justify European cultural hegemony and the paternalism of imperial government. As with other manifestations of African illness, kwashiorkor was explained in terms of deviance from metropolitan ideals.[123] Even Cicely Williams had used the existence of kwashiorkor to explain that 'the idea that the "simple savage" has instinctive knowledge in caring for her children is without foundation'.[124]

It took two decades for 'kwashiorkor' to be accepted into the medical lexicon. When it was, the medicalised use of the word erased much of its original meaning at the same time as adding new import. A 1949 editorial in *The Lancet* explained that '"kwashiorkor" has the merit of neutrality: it offers no explanation and its use prejudices no issue'.[125] The neutrality of the word was, however, sited entirely in the otherness of African language and its apparent incoherence, something which, ironically, entirely undermined any such neutrality. For the Ga, 'kwashiorkor' had a spiritual meaning and was not often said aloud. Williams had been stationed in the Gold Coast for three years before she was told the local name for a condition she had been seeing with some regularity.[126] In 1960s Uganda, the developmental psychologist Mary Ainsworth expanded John Bowlby's 'attachment theory' of child development to explain kwashiorkor in relation to *anorexia nervosa*, caused by the child's perceived abandonment after the abrupt cessation of breastfeeding.[127] Similar psychosocial definitions also underpinned Ga understandings of kwashiorkor. One doctor explained that kwashiorkor 'applies to the psychological condition ... in general conversation, if a child is crying, one might say to it, "what is your mother pregnant, are you getting kwashiorkor?"'[128] In the 1930s, and apparently independent of Williams, the anthropologist Margaret Field described '*kwasiɔkɔ*' as 'a special kind of jealousy. Young children and babies can perceive far more than grown people and the first child soon begins to know that there is another one coming.'[129] When the second baby is born, the first 'resents the withdrawal of the mother's attention ... and may even die from sheer chagrin.' Children at risk were to be 'treated with great patience, understanding, and humour'.[130] In this context, kwashiorkor seems to have more properly suggested a broken taboo. Indeed, in the early 1960s, Akan respondents further north explained that 'intercourse may affect the quality of the mother's milk and it is said that many children die as a result of this ... If such a thing happens, public opinion turns against the parents, especially the father; people say that he cannot control himself.'[131] Whatever the exact definition, kwashiorkor was part of a complex system of social welfare based around religion, spirituality, and those communalistic ideas of health which were often discarded within colonial medical discourse.[132]

Under European government, indigenous knowledge was, by turns, appropriated, discredited, and replaced by biomedical frameworks which exalted scientific understandings of illness and promoted technical approaches to its relief.[133] Worboys has suggested that colonial interest in deficiency was notable because it 'did not involve the creation of an exceptionalist, tropical nutritional science'.[134] Yet such conclusions are not true when considering kwashiorkor. Following the popularisation of the Ga word, both the history and the terminology of the disease have implicitly tied protein deficiency to the African continent. In their authoritative 1952 continent-wide survey for WHO, Brock and Autret explained that kwashiorkor is 'a nutritional syndrome (or syndromes) found among indigenous Africans', later explaining that 'any clinical syndrome which includes these five characters and occurs in Africa can undoubtedly be called kwashiorkor'.[135] Although they acknowledged that kwashiorkor may occur elsewhere, an African origin had become a core part of its pathology.

The conceptualisation of kwashiorkor as inherently African complemented an ahistorical understanding of the disease. Yarom and McFie's 1963 conclusion, that 'kwashiorkor has always been prevalent in the Kasai Province of South-East Congo', denied the disease any history in the Congo, let alone a history relevant to its relief.[136] This was part of a more general pattern that continues to promote Africa as a place of perpetual want. Speaking in Johannesburg in 1979, Jack Davies, the pathologist most closely concerned with the early biology of kwashiorkor, explained that the history of Africa had always been marred by 'inadequacies of diet'. Davies went on to explain that 'most of the foods which constitute the current dietary staples of African people have been developed elsewhere ... it has puzzled some investigators as to just what were the dietary staples prior to the introduction of these foods'.[137] The promotion of kwashiorkor both as the world's gravest nutritional concern and as a uniquely African tropical disease sits comfortably within this narrative. Framing deficiency as Africa's natural lot obstructs any critical appreciation of nutritional change. It also contributes to the fetishisation of an ahistorical form of African poverty entirely dissociated from the effects of colonial rule.

Considered 'so common that many doctors would regard it as almost normal', endemic kwashiorkor offered scientific and eugenicist justifications for colonial authority.[138] Playing on long-held assumptions regarding the idleness of African populations, a continent-wide deficiency of protein went some way towards explaining African underdevelopment.[139] In the Gold Coast, Purcell had explained that 'the men of Akim are generally regarded as being weak-willed, lazy and cowardly ... such inferiority may be attributed to their diet'.[140] Brock and Autret's 1952 WHO report extended similar speculations across the continent, stating that 'it would not be too far-fetched to attribute to that protein deficiency, at least in part, the backwardness of the African people'.[141] Even in 1979, Davies would ask his Johannesburg audience, 'how much did this nutritionally-induced apathy contribute to the docility of Negro slaves?'[142]

If protein deficiency naturalised African underdevelopment, Whiggish understandings of economic and technological modernisation offered a reprieve. Working from the assumption that 'cow's milk [is] normally the most convenient source of protein for the child during the post-weaning period', colonial veterinary services promoted the intensification of livestock cultivation.[143] Although the morbidity and mortality of livestock improved, limited tangible success left significant room for imported animal protein.[144] Building on the model developed by Bovril, Oxo, and other nineteenth-century nutraceuticals, similar solutions were sought to fill gaps in colonial diets and ply colonial markets. In a 1929 'index to the literature of food investigation', 27 pages detail scientific advances in the manufacture, preservation, and distribution of meat and animal products, 18 explore fruits and vegetables, and 4 consider grains, crops, and seeds. 'At the charge of the Empire Marking Board', these pamphlets were 'distributed gratis to the Colonial Governments'.[145] It was not long before the proliferation of tinned meats, at the expense of fresh local ingredients, were 'becoming so popular as to constitute a real menace to public health'.[146]

The promotion of breastmilk substitutes were part of this broader trend. In the Gold Coast, Purcell explained that 'the condition of the infants indicate strongly that breastmilk is often of poor quality'. However, at the Oda Weighing Clinic, bottle-fed Baby Kofi 'differed from all the other babies in that he was plump, robust and constantly cheerful … The healthy gleam of his eyes was sufficient to distinguish him from the other babies, all of them breast-fed.'[147] In 1937, only two years prior to her 'milk and murder' speech, even Cicely Williams would recommend that 'milk should be given with every feed until a child is eighteen months old and every day till he is ten years old'.[148] In fact, Williams was so optimistic about the potential for artificial feeding that she sought to acquire an official endorsement of Nestlé's tinned milk.[149]

Williams's early faith in the potential of infant formula was cultured by European and imperial discourses regarding the relative value of food. Although the science of nutrition pledged an objective valuation of diet, its conclusions were moulded by the biopolitics of nutrition as well as earlier histories of class and cuisine, hunger, humanitarianism, and *noblesse oblige*. Born from these conventions, the construction of kwashiorkor was taken to result from the deviant diets and food cultures encountered by Europeans in Africa. Made endemic both by the pressures of colonisation and the reification of nutritionist consensus, kwashiorkor was cast as a pervasive and timeless burden of African otherness. Working out of atypical rainforest food economies, research into malnutrition only offered partial insight into the aetiology and epidemiology of African deficiency during this period. Unlike the more problematic politics of hunger and undernutrition, malnutrition actively bolstered the racialised hierarchies which lay at the foundations of empire. While worthy and well intentioned, scientific interest in kwashiorkor helped naturalise narratives of African exceptionalism and European authority over African health. Such singular narratives have proved hard to shift. This does not mean to deny the burden of kwashiorkor during these years, or even the uniqueness of African food environments, but instead seeks to stress that both malnutrition and African alterity have long conceptual histories – stories spun in view of a metropolitan audience and, at times, for imperialist ends.

Notes

1 See, for instance, Nancy Rose Hunt, *A Colonial Lexicon of Birth Ritual, Medicalization, and Mobility in the Congo* (Durham, NC: Duke University Press, 1999); Jean Allman, 'Making Mothers: Missionaries, Medical Officers and Women's Work in Colonial Asante, 1924–1945', *History Workshop*, 38.1 (1994), 23–47. This chapter is a revised version of John Nott, '"No One May Starve in the British Empire": Kwashiorkor, Protein and the Politics of Nutrition Between Britain and Africa', *Social History of Medicine*, 34.2 (2021), 553–76.

2 Gold Coast Government, *Gold Coast Nutrition and Cookery* (Edinburgh: Published for the Gold Coast Government by T. Nelson and Sons, 1953), pp. 270–1.

3 Gold Coast Government, *Gold Coast Nutrition and Cookery*, p. 280.

4 For economic and social changes to domestic reproduction under colonial rule, see Claude Meillassoux, *Maidens, Meal and Money: Capitalism and the Domestic Community* (Cambridge: Cambridge University Press, 1981); Jean Comaroff and John L. Comaroff, 'Home-Made Hegemony: Modernity, Domesticity, and Colonialism in South Africa', in *African Encounters with Domesticity*, ed. by Karen Hansen (New Brunswick, NJ: Rutgers University Press, 1992), pp. 37–74; for the nutritional effects, see Moore and Vaughan, *Cutting Down Trees*; Nott, 'Malnutrition in a Modernising Economy'.

5 In the area around Kampala, for instance, the proportion of children receiving supplementary bottle feeds before six months of age increased from 14 per cent in the early 1950s to 42 per cent only 10 years later. At the same time, the amount of formula needed to replace breastmilk for one child cost a third of a labourer's salary. See D.B. Jelliffe, 'Pediatrics in Uganda', *Clinical Pediatrics*, 4.1 (1965), 55–61; D.B. Jelliffe and F.J. Bennett, 'Cultural and Anthropological Factors in Infant and Maternal Nutrition', *Federation Proceedings*, 20 (1961), S185–7.

6 H.F. Welbourn, 'Bottle Feeding: A Problem of Modern Civilization', *Journal of Tropical Pediatrics*, 3.4 (1958), 157–66; Nott, 'Malnutrition in a Modernising Economy'.

7 Cicely D. Williams, *'Milk and Murder': Reprint of a speech given to the Singapore Rotary Club, 1939* (Penang, Malaysia: International Organization of Consumers Unions, 1986), p. 5.

8 Jelliffe, 'Commerciogenic Malnutrition?'.

9 On the scale of nutrition mortality in contemporary contexts, see Black et al., 'Maternal and Child Undernutrition and Overweight'. For the current relationship between breastmilk substitutes and malnutrition, see Ellen G. Piwoz and Sandra L. Huffman, 'The Impact of Marketing of Breast-Milk Substitutes on WHO-Recommended Breastfeeding Practices', *Food and Nutrition Bulletin*, 36.4 (2015), 373–86. For the historical context of these trends, see Lola Wilhelm, '"One of the Most Urgent Problems to Solve": Malnutrition, Trans-Imperial Nutrition Science, and Nestlé's Medical Pursuits in Late Colonial Africa', *The Journal of Imperial and Commonwealth History*, 48.5 (2020), 914–33; Tehila Sasson, 'Milking the Third World? Humanitarianism, Capitalism, and the Moral Economy of the Nestlé Boycott', *The American Historical Review*, 121.4 (2016), 1196–224.

10 Cicely D. Williams, 'A Nutritional Disease of Childhood Associated with a Maize Diet', *Archives of Disease in Childhood*, 8 (1933), 423–33 (p. 432); Williams, 'Kwashiorkor'.

11 For the history of nutritional science, see, among others, Harmke Kamminga and Andrew Cunningham (eds), *The Science and Culture of Nutrition, 1840–1940* (Amsterdam: Brill Rodopi, 1995); Kenneth J. Carpenter, *Protein and Energy* (Cambridge: Cambridge University Press, 1994); E.C. Spary, *Feeding France: New Sciences of Food, 1760–1815* (Cambridge: Cambridge University Press, 2014).

12 The relationship between capitalism and taste-making in the history of sugar is evocatively detailed in Mintz, *Sweetness and Power*.

13 This history is the primary focus of Tappan, *Riddle*.

14 For the economic history of nutrition in southern Uganda, see Nott, 'Malnutrition in a Modernising Economy'; Kuhanen, *Poverty, Health, and Reproduction*.

15 This argument is made in greater detail here: Rijpma, *Livingstone*, p. 437.

16 See, for instance, Brantley, *Feeding Families*; James Vernon, *Hunger: A Modern History* (Cambridge, MA: Harvard University Press, 2007).

17 The exceptionalism of African poverty has been touched on here: Michael Watts, 'Entitlements or Empowerment? Famine and Starvation in Africa', *Review of African Political Economy*, 51 (1991), 9–26; for the exceptionalism of African health, see Jean Comaroff, 'The Diseased Heart of Africa: Medicine, Colonialism and the Black Body', in *Knowledge, Power, and Practice: The Anthropology of Medicine and Everyday Life*, ed. by Shirley Lindenbaum and Margaret M. Lock (Berkeley, CA: University of California Press, 1993), pp. 305–29.

18 Mkhwanazi, 'Medical Anthropology in Africa'.

19 Steven Feierman and John M. Janzen (eds), *The Social Basis of Health and Healing in Africa* (Berkeley, CA: University of California Press, 1992).

20 In this respect, this chapter speaks to Helen Tilley's arguments against a uniform 'imperial science'. See Helen Tilley, *Africa as a Living Laboratory: Empire, Development, and the Problem of Scientific Knowledge, 1870–1950* (Chicago, IL: University of Chicago Press, 2011).

21 Tripp Rebrovick, 'The Politics of Diet: "Eco-Dietetics," Neoliberalism, and the History of Dietetic Discourses', *Political Research Quarterly*, 68.4 (2015), 678–89.

22 William Drennan, 'To Ireland', in *The Monthly Magazine*, ed. by John Aikin and Benson Earle Hill (London: R. Phillips, 1796), p. 404.

23 Steven Shapin, 'How to Eat Like a Gentleman: Dietetics and Ethics in Early Modern England', in *In Right Living: An Anglo-American Tradition of Self-Help Medicine and Hygiene*, ed. by C. Rosenberg (Baltimore, MD: Johns Hopkins University Press, 2003), pp. 21–58; Rebrovick, 'Politics of Diet: "Eco-Dietetics"', p. 681.

24 See, for instance, Galen, *Galen on Food and Diet, Translation and Notes by Mark Grant* (London: Routledge, 2000).

25 Scrinis, *Nutritionism*.

26 Carpenter, *Protein and Energy*, pp. 17–54.

27 Carole Shammas, 'The Eighteenth-Century English Diet and Economic Change', *Explorations in Economic History*, 21.3 (1984), 254–69.

28 John Komlos, 'Shrinking in a Growing Economy? The Mystery of Physical Stature during the Industrial Revolution', *The Journal of Economic History*, 58.3 (1998), 779–802.

29 Kenneth J. Carpenter, 'A Short History of Nutritional Science: Part 2 (1885–1912)', *The Journal of Nutrition*, 133.4 (2003), 975–84.

30 George F. Shee, 'The Deterioration in the National Physique', *Nineteenth Century*, 52 (1903), 797–805.

31 Richard Soloway, 'Counting the Degenerates: The Statistics of Race Deterioration in Edwardian England', *Journal of Contemporary History*, 17.1 (1982), 137–64 (p. 142).
32 G.R. Searle, *The Quest for National Efficiency: A Study in British Politics and Political Thought, 1899–1914* (Oxford: Blackwell, 1971).
33 James Vernon, 'The Ethics of Hunger and the Assembly of Society: The Techno-Politics of the School Meal in Modern Britain', *The American Historical Review*, 110.3 (2005), 693–725; these were pan-European concerns which caught the attention of the continent's foremost scientists; see Justus von Liebig, *Animal Chemistry, or Organic Chemistry in Its Applications to Physiology and Pathology* (London: Taylor and Walton, 1842).
34 Michel Foucault, *The History of Sexuality. Vol. 1: The Will to Knowledge* (London: Penguin, 1979), pp. 135–45.
35 Robyn Smith, 'The Emergence of Vitamins as Bio-Political Objects during World War I', *Studies in History and Philosophy of Biological and Biomedical Sciences*, 40.3 (2009), 179–89.
36 Celia Petty, 'Primary Research and Public Health: The Prioritisation of Nutrition Research in Inter-War Britain', in *Historical Perspectives on the Role of the MRC: Essays in the History of the Medical Research Council of the United Kingdom and Its Predecessor, the Medical Research Committee, 1913–1953*, ed. by J. Austoker and L. Bryder (Oxford: Oxford University Press, 1989), pp. 83–108.
37 Philip D. Curtin, *Death by Migration: Europe's Encounter with the Tropical World in the Nineteenth Century* (Cambridge: Cambridge University Press, 1989), pp. 125–9.
38 Cynthia Brantley, 'Kikuyu-Maasai Nutrition and Colonial Science: The Orr and Gilks Study in Late 1920s Kenya Revisited', *The International Journal of African Historical Studies*, 30.1 (1997), 49–86.
39 J.B. Orr and J.L. Gilks, *Studies of Nutrition: The Physique and Health of Two African Tribes* (London: HMSO, 1931), p. 12.
40 Report by Hon W.G.A. Ormsby-Gore on his Visit to West Africa, quoted in G.E. Metcalfe, *Great Britain and Ghana: Documents of Ghana History, 1807–1957* (London: Thomas Nelson & Sons for the University of Ghana, 1964), p. 613.
41 LSHTM/0809/Nutrition/03, Volta River Project – Ghana.
42 PRAAD/A/ADM/11/1/1294, F.M. Purcell, 'Report'.
43 PRAAD/RG/3/5/600, Meat Supply Survey, Gold Coast, 1940, A. Fulton, 'Survey of Meat Supplies and Distribution in the Gold Coast'.
44 See Edward W. Said, *Orientalism* (London: Routledge & Kegan Paul, 1978).
45 Douglas M. Haynes, *Imperial Medicine: Patrick Manson and the Conquest of Tropical Disease* (Philadelphia, PA: University of Pennsylvania Press, 2001), pp. 140–51.
46 W.E. McCulloch, *An Inquiry into the Dietaries of the Hausas and Town Fulani of Northern Nigeria, with Some Observations of the Effects on the National Health, with Recommendations Arising Therefrom* (Lagos, Nigeria: Government Printer, 1930); M. Fortes and S.L. Fortes, 'Food in the Domestic Economy of the Tallensi', *Africa*, 9.2 (1936), 237–76.
47 Quoted in Arnold, '"Discovery" of Malnutrition', pp. 12–13.
48 E. Burnet and W.R. Aykroyd, 'Nutrition and Public Health', *League of Nations: Quarterly Bulletin of the Health Organisation*, 4.2 (1935), 323–474 (p. 452).
49 The National Archives, Kew (TNA) /CO/859/14/6, G.C. Eastwood, Joint Secretary to the Committee on Nutrition in the Colonial Empire, draft circular, 8 November 1939.
50 Malcolm Hailey, 'Nutrition in the Colonies', *The Times* (London, England, 26 July 1939), p. 15.
51 TNA/CO/323/1571/5, 'Nutrition in the British Colonial Empire: Summary of Replies', November 1937.
52 Emily Klancher Merchant, 'The Imperial Politics of (Mal)Nutrition in Colonial Gold Coast' (Unpublished working paper. Department of History, University of Michigan, 2005).
53 J.F. Brock and M. Autret, *Kwashiorkor in Africa* (Rome: FAO, Nutritional Studies, no. 8, 1952), p. 72.
54 H.F. Welbourn, 'The Danger Period During Weaning', *Journal of Tropical Pediatrics*, 1.1 (1955), 34–46; Valerie A. Fildes, *Breasts, Bottles and Babies: A History of Infant Feeding* (Edinburgh: Edinburgh University Press, 1985), pp. 365–6.
55 Fildes, *Breasts, Bottles and Babies*, pp. 390–3.
56 Edwin Clarke, 'Whistler and Glisson on Rickets', *Bulletin of the History of Medicine*, 36.1 (1962), 45–61 (p. 48); John Graunt, *Natural and Political Observations Mentioned in a Following Index, and Made upon the Bills of Mortality* (London: Thomas Roycroft, 1662).

57 Stephen Nicholas and Deborah Oxley, 'The Living Standards of Women during the Industrial Revolution, 1795–1820', *The Economic History Review*, 46.4 (1993), 723–49 (p. 730).
58 See, for example, Hugh Smith, *Letters to Married Women* (London: C. and G. Kearsly, 1767); George Armstrong, *An Essay on the Diseases Most Fatal to Infants* (London: T. Cadell, 1771); Richard Baron Howard, *An Inquiry into the Morbid Effects of Deficiency of Food, Chiefly with Reference to Their Occurrence amongst the Destitute Poor* (London: Simpkin, Marshall and Co., 1839); Eustace Smith, *On the Wasting Diseases of Infants and Children* (London: J. & A. Churchill, 1868).
59 This argument is made in greater detail here: Rijpma, *Livingstone*, p. 437.
60 A. Czerny and A. Keller, *Des Kindes Ernährung, Ernährungsstörungen Und Ernährungstherapie* (Leipzig: Franz Deuticke, 1906).
61 C.E. Bloch, 'Diseases of Infants Due to Prolonged Feeding with Excess of Carbohydrates', *British Medical Journal*, 1.3139 (1921), 293–95; I.A. Abt, 'Injuries Produced by Starch', *Journal of the American Medical Association*, 61.14 (1913), 1275–7.
62 Goody, *Cooking*, p. 136.
63 Vincent J. Knapp, 'The Democratization of Meat and Protein in Late Eighteenth- and Nineteenth-Century Europe', *Historian*, 59.3 (1997), 541–51.
64 Jonathan Pereira, quoted in Knapp, 'The Democratization of Meat and Protein', p. 546.
65 Mark R. Finlay, 'Early Marketing of the Theory of Nutrition: The Science and Culture of Liebig's Extract of Meat', in *The Science and Culture of Nutrition*, ed. by Kamminga and Cunningham, pp. 48–74; for the earlier French history, see Spary, *Feeding France*, pp. 203–34; for analogous contemporary trends, see, for instance, Alice Street, 'Food as Pharma: Marketing Nutraceuticals to India's Rural Poor', *Critical Public Health*, 25.3 (2015), 361–72.
66 Golden, 'Development of Concepts', p. 2117S.
67 J.A. Nixon, 'Famine Dropsy as a Food-Deficiency Disease', *Bristol Medico-Chirurgical Journal*, 37.140 (1920), 137–48; A.D. Bigland, 'Oedema as a Symptom in So-Called Food Deficiency Diseases', *The Lancet*, 195.5031 (1920), 243–47.
68 R.A. Frisch, Lafayette B. Mendel, and John P. Peters, 'The Production of Edema and Serum Protein Deficiency in White Rats by Low Protein Diets', *Journal of Biological Chemistry*, 84.1 (1929), 167–77.
69 A. Keys et al., *The Biology of Human Starvation* (Minneapolis, MN: University of Minnesota Press, 1950), 921–65; R.A. McCance, 'The History, Significance and Aetiology of Hunger Oedema', in *Studies of Undernutrition, Wuppertal 1946–9*, ed. by Department of Experimental Medicine, University of Cambridge (London: HMSO, 1951), pp. 21–82.
70 Joseph Dupuis, *Journal of a Residence in Ashantee* (London: H. Colburn, 1824), v–vi.
71 T.M. Winterbottom, *An Account of the Native Africans in the Neighbourhood of Sierra Leone; to which is added an account of the present state of medicine among them* (London: C. Whittingham, 1803), p. 66.
72 Fortes and Fortes, 'Food in the Domestic Economy', p. 267.
73 F.M. Purcell, *Diet and Ill-Health in the Forest Country of the Gold Coast* (London: Lewis, 1939), p. 14.
74 M. Autret and M. Behar, *Síndrome Policarencial Infantil (Kwashiorkor) and Its Prevention in Central America* (Rome: FAO Nutritional Studies, no. 13, 1954).
75 L. Normet, 'La Bouffissure d'Annam', *Bulletin de La Société de Pathologie Exotique*, 3 (1926), 207–13.
76 R.A.W. Procter, 'Medical Work in a Native Reserve', *Kenya Medical Journal*, 3 (1926), 284–9.
77 J. Falkenstein, quoted in Sjoerd Rijpma, 'Malnutrition in the History of Tropical Africa', *Civilisations*, 43 (1996), 45–63.
78 Rijpma, *Livingstone*, pp. 436–7.
79 For the history of kwashiorkor's 'discovery', see H.C. Trowell, J.N.P. Davies, and R.F.A. Dean, *Kwashiorkor* (London: Edward Arnold, 1954); for a more critical history, see Tappan, *Riddle*, pp. 11–36.
80 See, for instance, Trowell, 'Infantile Pellagra'.
81 Brock and Autret, *Kwashiorkor in Africa*, p. 30.
82 Brock and Autret, *Kwashiorkor in Africa*, p. 21.
83 Trowell, 'Infantile Pellagra'.
84 H.C. Trowell, J.N.P. Davies, and R.F.A. Dean, 'Kwashiorkor – II. Clinical Picture, Pathology, and Diagnosis', *British Medical Journal*, 2.4788 (1952), 798–801.

85 Rhodes House, Oxford (RH)/MSS.Afr.S.1872, Box XX, J.N.P. Davies, *Personal Reminiscences*.
86 RH/MSS.Afr.S.1872, Box XXXV, H.C. Trowell, Interview, 1982.
87 RH/MSS.Afr.S.1872, Box XXXV, H.C. Trowell, Interview, 1982.
88 Tappan, *Riddle*, p. 15.
89 TNA/CO/323/1571/5, 'Nutrition in the British Colonial Empire: Summary of Replies', November 1937.
90 H.F. Welbourn, 'Backgrounds and Follow-Up of Children with Kwashiorkor', *Journal of Tropical Pediatrics*, 5 (1959), 91.
91 Nutrition Sub-Committee, *Review of Nutrition in Uganda: A Summary of Previous Work and an Appreciation of the Present Position* (Entebbe: Government Printer, 1945), pp. 3–5.
92 Wylie, *Starving on a Full Stomach*, 223.
93 Worboys, 'Discovery of Colonial Malnutrition', 220.
94 PRAAD/A/ADM/11/1/1294, F.M. Purcell, 'Report'.
95 TNA/CO/859/68/1, Nutrition research survey: Gold Coast, 1941–3, A.I. Richards, 'Notes on Dr. Purcell's reports on Nutrition in the Gold Coast, 1940', 17 September 1941.
96 PRAAD/A/ADM/11/1/1294, Purcell, 'Report'.
97 F.M. Purcell, 'The Gold Coast Government, the Colonial Office, and Nutrition: Facts of an Astonishing Colonial Episode, Letters to the Editor', *West Africa*, 4 December 1943, p. 1095. More information on the Purcell case can be found in: Jerôme Destombes, *Nutrition and Economic Destitution in Northern Ghana, 1930–1957: A Historical Perspective on Nutritional Economics*, Economic History Working Papers (London: Department of Economic History, LSE, 1999).
98 TNA/CO/859/115/3, Note by S. Culwick, 5 December 1943.
99 TNA/CO/859/68/1, Note by S. Culwick regarding the *West Africa* article, 21 July 1943.
100 'Colonies and Calories', *West African Review*, March 1946, 255–6.
101 'Nutrition in West Africa', *West African Review*, June 1946, 618–19.
102 TNA/CO/859/115/3, Letter from Sir Alan Burns, Governor of the Gold Coast, to Oliver Stanley, Secretary of State for the Colonies, 16 February 1944.
103 Vernon, *Hunger: A Modern History*, pp. 18–80.
104 TNA/CO/323/1570/7, Response from the Gold Coast government to a circular requesting 'A summary of information regarding nutrition in the Colonial Empire', 29 June 1938.
105 Worboys, 'Discovery of Colonial Malnutrition', p. 218.
106 A.I. Richards, *Land, Labour and Diet in Northern Rhodesia: An Economic Study of the Bemba Tribe* (London: Oxford University Press, 1939), p. 3; see also Monica Hunter, *Reaction to Conquest: Effects of Contact with Europeans on the Pondo of South Africa* (Oxford: Oxford University Press, 1936).
107 Worboys, 'Discovery of Colonial Malnutrition', pp. 221–3.
108 RH/MSS.Afr.S.1872, Box XXXV, Trowell, Interview, 1982.
109 Jennifer Tappan, '"A Healthy Child Comes from a Healthy Mother": Mwanamugimu and Nutritional Science in Uganda, 1935–1973' (unpublished PhD, Columbia University, 2010), pp. 99–106.
110 On this important point, see Tilley, *Africa as a Living Laboratory*. To this end, and as described by Coghe with respect to the Belgian Congo, the political history of nutrition described here was not necessarily consistent across other European empires, all of which had their own imperial anxieties. See Samuël Coghe, 'Between Colonial Medicine and Global Health: Protein Malnutrition and UNICEF Milk in the Belgian Congo', *Medical History*, 65.4 (2021), 384–402.
111 PRAAD/A/ADM/11/1/1294, F.M. Purcell, 'Report'.
112 J. Stanton, 'Listening to the Ga: Cicely Williams' Discovery of Kwashiorkor on the Gold Coast', *Clio Medica*, 61 (2001), 149–71; Sally Craddock, *Retired Except on Demand: The Life of Doctor Cicely Williams* (Oxford: Green College, 1983).
113 Williams, 'Kwashiorkor', p. 1151.
114 Cicely D. Williams, 'The Mortality and Morbidity of the Children of the Gold Coast' (unpublished MD thesis, University of Oxford, 1936), p. 35.
115 Williams, 'Kwashiorkor'; Hugh S. Stannus, 'Kwashiorkor', *The Lancet*, 226.5856 (1935), 1207–8 (p. 1207).
116 Trowell, Davies, and Dean, *Kwashiorkor*, 283.
117 R. Schoenmaeckers et al., 'The Child-Spacing Tradition and the Postpartum Taboo in Tropical Africa: Anthropological Evidence', in *Child-Spacing in Tropical Africa: Traditions*

and Change, ed. by H.J. Page and R. Schoenmaeckers (New York: Academic Press, 1981), pp. 25–71.
118 Hunt, *Colonial Lexicon*, pp. 237–8.
119 Allman, 'Making Mothers', p. 23.
120 Allman and Tashjian, *'I Will Not Eat Stone'*.
121 See, for example, Jean Allman, 'Rounding up Spinsters: Gender Chaos and Unmarried Women in Colonial Asante', *Journal of African History*, 37.2 (1996), 195–214; Ifi Amadiume, *Male Daughters, Female Husbands: Gender and Sex in African Society* (London: ZED Books, 1987); Margrethe Silberschmidt, *'Women Forget That Men Are the Masters': Gender Antagonism and Socio-Economic Change in Kisii District, Kenya* (Uppsala: Nordiska Afrikainstitutet, 1999).
122 For a more detailed discussion of the medicalisation of malnutrition, see Tappan, *Riddle*, pp. 37–67.
123 Vaughan, *Curing Their Ills*, 1–29.
124 Cicely D. Williams, 'Child Health in the Gold Coast', *The Lancet*, 231 (1938), 97–102 (p. 99).
125 Editorial, 'Kwashiorkor', *The Lancet*, 253 (1949), 188–9 (p. 188).
126 Craddock, *Retired Except on Demand*, p. 62.
127 Mary D. Salter Ainsworth, *Infancy in Uganda: Infant Care and the Growth of Love* (Baltimore, MD: Johns Hopkins Press, 1967).
128 Wellcome Library (WL)/PP/CDW/L.1, Cicely Williams's Papers G. Saunders to M. Autret, 9 October 1953.
129 M.J. Field, *Religion and Medicine of the Gã People* (Oxford: Oxford University Press, 1937), p. 165. Although publishing after Williams, it seems Field is unaware of Williams's work. She also has some experience in mental health, working at Maudsley Hospital 'on the Biochemical aspect of Mental Pathology' in 1927 (Field, *Religion and Medicine*, p. v).
130 Field, *Religion and Medicine*, p. 177.
131 Barrington Kaye, *Bringing Up Children in Ghana: An Impressionistic Survey* (London: George Allen & Unwin, 1962), p. 67.
132 Feierman and Janzen, *The Social Basis of Health*.
133 On the history of epistemic erasure in medicine, see, for instance, Clapperton Chakanetsa Mavhunga, *The Mobile Workshop: The Tsetse Fly and African Knowledge Production* (Cambridge, MA: MIT Press, 2018).
134 Worboys, 'Discovery of Colonial Malnutrition', p. 222.
135 Brock and Autret, *Kwashiorkor in Africa*, pp. 11, 30.
136 R. Yarom and J. McFie, 'Kwashiorkor in the Congo: A Clinical Survey of a Hundred Successive Cases in the Kasai Province', *The Journal of Tropical Pediatrics and Environmental Child Health*, 9 (1963), 56–63 (p. 56).
137 J.N.P. Davies, *Pestilence and Disease in the History of Africa* (Johannesburg: Witwatersrand University Press, 1979), pp. 4, 7–8; on the endurance of these stereotypes in academic literature, see Logan, *The Scarcity Slot*.
138 Brock and Autret, *Kwashiorkor in Africa*, p. 34.
139 Klas Rönnbäck, 'The Idle and the Industrious – European Ideas about the African Work Ethic in Precolonial West Africa', *History in Africa*, 41 (2014), 117–45.
140 Quoted in Trowell, Davies, and Dean, *Kwashiorkor*, p. 243.
141 Brock and Autret, *Kwashiorkor in Africa*, pp. 32–3.
142 Davies, *Pestilence and Disease*, p. 8.
143 Brock and Autret, *Kwashiorkor in Africa*, p. 58.
144 K. David Patterson, 'The Veterinary Department and the Animal Industry in the Gold Coast, 1909–1955', *The International Journal of African Historical Studies*, 13 (1980), 457–91. The relationship between nutrition and the development of both human and animal capital deserves more work, especially given the recent 'animal turn' in historiography. An interesting exception is Jonathan Saha, 'Milk to Mandalay: Dairy Consumption, Animal History and the Political Geography of Colonial Burma', *Journal of Historical Geography*, 54 (2016), 1–12.
145 PRAAD/A/CSO/11/1/337, Index to the Literature of Food Investigation, 1933.
146 M.J. Field, 'Gold Coast Food', *Petit Propos Culinaires*, 42 (1931), 7–21 (p. 10); on efforts to localise food production in the Gold Coast, see Jonathan E. Robins, '"Food Comes First": The

Development of Colonial Nutritional Policy in Ghana, 1900–1950', *Global Food History*, 4.2 (2018), 168–88.

147 Purcell, *Diet and Ill-Health*, p. 15.

148 WL/PP/CDW/B.1/3, Cicely Williams's Papers, Gold Coast Handbook of Nursing, Children's Section, Accra, 1937.

149 PRAAD/CSO/11/6/4, Infant welfare centres – Principles, 1931–2, C.D. Williams to Deputy Director of Health Services, 18 January 1932.

3
Food and health in the nineteenth century

On an 1817 visit to see the *Asantehene*, the paramount ruler of Asante, the British diplomat Thomas Bowdich and his retinue arrived around breakfast time. Greeting them in the marketplace and, after 'enquiring anxiously if we had breakfasted', the *Asantehene*, Osei Bonsu, 'ordered refreshment'. 'After some conversation we were conducted to a house prepared for our reception, where a relish was served (sufficient for an army) of soups, stews, plantains, yams, rice, &c. (all excellently cooked) wine, spirits, oranges, and every fruit.' Only a few hours later, at 'about two o'clock', 'dinner was announced':

> We had been taught to prepare for a surprise, but it was exceeded … The large silver waiter supported a roasting pig in the centre; the other dishes on the table were roasted ducks, fowls, stews, pease pudding, &c. &c. On the ground on one side of the table were various soups, and every sort of vegetable; and elevated parallel with the other side, were oranges, pines, and other fruits; sugar-candy, Port and Madeira wine, spirits and Dutch cordials.

Unsurprisingly, of this remarkable feast, Bowdich wrote that 'we never saw a dinner more handsomely served, and never ate a better'.[1] Clearly the nineteenth-century Asante, or at least some people in nineteenth-century Asante, ate very well indeed. Although obviously not representative of the average Asante diet (and not least because of how drunk everyone would have been by lunchtime), the nature of African eating and the relative sufficiency of African food economies before and after colonisation has been a long-standing point of contention in African historiography.

Beyond contention is the depth, breadth, and speed of the social and economic transformations wrought by colonisation. The imperial invasion brought urbanisation and industrialisation, cash-crop agriculture, more globalised markets, and massive structural changes to the social threads which had ensured food security across Africa. Over the course of the late nineteenth and early twentieth centuries, the relationship between land, labour, food, and family adjusted to a new economic paradigm. While historical debate has tended to focus on the continent's susceptibility to famine relative to the immediate precolonial period, colonisation also affected diets, and nutrition as distinct from famine, both in terms of sub-clinical deficiency and clinically manifested disease.[2] This history remains less clear, and has received much less attention.

In the early twentieth century, some took that hunger and poor diet were a timeless, unavoidable burden of African ecology. As the previous chapter suggests, this naturalisation of dietary deficiency was useful to – and actively cultivated by – colonial administrators both in Whitehall and in West Africa. Others, however, came to promote what the economic historian A.G. Hopkins described as the 'myth of Merrie Africa' where, prior to colonisation, people lived in abundance, pursuing lives of leisure which appear to have mainly consisted of 'interminable dancing and drumming'.[3] According to this view, communalism and widespread kin-based systems of social security excluded poverty from the precolonial continent. As one Lagos newspaper explained in 1913, 'the rules and regulations of every African Community leave no ground for idle women, prostitutes or vagabonds, and create no possibility for the existence of waifs and strays ... no Barnardo's Homes, no Refuge for the Destitute grace the cities; because the conditions producing them are absent.'[4] This mythologised view, which was prominent well into the postcolonial period, presented the idea that African food insecurity was rooted solely in recent histories of European exploitation, in the chaos of the slave trade, and in the social deterioration which accompanied colonial capitalism.

Anthropologists working under various colonial governments certainly described the negative social impact of European authority. Max Gluckman, for instance, considered central Barotseland a place of abundance when he visited in 1940. On his return, only two years later, he struggled to find enough food for his researchers. By 1947, he described what was then Rhodesia's central plain as suffering from near famine conditions, a situation he ascribed to colonial meddling in the local economy.[5] Earlier, in the 1930s, Audrey Richards had asserted that industrialisation and the flood of European goods had depleted Northern Rhodesia's rural labour force, undermining food production as well as the draw of a rural lifestyle. The resulting, rapidly growing urban population was 'inadequately accommodated, cut off from contact with their land and the educational agencies to which they were formerly subject, and existing in conditions of extreme poverty'.[6] An idealised view of precolonial health fits into this broader historical construction. In terms of nutrition, Weston A. Price used the absence of dental malformations in East African populations in the 1930s to suggest the superiority of 'primitive' precolonial diets, informing influential Marxist thinkers such as Josué de Castro and Walter Rodney in the process.[7] Richards too thought it 'small wonder that the medical officers report that the physique of natives, whether in the town or the country, is actually deteriorating and that the proportion of definite malnutrition is on the increase'.[8]

The impact of colonial rule has also been seen to extend beyond social and economic disruption and to affect the ecological underpinnings of African food supply. Cash-cropping diminished the carrying capacity of the land, with soil fertility declining in a process which skewed delicate environmental balances across the continent. Land shortages increased as population densities rose, while colonial rule diminished peasant agency over agriculture, restricting the capacity for the self-regulation which had previously secured soil fertility.[9] Of Northern Rhodesia, the historian Leroy Vail explained that the growth of export agriculture presented 'a major ecological catastrophe', one where 'the people dwelling in some of the most fertile and hospitable land … were [now] impoverished and disease ridden'.[10]

So, is Merrie Africa simply myth? Less simplistic takes on this thinking are certainly not without their more modern advocates. Sjoerd Rijpma, for instance, has used the writings of David Livingstone and other early European doctors exploring Africa to suggest that poverty, malnutrition, and famine were indeed limited, at least as compared with the period after 1880. Instead, Rijpma proposes that these accounts describe a continent which was generally well fed, and where social and sexual traditions had evolved to protect children from malnutrition. Birth rates were low, encouraged by taboo as well as polygyny; societies reflected and functioned in accordance with the bounds of their local ecology; and nutritional illness was rare, at least in comparison with the colonial period.[11] As elsewhere in the world, food insecurity was said to result from the social disruption which followed war, slave raids, or epidemics of disease, events which often had their roots in relatively recent interactions between indigenous populations and Arab or European traders.[12] Here the health and wellbeing apparent in the centre stood in contrast to the disarray on view at the coast. In *Missionary Travels*, reflective of a period between 1840 and the mid-1850s, Livingstone noted that many illnesses common in England were absent from Africa and that 'in the more central parts the people were remarkably kind and civil and free from disease'.[13] Closer to the coasts, on the other hand, epidemic disease was brought in by ship, while the pull of trade goods and foreign wealth stoked social disintegration, slaving, and conflict.[14]

Amanda Logan's recent archaeological analysis of Banda, on the edge of the Asante forest, adds temporal depth to these arguments, employing a rich seam of archaeological evidence in order to detail local resilience to drought and socio-political crises prior to the intense upheaval of the eighteenth and nineteenth centuries.[15] Elsewhere, economic historians have utilised anthropometric data in an attempt to provide an empirical basis for discussions of health and nutrition in the nineteenth century and earlier. By considering discrepancies in adult height, several studies have found that comparable food and disease environments led to remarkably similar statures on all three Old World continents in the late eighteenth and early nineteenth centuries.[16] The working hypothesis is that improvements in European health and nutrition in the later nineteenth century meant that average European heights rose relative to those of their African counterparts.[17] Supplementing more complex social histories of African poverty, the innovative use of these biological data suggests that Africa was not a nutritional backwater in the years before more direct European involvement in African affairs.

Whether such conclusions should be stretched across a diverse continent is unclear. However well-researched or well-meaning, historical generalisations are prone to ignore spatial deviations which do not fit narrative arguments.[18] Prior to the colonial invasion, Ghana was a patchwork of economies bounded by ecology and reinforced by ethnopolitics and military prowess. The north–south discourse in modern Ghanaian politics has its foundations in these precolonial distinctions. The less forgiving ecology of the Northern savannah – defined by low soil fertility, short growing seasons, and periods of sporadic drought – is readily contrasted with the alluvial soils, consistent rainfall, and agricultural security of the Southern forests. In these distinct environments, food and wealth interacted in markedly different ways, complicating pan-African histories of hunger. In Asante, for instance, studies which associate poverty with hunger are problematic, while they are less so for savannah societies. Cultural signifiers of wealth and poverty evolved in largely incomparable societies and in reaction to the demands of localised environments. If poverty, as it could be understood in the nineteenth-century savannah, was largely absent in Asante, the more recent history of poverty in the country is all the more interesting, as the Gold Coast – an entirely new geography – was transformed under the aegis of colonial capital.

Poverty and nutrition

Although the history of nutrition has enjoyed considerable recent interest, much of this work stands apart from the conceptual problems necessary to understand malnutrition in a historical context. In view of the complex aetiology of malnutrition, habitually defining malnutrition as 'a sensitive indicator of poverty', or a facet of food insecurity, is overly simplistic.[19] As an often-fleeting biological standard, adequate nutrition, or good nutritional status, cannot necessarily indicate long-term food security. Meanwhile, although nutrition security cannot be achieved without food security, it is also dependent upon good health and adequate care. To assume that nutrition can be used as a yardstick for poverty or food insecurity, without first comparing regional and ecological differences in the nature of poverty, food supply, and nutrition, is to sweep over important spatial differences in the aetiology of malnutrition and skirt around those social and cultural determinants of nutritional status which are affected by geography and cultural norms, and which can act independently of wealth.

We should also keep in mind that nutrition is not driven by inputs alone. Labour demands and the effects of ill-health are spatially and temporally dependent, and are important determinants of community nutrition. For instance, economic developments which may generate wealth, such as the expansion of labour-intensive mining or of cash-cropping sectors, will also increase demands for food. Similarly, the disease environment influences localised patterns of malnutrition but does not necessarily interact with poverty in a linear fashion. For instance, roads and train tracks brought influenza and smallpox but also wealth and development.[20]

In some respects, however, the ready conflation of poverty and malnutrition is fairly apposite. In places where food insecurity is widespread, equating poverty with an absolute lack of food is often understandable. This 'absolute' poverty, being a failure to maintain physical efficiency, is explicitly concerned with the acquisition of food. It is this approach that John Iliffe took in his comprehensive history of African poverty. Working out from older histories of European poverty, Iliffe defines the 'poor' as those who are obliged to struggle continuously to preserve themselves and their dependants from physical want, while the 'very poor', or 'destitute', are those who 'have permanently or temporarily failed in that struggle and have fallen into physical want'.[21] Iliffe goes on to explain poverty as either structural – 'long term poverty of individuals due to their personal or social circumstances' – or conjunctural – 'temporary poverty into which ordinarily self-sufficient people may be thrown by crisis'.[22] In the labour-scarce, land-rich generalisation of precolonial Africa, structural poverty resulted from a dearth of labour and an inability to exploit abundant land.[23] The structural poor included the elderly or infirm who lived without familial support, as well as members of weak or insubstantial households. In land-scarce societies, by contrast, poverty results from an inability to acquire requisite land or sell one's labour for a requisite wage. Conjunctural poverty may afflict an individual through illness, a region through drought, or a nation through war.

Absolutist definitions of either structural or conjunctural poverty assume a failure of acquisition which, of course, remains both spatially and temporally dependent. In subsistence economies, the basic content of diet is still largely defined by ecological niche. However, diets are buoyed and deficiencies averted with the addition of non-staple foodstuffs which are more likely to be acquired by purchase, barter, foraging, or hunting. The availability of such supplementary foods is often determined by personal or local degrees of wealth. Even those dietary augmentations less reliant on capital – hunting or foraging, for instance – require a degree of wealth in labour. In this respect, the analysis of protein-energy malnutrition relates to the study of famine, food security, and food acquisition. Due to different modes of production and acquisition, the poorest strata in even food-secure environments might endure nutritional deficiencies other than total-calorie shortages as a result of their inability to obtain more nutritious foods. While individuals or families may escape frank starvation through charity, remittances, or their own hard work, the route to a balanced diet is not necessarily so readily available. Malnutrition may then derive from an inability to obtain a basket of foods which combine to form a wholly sufficient diet.

By co-opting sensitive approaches to the analysis of famine, we can begin to consider malnutrition as a symptom of absolute poverty.

Central to most modern analyses of hunger, Amartya Sen's 'entitlement approach' has directed attention away from supply-side theories of famine by promoting the idea that famine mortality generally results from demand failure. Entitlement analyses have helped to explain why, even in clear-cut supply-side failures, or food-availability decline (FAD) famines, particular demographics are more or less prone to hunger.[24] For instance, the 1944 Dutch Hongerwinter, caused by Nazi food blockades, promoted an atypical blanket decline in food availability. However, individuals with social and economic influence were able to secure 'extra-legal resources [which] doubled the extremely meagre official ration'.[25] If famine mortality is determined by socioeconomic intricacies and group-specific demand failures, then it is reasonable to assume that malnutrition may be too. In fact, frank starvation is only the most extreme failure of entitlement. By contrast, the Kampala-based MRC Nutrition Unit acknowledged that 'changes in the family's economic position, brought about by losses through theft, or the failure of a crop, although causing no more than a temporary lowering of living standards, may become a major disaster for a young child'.[26] Approaching clinical malnutrition, in terms of both quantity and quality, as a symptom of entitlement failure grants a flexible apparatus to discuss malnutrition as an absolutist shortfall at the microeconomic level.

Although poverty clearly interacts with malnutrition in an absolutist sense, food markets, diets, and childrearing practices are heavily influenced by the sociocultural environment as well. While malnutrition is symptomatic of physical want, it is a subconscious deficit which manifests in ill-health, rather than in any conscious desire for particular foods. Increasing income, therefore, does not necessarily foreshadow an immediate improvement in nutritional health. For instance, an apparent 'nutrition transition' in lower- and middle-income countries has correlated increasing income among the poor with a detrimental shift in the source of calories from complex carbohydrates to high-fat and high-sugar foods, as well as a corresponding increase in diet-related non-communicable disease (see also Chapters 7 and 8).[27]

With this in mind, how should we consider the relationship between poverty and malnutrition in food- and nutrition-secure parts of Africa? How has poverty related to those nutritional deficiencies caused by infant feeding, the use of breastmilk substitutes, or the consumption of processed food in general? These deficiencies are not exclusively derived from an absolute inability to acquire a particular basket of foods. Any attempt at historicising malnutrition has to therefore temper and discuss the economics of nutritional deficiency in view of shifting, localised food cultures, domestic economies, and medical anthropologies – or what some nutritionists once termed 'cultural blocks'.[28] This fits food economics into the anthropological study of diet, a subject which received considerable interest throughout the twentieth century.[29]

Since the historical epidemiologies of various deficiencies relate to spatially specific environments, we also have to consider the economic determinants of malnutrition in their distinct geographical and historical contexts. For instance, in African settings, several studies of urban–rural differences in protein-energy malnutrition have found that rural nutrition trails behind that in urban areas, even after controlling for socioeconomic status and related covariates.[30] Parental knowledge, medical access and understanding, food availability, food preferences, childrearing practices, and patterns of fertility vary markedly across and inside countries. Any medical history of malnutrition clearly has to first consider such spatially dependent social differences before inserting them into the wider historical narrative. Such a history has to question the relationships between environment, poverty, and malnutrition, and to ask how these relationships have changed with time.

Absolutist ideas of malnutrition can clearly only take us so far. Poverty, however, can also be thought of as a relative problem. Peter Townsend has been most prominent in promoting the idea that poverty is relative to place and time and that any definition of poverty must arise from the social reality of the society in question. In this sense, poverty arises when a group or individual lacks the means to obtain the diets, living conditions, and amenities which are the social prerequisites for an ordinary existence in their respective societies.[31] As Townsend explains, this means that:

> People's needs, even for food, are conditioned by the society in which they live and to which they belong, and just as needs differ in different societies so they differ in different periods of the evolution of single societies. Any conception of poverty as 'absolute' is therefore inappropriate and misleading.[32]

Relative ideas of poverty are not necessarily concerned with food in the sense of fundamental want. Instead, there is a conscious understanding of one's own poverty. Individuals can be healthy and well-nourished but, if their material lives lag behind those of their neighbours, they can still be considered and can consider themselves poor. Conversely, food is factored into household economies in view of a number of other demands. Here, good nutrition may be consciously or subconsciously sacrificed in the face of another, more pressing need. Such definitions of poverty become even more interesting in the context of globalisation and after the social amalgamation of colonial rule stretched understandings of social prerequisites across diverse and previously distinct societies.

This book is not in a position to speak to the strength of any one definition of poverty. However, it does seek to utilise and modify various understandings of poverty – none of which were developed with a mind to nutrition – in order to discuss how diet interacts with poverty, and how the history of African poverty has affected the nature of Ghanaian diets. Although the microeconomics of poverty and famine are essential to our understanding of malnutrition, nutrition does not interact with economics in a linear fashion. Nutritional status, as well as the aetiology and epidemiology of individual clinical deficiencies, are first mediated by the social and cultural environment of a given time and place. In order to formulate a history which can contribute to the understanding of continental patterns of nutrition, hunger, and poverty, we have to walk modern ideas of nutritional science through the distinct histories of distinct societies. In Ghana, this requires us to first think about the various ways in which poverty and nutrition interacted in the period immediately prior to colonisation.

Poverty amid plenty: nutrition, class, and family in nineteenth-century Asante

In nineteenth-century Asante, there was no real destitution, certainly not in terms of frank starvation. The same social and agricultural systems which afforded Asante its powerful political position also provided relative freedom from hunger. Diaries and chronicles from early Europeans visiting the Gold Coast forest were replete with descriptions of the country's 'spontaneous abundance'.[33] In the late nineteenth century, T.B. Freeman wrote:

> In these bright and sunny regions nature is also bountiful in its supplies of suitable vegetables and fruits – the yam, cassada, Indian corn, sweet potato, cocoa-bulb … millet, rice, sugar-cane, ginger, tomato, onion, ground-nut, orange, lime, plantain, banana, sour-sop, custard apple, and last not least, the noble pineapple, all flourish in Asantee, under ordinary cultivation.[34]

Lying between Asante and the sea, the Fante forest was also a place in which 'yams, bananas, plantains and papas [sic] flourished without culture … in a state of natural perfection'.[35] In Axim, too, Burton and Cameron were struck by the fact that 'they are never pinched for food, and they have high ideas of diet'.[36] Later in the century, George Macdonald, then the colony's Director of Education, wrote that Asante agriculture supplied 'the natives with such a continuous succession of crops, that famine and want of food are absolutely unknown'.[37] Although most obvious in the diets of the elite, a remarkable culinary diversity, which has only recently received the attention of historians, was available to almost everyone in nineteenth-century Asante.[38]

The richness of Asante food culture reflects the incredible productivity of the rainforest economy. Although, at times, social disruption could curtail some of the more diverse forest products, even this did not necessarily precede widespread food insecurity. Freeman, for instance, describes the Akan Adansi, who had 'kept up a more or less chronic war with their more powerful neighbours, in which they had generally been worsted'. Yet 'in every village there was a large plantation of plantains and another of pawpaw trees. These appeared to be common property, and their fruits together with that gathered from the oil-palms in the forest seemed to form the principal and almost the only sustenance of the inhabitants.'[39] Despite being a 'country where not a living soul was to be met with, all the inhabitants having been either killed, captured, or driven out by the conquering Ashantis', even Adansi food production had not entirely collapsed.[40] The historian Tom McCaskie has gone so far as to say that 'in the entire corpus of Asante tradition and European commentary, the only accounts of severe food shortages, widespread hunger and regional or sectoral famine are associated with the virtual collapse of subsistence agriculture affected by the five years of civil war in the 1880s'.[41]

This is largely because food farming was remarkably straightforward. Since, as Hopkins famously explained, land was 'not scarce enough to acquire a market value', land tenure was such that 'a subject could clear any part of the bush for building a house or making a plantation, without paying rent to the king or chief'.[42] Clearing the dense tropical forest, however, required a fairly large input of human labour to swing axes, cutlasses, and billhooks. The farms which followed this initial exertion were oriented around the long-term, stable intercropping of high-yielding foodstuffs, primarily yam, plantain, cocoyam, and cassava. Maize was popularised as a storable food between 1800 and 1900, but its cultivation fell away with the decline of the Asante military tradition.[43] In general, though, it was remarkably easy to provide basic sustenance to large numbers of people. Asante's food economy can, therefore, be tacked onto what Gareth Austin has called the kingdom's '"broad" forest rent', the agroeconomic benefits derived from capturing forest agriculture, generally defined as supply-side savings and a lowered cost of production. As a source of wealth not necessarily achieved through market competition, the opportunities derived from forest rent were a boon to Asante production.[44] The counterpoint to this, and a further broadening of the concept, was the remarkably low cost of social reproduction proffered by the forest food economy.

Social reproduction was also at least partially insured by Asante's political centralisation. Deriving divine authority from the *Asantehene*, the state exercised some control over food supply too. For instance, fishing in Lake Bosumtwi was partially regulated from the centre, with the use of the more efficient seine nets forbidden in favour of simple cane baskets set in shallow water. However, as colonial authority usurped traditional authority, by the early 1940s it was noted that 'this prohibition is widely disregarded [and that] there is no doubt the use of the seine net has led to over-fishing'.[45] More famously, the *odwira* yam festival was used to standardise the harvest of Asante's favoured bulk food. Draconian punishments for harvesting new-season yams prior to the start of the festival suggest that the regulation of food supply and the reinforcement of food security were understood as a valuable facet of state security.[46]

With this in mind, it is difficult to discuss an absolute form of poverty based around hunger or conscious need. In the pre-cocoa past, poverty was usually paired with social isolation:[47]

> The poor man has no friend.
> On the day of poverty it is then you perceive who is a friend.[48]

Hunger, in this environment, could be alleviated through the richness of the local economy, through borrowing, or hunting and fishing:

> Of (the two) hunger and debt, debt is preferable.
> When a man is in want, he sleeps in the forest (i.e. to hunt and fish).[49]

With so many routes out of poverty and away from hunger, the poor were improvident, foolish, or mad:

Poverty is madness.
Poverty is stupidity.[50]

In nineteenth-century Asante, the strength of the traditional subsistence economy cannot be overstated. In 1817, Bowdich explained the process by which the fertile environs of Kumasi could easily feed the city's large permanent population:

> The higher class could not support their numerous followers, or the lower their large families in the city, and therefore employed them in plantations … generally within two or three miles of the capital, where their labours not only feed themselves, but supply the wants of the chief, his family, and more immediate suite. The middling orders station their slaves for the same purpose.[51]

As a whole, the kingdom was said to have the capacity to support a standing military which constituted as much as one-fifth of the entire population.[52] Despite Kumasi's size (several tens of thousands of people at any one time), Freeman found it 'possessing nothing deserving the name of a market'.[53] There was no way that what few foods were sold could have supported this urban population; instead, Kumasi operated as 'a closed system' where a class of rural labourers were employed to support themselves as well as their kin or masters in the city.[54]

In the precolonial nineteenth century, poverty was largely linked to social status. Taking Ivor Wilks's definition of the Asante 'proletariat', it was the labour of 'the *ahiafo* or under-privileged, a group including elements from both the free and unfree population', which allowed the survival of these 'superior' or 'middling' orders. The ranks of the *ahiafo* were swelled by the constant arrival of enslaved people and supplemented by those Asante whose positions were in decline, pawns whose freedom was surrendered in debt or disgraced officials stripped of their property.[55] Inequalities in wealth left standards of living for the Asante poor far below that of the upper or middling classes.[56] Polygyny was the rule among the middle and higher classes, but free Asante *ahiafo* seldom had more than one wife, most slaves remaining unmarried.[57] It was also said that, among the rich, 'every house had its cloacae [toilet], besides the common ones for the lower orders without the town'.[58] Unsurprisingly, the rich in Asante were noted as 'nice and cleanly', while the 'poorer sort of Ashantees and slaves, arising from their neglect of cleanliness', were particularly prone to disease.[59]

Despite marked inequality, neither Akan *ahiafo* nor the *nnɔnkɔfɔ* (singular *ɔdɔnkɔ*), enslaved people from outside Asante, went hungry in the kingdom. In fact, Asante's relatively small population combined with the forest's massive potential carrying capacity to drive a thirst for labour and social expansion. As European demand for slaves declined – with British enforcement of abolition arriving in the early nineteenth century – Asante increased its internal consumption of slaves in order to profit from a shift towards 'legitimate agriculture'. Enslaved people, as well as Asante pawns and *corvées*, provided the labour necessary to reinvigorate and profit from the production and exportation of gold, rubber, kola, and palm oil.[60] Although unfree, slaves had clearly defined rights, while owners had similarly defined duties of care. According to C.H. Armitage, then Commissioner for the Southern District of Ashanti, 'these natives on entering their "master's" house immediately become one of the family and usually adopt the family name. They work in the interests of the family and share in its success and prosperity.'[61] Generally, the demands of the forest economy shaped slaveholding into an increasingly assimilative process where slaves 'might marry; own property; himself own a slave; swear an "oath"; be a competent witness; and ultimately might become heir to his master'.[62] The children of slaves were born free and, according to the anthropologist and administrator Captain R.S. Rattray, 'an Ashanti slave, in nine cases out of ten, possibly became an adopted member of the family, and in time his descendants so merged and intermarried with the owner's kinsmen that only a few would know their origin'.[63] Asante law also worked to prohibit those privy to such knowledge from mentioning any slave lineage.[64] In the later 1800s, the paramount chief of Kokofu was destooled by the elders 'for being fond of disclosing the origin of his subjects'.[65] Slaves were usually acquired by individuals or families, but, given the 'fettered multitude which could no longer be driven off to the coast directly', chiefs could also use whole communities of slaves 'to create plantations in the more remote and stubborn tracts'.[66] Ultimately, it was the strength of the subsistence economy that facilitated and promoted this assimilative form of slave agriculture. The food environment encouraged families to modify their domestic structures, to exploit the ecological advantage of the forest, and to expand and diversify their production. As Austin has explained, slaves were the most cost-effective *choice* to this end, but they may also be seen as a productive extension of the family.[67]

Although food insecurity was essentially unknown, it is more difficult to say how Asante's social expansionism interacted with other determinants of malnutrition. While we should be wary about referencing colonial anthropology as evidence of precolonial practice, we can speculate about the nature of nutrition in earlier periods using later information as our basis. In colonial Asante, infant nutrition was secured primarily through prolonged breastfeeding. Even in the 1940s, Russell reported that 'breastfeeding is universal, and is continued for eighteen months, two years, or longer, unless the mother becomes pregnant again'.[68] Lactational amenorrhea – the temporary period of postnatal infertility that results from exclusive breastfeeding – could be effective for around six months, and gave mothers some respite from a cultural tendency towards high fertility.[69] Children were also not immediately or abruptly weaned with the onset of another pregnancy. Instead, 'most women reported that they nursed the babies until the second or third month of the next pregnancy', giving the nursing baby some time to adjust to the change of diet and the loss of maternal attention.[70]

However, any conscious form of birth control was limited and perhaps even discouraged in an environment where the standard puberty rite contained the prayer 'may the elephant give you her womb that you may bear ten children'.[71] Well into the twentieth century, if such prayers bore fruit, 'a mother of ten boasts of her achievement and is given a public ceremony of congratulation'.[72] Post-partum sexual abstinence was, as a result, particularly short among the Asante, perhaps only six months for the first child and only 40 days for each subsequent birth.[73] Writing in the 1950s, the anthropologist Meyer Fortes reported a universal post-partum abstinence of 80 days, and that 'denial of sexual satisfaction is an infringement of marital rights in Ashanti law and any other method of contraception would be regarded by a wife as a slur on her womanhood'.[74] Further south, among the Akan Akuapem and the coastal Ga there was at least some socially acknowledged relationship between short birth spacing and high child mortality – perhaps a result of the less secure food environment – yet the post-partum taboo still rarely exceeded six months.[75] Post-partum abstinence was also lengthened in polygynous, generally wealthy households.[76] In the cultural and economic setting of eighteenth- and nineteenth-century Asante, high fertility was hugely advantageous to the mother and to the wider matrikin, where children were an essential source of labour. More importantly, the matrilineal orientation of Akan families meant 'the influence of a lineage in public affairs is proportional to its numbers' and that children were directly relevant to the power and status of the family.[77]

Despite what might be considered a cultural propensity for kwashiorkor, there is little reliable evidence for widespread deficiency in precolonial sources. This is not to say, though, that kwashiorkor was not regularly seen. In the same way that Williams found the Ga unforthcoming about their understanding of kwashiorkor, Fortes understandably encountered 'reluctance, bordering on dread, to speak about dead children', causing the Asante, 'even more than most peoples, to ignore their dead children'.[78] Where nutritional disease and death from such diseases did exist, its presentation was unlikely to be readily alluded to in the presence of foreign anthropologists. Yet later research suggests that kwashiorkor was certainly recognised by Akan peoples and, as elsewhere, was framed within a social understanding of illness. Deriving from *hõṅ*, meaning 'to swell', in 1940s Akim, Purcell described a form of oedematous malnutrition, 'known everywhere as "*ahonhon*"'.[79] Around the same time, in Asante proper, Russell explained that 'illnesses of the displaced baby is so common that there is a general belief among the people that the unborn child exerts a direct and malign influence upon his brother'.[80] Among the Akuapem, in the early 1960s, it was further understood that 'intercourse may affect the quality of the mother's milk and it is said that many children die as a result of this … If such a thing happens, public opinion turns against the parents, especially the father; people say that he cannot control himself, that he is a wicked and greedy person.'[81] Though clinical deficiency was probably readily recognised prior to colonisation, it is more difficult to suggest how much of a problem it posed. However, it is also difficult to imagine that Asante women would subscribe to a reproductive culture which saw an obvious correlation between pregnancy and the death or conspicuous illness of their older children, especially given the degree of power wielded by women in the precolonial kingdom.

In 1964, and amid the global obsession with protein deficiency (see Chapters 2 and 7), John Whiting advanced the hypothesis that, around the world, those populations with longer birth spacing would also be the areas with lower-protein diets.[82] Though not much discussed today, perhaps Asante's food environment alleviated the dangers which could be associated with such enthusiastic pronatalism. In terms of the general structure of Akan diets, there seems to have been limited change over the course of the nineteenth century. *Fufu* is a ubiquitous staple in Asante, while *banku* or *kenkey* traditionally dominate among the Fante and Ga further south. *Fufu* is usually made from pounded plantain, yam, cocoyam, or cassava. *Banku* and *kenkey* are generally made from fermented maize flour, although sometimes cassava flour is also used. All three are sticky, starchy balls of dough, with distinct flavours and, importantly, textures, and which require considerable time and skill to prepare. These starchy bases are eaten with one of any number of soups, determined according to taste, tradition, and seasonal access to ingredients. In the early nineteenth century, Bowdich had described these soups in some detail: 'the food of the higher orders is principally soup of dried fish, fowls, beef or mutton (according to the fetish), and ground nuts stewed in blood. The poorer class make their soups of dried deer, monkey's flesh, and frequently of the pelts of skins.'[83] Although the quality of individual diet was clearly dictated by class, if this is an accurate representation of Asante diet, later accounts which emphasised the lack of animal protein seem unlikely to be representative of the nineteenth century.[84]

Bush meat apparently went some way to make up for the lack of livestock, unsuitable to life in the often tsetse-infested forest. 'The oxen, sheep and fowls' which were kept were described by Macdonald as 'all lean, dry and tough, requiring an amount of energy, appetite and determination to eat them that a sound man seldom possesses'.[85] Livestock were infrequently slaughtered in any case, most people preferring to keep their animals as a form of reproducing capital rather than a ready source of food.[86] However, snails were collected in 'colossal' quantities, providing 'one of the most important articles of food amongst the forest people'. Following the rains, 'whole villages – men, women and children – migrate into the forest' for these ends.[87] In Akokoaso, in the 1930s, the seasonal supply of dried fish from the coast complemented the seasonal supply of snails, evening out animal produce across the year. Here dried fish, snails, and bush meat were, in that order, the three most commonly consumed forms of animal produce, far outstripping livestock consumption.[88] However, these ratios may well have changed, even fairly recently. In the 1840s, elephants were still being successfully hunted for food along the Bosompra River, and game hunting was an intensive and valuable economic activity in north and west Asante as late as the 1920s.[89] However, this intensity meant that, even prior to the nineteenth century, the amount of game available in the forest was in the midst of a long and steady decline. In the 1890s, Macdonald acknowledged that 'the animal life of the colony has much changed during the last two centuries, and at the present day you may travel through the length and breadth of the land without finding occasion to use your gun'. In 1894, 168,045 skins were exported; two years later, the number had fallen to 67,660.[90] In contrast to Bowdich's earlier description, by the late nineteenth century it was said that 'the ordinary diet of the bulk of the population was … very simple in nature', something which can, perhaps, be seen as a fairly recent change.[91]

An absence of hunger obviously does not mean that poverty was absent, but it does mean that our understanding of poverty, especially in relation to food, has to move past a conceptualisation based entirely around physical forms of want. As a start, we could consider nutrition more generally since, although total-calorie deficiencies were largely absent, nutrition security was not necessarily so straightforward. On the 1817 mission to Kumasi, Bowdich described dietary patterns which were dependent on socioeconomic status. His assistant-surgeon, H. Tedlie, also recorded that craw-craw, a painful itch symptomatic of onchocerciasis, or river blindness, 'is most commonly met with in children, few of the Dunko [*nnɔnkɔfɔ*] slaves are without it, from their poor diet and extreme dirtiness'. Several other illnesses were also seen to primarily affect children, enslaved people, and the poor. It can probably be assumed that these were conditions often exacerbated by malnutrition.[92]

As a failure of social reproduction, malnutrition is born from shortcomings in either the domestic economy or the food economy. These failures can be localised, sectoral, or both. Poverty, here, interacts with malnutrition when maternal time is too constrained to provide the requisite amount of protection to children, or when parental labour fails to provide enough nutritious foodstuffs. Given that coercion and inequality were an inherent part of precolonial Asante production, this was a problem primarily for the poor, free or unfree, Akan or *nnɔnkɔfɔ*. As Bowdich explained of enslaved people in Asante:

> Their labour was first to produce a proportionate supply to the household of their Chief, and afterwards an existence for themselves: of the greater part of the necessaries for the latter, they had been pilfered in common with the poorer class of Asantees (nominally but not virtually free), under various pretences, either in their distant plantation or on the arrival at the markets, by the public servants of the King and the Chiefs.[93]

We can, then, assume that the social epidemiology of malnutrition in nineteenth-century Asante was largely dictated by wealth. The *ahiafo*, though fed and watered, found their economic agency drained by the demands of Asante's upper classes and their involvement in the expanding extra-subsistence economy. Although it is impossible to suggest the degree to which these demands affected nutritional status, it was the *ahiafo* that had the least opportunity to provide their children with sufficient food or necessary care. In this respect, malnutrition interacted with an absolutist form of structural poverty unrelated to food insecurity.

However, for free Asantes, emergent forms of capitalist production tied poverty to a lack of capital distinct from basal subsistence.

Debt flourished among Asante's proto-capitalists and, as part of their struggle up the social ladder, even free citizens could find themselves in debt bondage, sold to a family creditor until the debt was repaid.[94] Simplistic land-rich/labour-scarce models of Asante economics are then 'overly aggregative' for nineteenth-century Asante, since, among other things, they ignore the supply of capital as an important short-term determinant of output.[95] The diversification of production and the intensified pursuit of extra-subsistence production cultivated a more demanding, relativistic understanding of poverty. For both the free and unfree in Asante, dietary compromises and malnutrition resulted from an absolute form of poverty. For free Asante, however, this could be sparked by conjunctural crisis, or a relative form of want largely disconnected from physical need.

Poverty in the nineteenth-century savannah

The area north of Asante was both less interesting and less visible to Europeans on the Gold Coast. Asante already controlled the trade in slaves, gold, kola, palm oil, and animal skins, reducing the need for exploration further north. The political and military power of nineteenth-century Asante also proved a formidable bulwark against European trade with Asante vassals in the savannah. As a result, the precolonial history of the North is much less accessible than Asante's. Northern historiography instead looks to the Arabic world, to the ancient empires of Ghana, Mali, and Songhai, and to the trans-Saharan trade route. The Arabic literature emanating from Northern Ghana or discussing the savannah states is generally concerned with the political and religious history of the various kingdoms, rather than the details of savannah life.[96] More socially oriented descriptions from missionaries and traders, principally from the flourishing Gonja slave market at Salaga, begin to appear after the decline of Asante power in the 1870s.[97] However, the first extensive accounts arrive in the early twentieth century, accompanying the expansion of colonial authority over the North.[98]

On account of the long and bloody history of savannah slaving, Europeans arrived in an area decimated by decades of intermittent raiding. Beginning in earnest in the mid-eighteenth century, the Gonja and Dagomba began raiding less well-armed ethnic groups in order to pay the Asante tribute, in the case of the Gonja, or to repay war debts, in the case of the Dagomba. Gonja and Dagomba's raiding declined following Asante's 1874 defeat at the hands of the British, but the zenith of raiding in the north-east came with the leadership of the notorious Zabarima leader, Babatu, and only ceased following the advance of a French column in 1896. The next year, the last of the Gold Coast's slave-raiders were brought to heel with the northward expansion of British forces.[99]

The prevalence of slave-raiding meant that the first European forays into the Northern Territories coincided with a period of massive social instability. Any discussion of the nineteenth-century environment has to take into account that this was a time where even powerful Northern kingdoms were subject to the demands of Asante imperialism. In Gonja, for instance, it was said that 'no man could say he possessed anything of his own. His wives, his children, his property, were all at the mercy of passing Ashantis.'[100] On his 1876 visit to Salaga, one British agent wrote, 'I myself saw the ruins of several large villages in the county through which I passed, and on inquiring the cause of the desolation, the reply in every case was, "the Ashantees sold all the inhabitants".'[101] Given the breadth of the disruption caused by slavery, we have little real idea as to what the social and economic standard of the West African savannah was like before the social chaos which succeeded Asante expansionism and the growing demand for slave labour in the Americas.

Keeping this in mind, and in spite of the relative dearth of written evidence, the later folk tradition allows us to make some assumptions about the nature of poverty, wealth, and hunger in the precolonial North, aspects of which diverge significantly from that seen in the forest. However, Ghana's savannah society is formed from numerous ethnic groups, all of which have unique social structures, economies, and histories, all often more distinct in the nineteenth century than they are today. Any assumptions drawn simply from geographical proximity cannot be considered especially robust. That said, Northern ecologies and economies are relatively homogeneous and, with broad strokes, we can at least try to describe how poverty, wealth, and hunger interacted with this specific environment.

Given the muddied history of savannah subsistence, it is also difficult to speak to the historical depth of Northern hunger. Traditionally, the Northern diet was based upon grains and supported with legumes, nuts, roots, and produce from an array of domestic and wild animals. As is the case today, harvests were in June and July for early millet and in November for guinea corn and late millet. Supplementary crops are gathered in the interceding months, but, by at least at the start of the colonial period, by 'the end of the dry season there is usually great scarcity ... which is tided over by storing the grain, but is most frequently a period of semi-starvation'.[102] Recurrent scarcity was exacerbated by vagaries in the rainfall pattern, or in the failure of one or both rains.

Hunger was certainly no stranger at this point. In the north-eastern corner of the Protectorate, a 1910 report noted that 'there is said to have been a famine in Frafra fifteen or sixteen years ago [1890s], when children were sold for a calabash of corn, or a goat'.[103] Writing in the late 1910s, the administrator-cum-anthropologist Allan Wolsey Cardinall described the extensive religious relationship Northern peoples had with the rain. Fragile, rain-dependent food economies evolved a tradition in which 'rain is in possession of a man just as is the earth. He is *duatu*, *saa-dana*, *ngwaro nyona* in Kassena, Nankanni, and Builsa.'[104] Cardinall found that 'few things are inedible. Except for one's totem, all meat is devoured, fowl, flesh, and fish.' Hunger was held at bay with a flexible approach to diet, but famine foods were also well known:

> Snakes and caterpillars ... the shea-butter pest, frogs, and even lizards make their way to the local stomachs ... One Nankanni brought me twenty-two edible weeds from a field in front of my house at Zuaragu [Zuarungu]. Once the first rains begin, the shea-butter, baobab, locust-beans and other fruits mature and help to carry on till the early crop of millet.[105]

Cardinall's pitying tone, here at times drifting towards disgust, was not uncommon in European reports of African dietaries (see Chapter 2), nor is his ungenerous analysis of Northern cuisine. Another interpretation might instead emphasise the rich resourcefulness, emplacedness, and flexibility of savannah cooking.[106] Still, the potential insecurity of savannah food production undoubtedly encouraged a culture of prudence and relative restraint:

> To taste regularly brings too much eating.[107]

In this environment, there was a constant underlying threat of cyclically manifested poverty:

> If poverty nests on your head try to get rid of it for, should it penetrate your house, you will be unable to get rid of it.[108]

In the Northern folk tradition, the avoidance of hunger is usually explained in terms of the relative strength of the relationship between food and family. For instance, hunger among the Dagaaba was circumvented through the communalism afforded by extended ideas of family:

> If an orphan kid does not suck the breasts of several goats, it cannot survive.[109]

Social isolation interacts with social and spiritual destitution. Individualism appears at a crossroads between hunger and mortality, if not specifically poverty:

> The tortoise says it has no relatives; for this reason it carries its own coffin along, so that when it dies it becomes its grave.[110]
> The grave of an unattached person is very wretched.[111]
> Lone eater, lone death.[112]
> He that eats alone dies alone.[113]

Food security was underwritten by communal ties, but food insecurity remained endemic. Without the agroeconomic security and forest rents enjoyed further south, savannah subsistence precluded the class stratification which at least partially defined nutritional status in Asante. Among the Tallensi, for instance, Fortes found an 'absence of both material and institutional possibilities for capital accumulation or for technical advance'.[114] Apart from chiefs and the few other spiritual leaders entitled to communal labour, few in the nineteenth-century North could be considered wealthy.[115]

Yet an absence of wealth does not necessarily indicate the pervasion of poverty. Indeed, the Gonja land which surrounded Salaga had the capacity to produce more than enough food for a city whose semi-urban population could swell into the tens of thousands given the season. One late nineteenth-century visitor explained that 'the high plateau is covered with low savannah grass (giving fine pasture) and two-foot-high shrubs, and is fruitful enough to bear cultivated maize, millet and yam fields, and to serve the needs of the town in provisions of all kinds.'[116] Even with the city in rapid decline, late nineteenth-century Salaga remained a place where 'even the blind found a useful occupation in basket-making'.[117] The Gonja countryside was known to be 'well suited for growing yams, legumes and tropical grains … sheep and goats are abundant in and around Salaga, and there are also large numbers of horses and donkeys'.[118] As Yendi earlier in the century, Salaga was home to a sprawling market, where meat, milk, game, and sundry other foods could be readily purchased.[119] Although Salaga is a special case for many reasons, even into the 1960s the Dagomba system of agriculture, 'which has altered little', 'ensures not only an ample food supply for the cultivating family but also a surplus for sale', and was 'capable of supporting a considerable degree of urban development and of providing the cultivator with a satisfactory income'.[120] With few expensive inputs – aside from physical labour – even the poor, isolated farmer did not necessarily suffer chronic hunger:

> There is someone who eats and is satisfied but has no wife to grind [grain].[121]

Neither did the greater degree of food insecurity or poverty, at least as relative to the South, equate with malnutrition. Anthropometric analyses of Northern Ghanaian and Burkinabe soldiers in the nineteenth-century Dutch military – most of whom were enslaved before their coerced recruitment on the coast – show that savannah recruits were of similar height to their Dutch counterparts. Although shorter than individuals from sparsely populated countries with good access to animal protein (the USA, Argentina, and Australia, for instance), even these formerly enslaved people do not appear to have grown up in a state of chronic undernutrition. Perhaps benefiting from agricultural innovation and the adoption of new world crops, such as maize, groundnuts, and cassava, these soldiers were, on average, about 1.6 centimetres taller than other West African freedmen during the 1800s.[122]

Family, famine, poverty, and wealth

Unlike in the food-secure economies of the Southern forest, family in the North was the primary means to escape famine and the primary route to security, if not affluence. In the 1930s Victor Aboya, a Nankanse man, explained the relationship between wealth, famine, and family:

> If you have not got a son, when you become old and are only able to drag your buttocks along the ground, and have still to work for yourself, what will you do? You will eat only pity; you will fall down [i.e. die] like some light thing and they will not even know that someone is dead ... When a man has many sons, corn cannot fail in his house ... when this farm fails, that one does not. On account of this, they do not ever fail to have corn. Such people are better off than

> their neighbours. Starving people's best goats, sheep, the biggest of the heifers, find their way to their place in exchange for corn.[123]

Clearly, where food supply was defined by the family, nutrition was generally determined by the efficacy of family labour. Cattle were a wise investment but, when access to familial labour ensured food security via the supply of staple grains, children were a better one.

The Northern family was a flexible, fluid construction which could be adapted according to the relative and shifting demands of individual societies. In the North, selling children was not unheard of in times of famine. Similarly, in Asante, family members were said to have been sold to assuage the burden of debt.[124] Whereas families in Asante were usually expanded with slaves and pawns, dependants in the North could be shorn if they could not be fed and housed. Writing in 1910, one administrator in the north-east found that, following a Nankani famine in the 1890s, 'disputes are still brought in for settlement, over the ownership of young women, owing to the sales of children which took place at that time'.[125] Less dramatically, Cardinall reports that 'adoption would be abhorrent, but [in times of particular hardship] a custom exists for a son to give his eldest male and female children to the grandfather on the father's side, and another custom of exchanging the ownership of the eldest children between two brothers'.[126] These practices supported the adoption of those older children whose labour is more valuable, rather than those more dependent younger children. Either as a boon to household production or as a potential drain on limited resources, the adoption of children could be used to relieve the pressure placed on precarious household economies without depleting human capital from the wider kinship group.

In this environment, where the extension of the family was the best method to ensure food security, religious and cultural practices evolved to promote investments in only productive human capital. Infanticide, for instance, was apparently 'prevalent everywhere' and was both socially reinforced and practised in collaboration with the community.[127] Cardinall, for instance, explained that 'almost invariably a deformed child is a devil, twins sometimes are … once the father is certain that his wife has brought forth a devil, he proceeds to the devil-killer.'[128] In an often-precarious subsistence economy, the relative worth of human capital is more sharply realised than in areas which enjoy a greater level of food security. Raising disabled children who, when grown, were often less able to contribute to the domestic economy could be recognised as an improvident investment in the household. Twins, likewise, are a greater drain on maternal time and energy during nursing and on often scant household resources during infancy.[129] Both twins and disabled children are also markedly more likely to die before.[130] Register data from rural Finland in the eighteenth and nineteenth centuries actually suggests that 'the survival of twins was so low that twin deliveries were no more productive than singleton deliveries'.[131] Traditions regarding sexual abstinence after birth or during breastfeeding also limit a mother's ability to conceive again, perhaps for several years. In the savannah – where the physical extension of the family is central to the economic survival of the family – cultural processes evolved to condone, both socially and spiritually, the safest investments in human capital. For instance, in the far north-east, Tauxier noted that, if 'the Kassouna-Boura women give birth to evil spirits', those children 'would later kill their father or mother'.[132] In the borderline economies of the North such an assumption was not exclusively superstition but a metaphor with some basis in the hard realities of savannah existence.

As part of this considered investment in children, communities living in the savannah generally enforced lengthy post-partum taboos regarding sex or cohabitation. In order to ensure that breastfeeding could continue without interruption from another pregnancy, 'women generally have intercourse with a man only after two years, because they are convinced if they become pregnant again before the child can eat native food they will die'.[133] Polygyny was fairly common though, and seen as a response to this tradition. Yvonne Fox, the wife of a colonial administrator in the Northern Territories, explained that 'men had to resort to many wives and at that time several chiefs boasted a "harem" of fifty women'. In contrast with the cult of fertility seen in Asante, in the North high fertility was considered detrimental to the family. Fox recalls that when 'a White Father once mentioned to a chief that he was one of a family of nineteen children. The African's comment was to the effect that his mother must have been a goat.'[134]

In contrast with the North, the Southern economy had the flexibility to incorporate less-productive dependants into the community. Among the Ga, for instance, the security of twins and the disabled was socially reinforced by their sacred position. In the 1930s, Field explained that their 'displeasure is greatly dreaded' through fear of otherworldly repercussions. The extent to which social ties could support particularly dependent children was such that 'idiots, *I am told*, are born only into chief's families'.[135] In Asante, Rattray found that infanticide did exist for some physical deformities.[136] However Fortes, writing later, explained that generally:

> Twins are welcomed and honoured. Special ritual observances distinguish them and their mother. Girl twins become the wives of the chief of their mother's chiefdom and boys become his personal attendants. Deformed and abnormal children, such as dwarfs, hunchbacks and albinos, are also taken into the chief's service.[137]

Further south, chiefs, in their role as representatives of the community, had an established duty of care over their most vulnerable kin. While individual families may not have had the capacity to incorporate the survival of their most dependent children, the wider economy did. Again, among the Ga, community support secured the wellbeing of the disabled: 'not only do his family care for him but all the neighbours help to keep an eye on him. If he shambles into any compound he will probably be given food, and if he eats it messily his face will be cleaned for him before he is sent home.'[138] Unlike in the South, the fragile food environment in the savannah precluded the inclusion of these less-productive dependants. Families were still actively built in view of the community but with familial security a more pressing concern.

Although family labour was important to the Asante subsistence economy, childlessness was less associated with poverty than with social stigma. In Asante the childless or infertile were viewed with a mixture of compassion, contempt, and suspicion. Childless women were incomplete, childless men laughable.[139] In 1927 Rattray wrote:

> Not so very many years ago the childless man or woman after death had great thorns ... driven into the soles of the feet ... At the same time the corpse was addressed with these words, *wonwo ba, mma sa bio* (you have not begotten-or borne-a child: do not return like that).[140]

Although individuals were certainly concerned about the support children could offer their elderly parents, this worry was secondary in an environment free from any real want of food. In Asante, family usually preceded wealth but childlessness did not necessarily precede hunger. Procreation was more than an economic concern or a strategy to stem poverty. It transcended fears regarding individual or familial survival and was instead considered a social duty, a contribution to both the power of the kingdom and the power of the lineage. Whereas family averted poverty in the North, family created wealth in Asante. As Wilks has explained, 'the Asante view of the position of the individual within society, as trustee of the legacy of the ancestors on behalf of the generations yet born, carried the implication that the good citizen was the one who worked to bequeath more to his successors than he had acquired from his predecessors. *Sika sene, biribiaransen bio*, runs a familiar maxim: "there is nothing as important as wealth".'[141]

It is impossible to give anything like an accurate epidemiology of nutritional illness in the nineteenth-century Gold Coast. Narrative accounts garner little useful information, while recent anthropometric analyses only grant a generalised view of nutritional status. Still, there are some speculations which we can forward. Kwashiorkor, or symptomatic manifestations of childhood malnutrition, were probably recognised everywhere and pathologised socially and in relation to the family. Total-calorie deficiencies were probably of greater concern in the North, where hunger could be epidemic and relief less forthcoming. Meat was more abundant than in the twentieth century and more regularly consumed everywhere, especially in the eighteenth century and before. Children were central to the survival and advancement of the family, and domestic structures worked to safeguard the health and nutrition of infants. Diet and nutritional status, in a generalised sense, were likely determined by social standing. Universal and prolonged breastfeeding, however, mitigated the damage caused by early weaning onto an insufficient adult diet, regardless of wealth. These cautious conclusions neither support nor deny the view of 'Merrie Africa', at least in terms of health and wellbeing. What they do deny, however, is the static homogeneity implied in such a view.

Across what was to become the Gold Coast, various modes and units of production had developed over the long course of history in order to prevent hunger and promote family survival in relation to localised environments which were subject to change. Amid the bounty of the forest economy, personal and familial poverty was rarely what Iliffe defines as 'conjunctural' – temporary poverty into which ordinarily self-sufficient people may be thrown by crisis – because of the ease with which most Asante could modify their food supply. Kinship ties mitigated the threat of conjunctural poverty at the personal or familial level. At the local level, conjunctural crisis could result from adverse political or climactic conditions; however, there is no cause to believe that such crises were anything but extremely rare in the immediate precolonial period. What poverty did exist largely resulted from social exclusion or isolation, poverty which comes under the banner of structural poverty, long-term poverty caused by an individual's personal or social circumstances. However, the centralised communalism of Asante society also assuaged the threat of consistent hunger, even for the lowest orders or for the physically incapacitated. Iliffe suggests that continent-wide changes under colonial rule meant that patterns of 'epidemic starvation for all but the rich gave way to endemic undernutrition for the very poor'.[142] Yet this argument does not fit Asante, where epidemic starvation was never a constant threat. Malnutrition perhaps correlated with social standing – in terms of the quality of food available – but any problem of quantity was likely the concern of an extremely small group of individuals existing at the absolute edge of society.

Although it is clearly misleading to suggest that famine and structural poverty were ubiquitous and timeless features of Northern life, the nineteenth-century savannah fits an archetype of African poverty which the forest does not. For instance, Jack Goody's generalisation of Africa as a place where relatively simple modes of production denied the development of an expanded class structure is more relatable when considering a generalised North.[143] Iliffe's arguments stand on firmer ground too. By the end of the nineteenth century, at least, economic marginality and the threat of conjunctural crisis had levelled most individual advantage, making long-term parasitism untenable for both the comparatively rich and the comparatively poor. Epidemic starvation was an endemic concern and the threat of food insecurity had undoubtedly shaped savannah culture. Family was articulated into the primary form of wealth, the primary form of famine relief, and the surest way to avoid conjunctural crises. Despite this, the extension of the Northern family was informed by a social acknowledgement of the precarious nature of child survival. The North's considered form of pronatalism, where families were regulated in view of the often-delicate food environment, stands in contrast with the thirsty social expansionism that the food security of the forest granted Asante kin groups. The ready distinction which can be made between these diverse spaces is especially important as we consider how they moved forward into a period where cash-earning and export economics swelled production and promoted economic integration across previously distinct geographies. Family structures changed in response to the demands and responsibilities of the new economy, reflecting changing forms of poverty and food security, and influencing diet and nutrition in turn. The coming decades resulted in a dramatic restructuring of the economic geographies and moral economies of these two distinct polities.

There is the common conflation of Jack Goody's famous argument – that limited class stratification across much of the continent had led to a relative absence of haute cuisine – with the idea that African cuisine is, by extension, an innately subordinate form of eating.[144]

As paeans to the foods and feasts enjoyed in nineteenth-century Asante make quite plain, hautifying the history of African cuisine should not be difficult, and recent additions to African food history have, in this vein, provided substantive challenge to the stereotyping of food in the African past.[145] However, such an approach also distracts from the fact that, in Goody's examples, the frivolity and excess of haute cuisine in Europe and Asia was derived from the exploitation of the Eurasian poor, and the violent social stratification which was progressively foisted onto colonised peoples across Africa. The resilient, diverse, and complex cuisines which emerge from a fuller and longer history of African foodways should instead be considered testament to the precolonial moral economies which also worked to protect health and wellbeing in disparate and sometimes challenging environments.[146] In other words, the relative absence of haute cuisine speaks to a degree of social equity which, as we will see, was eroded through exposure to colonial capital and greater integration into global markets.

Notes

1 T.E. Bowdich, *Mission from Cape Coast Castle to Ashantee: With a Statistical Account of That Kingdom and Geographical Notices of Other Parts of the Interior of Africa* (London: John Murray, 1819) pp. 114–15.
2 See, for instance, the important distinctions found between Watts, *Silent Violence*, and Iliffe, *Famine in Zimbabwe*.
3 A.G. Hopkins, *An Economic History of West Africa* (London: Longman, 1973), p. 10.
4 Quoted in Iliffe, *African Poor*, p. 3.
5 Max Gluckman, 'The Lozi of Barotseland in North-Western Rhodesia', in *Seven Tribes of British Central Africa*, ed. by Elizabeth Colson and Max Gluckman (Manchester: Manchester University Press, 1951), pp. 1–93; William Allan, *The African Husbandman* (Edinburgh: Oliver & Boyd, 1967), pp. 152–5.
6 Richards, *Land, Labour*, p. 3.
7 Weston A. Price, *Nutrition and Physical Degeneration: A Comparison of Primitive and Modern Diets and Their Effects* (London: P.B. Hoeber, 1939); Josué de Castro, *The Geography of Hunger* (Boston, MA: Little, Brown, 1952), p. 220; Walter Rodney, *How Europe Underdeveloped Africa* (Washington, D.C.: Howard University Press, 1974), pp. 236–8.
8 Richards, *Land, Labour*, p. 4.
9 William Beinart, 'Soil Erosion, Conservationism and Ideas about Development: A Southern African Exploration, 1900–1960', *Journal of Southern African Studies*, 11.1 (1984), 52–83.
10 Leroy Vail, 'Ecology and History: The Example of Eastern Zambia', *Journal of Southern African Studies*, 3.2 (1977), 129–55 (p. 129).
11 Rijpma, 'Malnutrition', pp. 56–7, 52.
12 Rijpma, *Livingstone*.
13 Quoted in Rijpma, *Livingstone*, p. 447.
14 For the Gold Coast, see James D. La Fleur, *Fusion Foodways of Africa's Gold Coast in the Atlantic Era* (Leiden: Brill, 2012).
15 Logan, *The Scarcity Slot*.
16 Richard H. Steckel, 'Heights and Human Welfare: Recent Developments and New Directions', *Explorations in Economic History*, 46.1 (2009), pp. 1–23; Joerg Baten and Matthias Blum,

'Growing Tall but Unequal: New Findings and New Background Evidence on Anthropometric Welfare in 156 Countries, 1810–1989', *Economic History of Developing Regions*, 27 (2012), S66–85.

17 Gareth Austin, Joerg Baten, and Bas Van Leeuwen, 'The Biological Standard of Living in Early Nineteenth-Century West Africa: New Anthropometric Evidence for Northern Ghana and Burkina Faso', *The Economic History Review*, 65.4 (2012), 1280–302.

18 Even Logan's excellent, nuanced *longue durée* history of food *security* in Banda – a somewhat liminal area between the rainforest and the savannah proper – tends to stretch convincing, and highly localised, arguments across time-spaces which are not plainly comparable.

19 Iliffe, *African Poor*, p. 161.

20 James W. Brown, 'Increased Intercommunication and Epidemic Disease in Early Colonial Ashanti', in *Disease in African History: An Introductory Survey and Case Studies*, ed. by K. David Patterson and Gerald W. Hartwig (Durham, NC: Duke University Press, 1978), pp. 180–207.

21 Iliffe, *African Poor*, p. 2.

22 Iliffe, *African Poor*, p. 4.

23 Hopkins, *Economic History*.

24 Sen, *Poverty*.

25 Zena Stein, *Famine and Human Development: The Dutch Hunger Winter of 1944–1945* (Oxford: Oxford University Press, 1975), pp. 47–51.

26 TNA/FD/12/273, Medical Research Council, Child Nutrition Research Unit (Formerly Infantile Malnutrition Research Unit), Kampala, Uganda, 1961. 'Infantile Malnutrition Research Unit: Progress Report, January 1962.'

27 Barry M. Popkin, 'The Nutrition Transition in Low-Income Countries: An Emerging Crisis', *Nutrition Reviews*, 52.9 (1994), 285–98; Shufa Du et al., 'Rapid Income Growth Adversely Affects Diet Quality in China – Particularly for the Poor!', *Social Science & Medicine*, 59.7 (2004), 1505–15.

28 D.B. Jelliffe, 'Social Culture and Nutrition: Cultural Blocks and Protein Malnutrition in Early Childhood in Rural West Bengal', *Pediatrics*, 20.1 (1957), 128–38.

29 Ellen Messer, 'Anthropological Perspectives on Diet', *Annual Review of Anthropology*, 13.1 (1984), 205–49.

30 Lisa C. Smith, Marie T. Ruel, and Aida Ndiaye, 'Why Is Child Malnutrition Lower in Urban Than in Rural Areas? Evidence from 36 Developing Countries', *World Development*, 33.8 (2005), 1285–305.

31 Peter Townsend, 'Poverty as Relative Deprivation: Resources and Style of Living', in *Poverty, Inequality & Class Structure*, ed. by Dorothy Wedderburn (Cambridge: Cambridge University Press, 1975), pp. 15–42 (p. 15).

32 Peter Townsend, *Poverty in the United Kingdom: A Survey of Household Resources and Standards of Living* (Berkeley, CA: University of California Press, 1979), p. 38.

33 Bowdich, *Mission*, pp. 273–4.

34 T.B. Freeman, 'Life and Travels on the Gold Coast', *The Western Echo* (Cape Coast, 6 March 1886), p. 8.

35 Dupuis, *Journal*, p. 6.

36 Richard Francis Burton and Verney Lovett Cameron, *To the Gold Coast for Gold: A Personal Narrative* (London: Chatto and Windus, 1883), p. 95.

37 George Macdonald, *The Gold Coast, Past and Present: A Short Description of the Country and Its People* (London: Longmans, Green & Co., 1898), p. 69.

38 James C. McCann, *Stirring the Pot: A History of African Cuisine* (Athens, OH: Ohio University Press, 2009); La Fleur, *Fusion Foodways*; Logan, *The Scarcity Slot*; Brandi Simpson Miller, *Food and Identity in Nineteenth and Twentieth Century Ghana: Food, Fights, and Regionalism* (Cham: Springer International Publishing, 2021), pp. 143–78. Margaret Field's 1931 pamphlet is the first to detail the rich diversity of Akan cuisine. See Field, 'Gold Coast Food'.

39 R. Austin Freeman, *Travels and Life in Ashanti and Jaman* (London: A. Constable & Co., 1898), p. 39.

40 Freeman, *Travels and Life*, pp. 37–9.

41 T.C. McCaskie, *State and Society in Pre-Colonial Asante* (Cambridge: Cambridge University Press, 1995), p. 29.

42 Hopkins, *Economic History*, p. 39; Macdonald, *Gold Coast*, p. 289.

43 McCaskie, *State*, p. 26.

44 Austin, *Labour*, pp. 10–12.
45 PRAAD/Kumasi (K)/ARG/6/14/7, Diet and Nutrition Surveys, 1940–7, E.H. Roach, Acting District Commissioner of Kumasi, to Chief Commissioner of Ashanti, 23/10/41.
46 McCaskie, *State*, pp. 144–51; Lynne Brydon, 'Rice, Yams and Chiefs in Avatime: Speculations on the Development of a Social Order', *Africa*, 51.2 (1981), 659–77; Kwame Arhin, 'The Financing of the Ashanti Expansion (1700–1820)', *Africa*, 37.3 (1967), 283–91.
47 For a similar folk analysis of poverty in southern Uganda, see Kuhanen, *Poverty*, p. 34; for the Northern Gold Coast, see Paul Shaffer, 'Seasonal Hunger in the Northern Territories of the Gold Coast, 1900–40', *Economic History of Developing Regions*, 32.3 (2017), 270–300. Proverbs and other linguistic evidence are relatively weak historical sources, largely because they are almost impossible to date. Yet they do offer valuable insight into the period immediately prior to their collection. See Rhiannon Stephens, 'Poverty's Pasts: A Case for Longue Durée Studies', *The Journal of African History*, 59.3 (2018), 399–409.
48 R.S. Rattray, *Ashanti Proverbs: The Primitive Ethics of a Savage People* (Oxford: Clarendon Press, 1916), pp. 159–60.
49 Rattray, *Proverbs*, pp. 146, 157.
50 Rattray, *Proverbs*, pp. 159, 158.
51 Bowdich, *Mission*, pp. 323–4.
52 Bowdich, *Mission*, p. 316.
53 T.B. Freeman, 'Life and Travels on the Gold Coast', *The Western Echo* (Cape Coast, 24 February 1886), p. 8. This was part of a broader pattern. Bowdich apparently 'never saw, or heard of a good public market in any part of the forest'. See Bowdich, *Mission*, p. 324.
54 McCaskie, *State*, p. 35.
55 Wilks, *Asante*, pp. 705–7.
56 Wilks, *Asante*, p. 443.
57 Bowdich, *Mission*, p. 317.
58 Bowdich, *Mission*, p. 306.
59 Bowdich, *Mission*, pp. 306, 318, 376.
60 Gareth Austin, 'Between Abolition and Jihad: The Asante Response to the Ending of the Atlantic Slave Trade, 1807–1896', in *From Slave Trade to 'Legitimate' Commerce: The Commercial Transition in Nineteenth-Century West Africa*, ed. by R. Law (Cambridge: Cambridge University Press, 1995), pp. 93–118.
61 Quoted in Austin, *Labour*, p. 117.
62 R.S. Rattray, *Ashanti Law and Constitution* (Oxford: Oxford University Press, 1929), p. 38.
63 Rattray, *Ashanti Law*, p. 42.
64 Rattray, *Ashanti Law*, pp. 81–2.
65 Austin, *Labour*, p. 119.
66 T.E. Bowdich, *The British and French Expeditions to Teembo: With Remarks on Civilization in Africa* (Paris: J. Smith, 1821), p. 18.
67 Austin, *Labour*, pp. 117–21.
68 Beatrice A.S. Russell, 'Malnutrition in Children under Three Years of Age in Ashanti, West Africa', *Archives of Disease in Childhood*, 21.106 (1946), 110–12 (p. 110).
69 See, for instance, Giovanni A. Tommaselli et al., 'Using Complete Breastfeeding and Lactational Amenorrhoea as Birth Spacing Methods', *Contraception*, 61.4 (2000), 253–7.
70 Faye Woodard Grant, 'Nutrition and Health of Gold Coast Children. II. Care and Physical Status of Children', *Journal of the American Dietetic Association*, 31.7 (1955), 694–702 (p. 697).
71 R.S. Rattray, *Religion and Art in Ashanti* (Oxford: Clarendon Press, 1927), p. 73.
72 Meyer Fortes, 'Kinship and Marriage among the Ashanti', in *African Systems of Kinship and Marriage*, ed. by A.R. Radcliffe-Brown and D. Forde (Oxford: Oxford University Press, 1952), pp. 252–84 (pp. 262–3).
73 Dennis M. Warren, *The Techiman-Bono of Ghana: An Ethnography of an Akan Society* (Dubuque, IA: Kendall/Hunt Pub. Co., 1975), p. 25.
74 Meyer Fortes, 'A Demographic Field Study in Ashanti', in *Culture and Human Fertility: A Study of the Relation of Cultural Conditions to Fertility in Non-Industrial and Transitional Societies*, ed. by Lorimer Frank (Paris: UNESCO, 1954), pp. 253–340 (p. 265).
75 Kaye, *Bringing Up Children*, pp. 67–9.

76 Kaye, *Bringing Up Children*, pp. 67–8.
77 Fortes, 'Field Study', p. 267.
78 Fortes, 'Field Study', p. 267.
79 Johann Gottlieb Christaller, *A Dictionary of the Asante and Fante Language Called Tshi (Chwee, Twi)* (Basel: Evangelical Missionary Society, 1881), pp. 188–9; PRAAD/A/ADM/11/1/1294, Purcell, 'Report', pp. 109–10.
80 Russell, 'Malnutrition', p. 110.
81 Kaye, *Bringing Up Children*, p. 67.
82 J.W.M. Whiting, 'Effects of Climate on Certain Cultural Practices', in *Explorations in Cultural Anthropology*, by W. Goodenough (New York: McGraw-Hill, 1964), pp. 511–44 (p. 521).
83 Bowdich, *Mission*, p. 319.
84 This also contradicts Goody's assessment of food and class in precolonial Africa: see Goody, *Cooking*.
85 Macdonald, *Gold Coast*, p. 69.
86 Russell, 'Malnutrition', p. 110.
87 A.W. Cardinall, *In Ashanti and Beyond* (London: Seeley, Service & Co., 1927), pp. 78–80.
88 W.H. Beckett, *Akokoaso: A Survey of a Gold Coast Village* (London: P. Lund, Humphries & Co., 1944), pp. 22–3.
89 McCaskie, *State*, pp. 27–9.
90 Macdonald, *Gold Coast*, p. 72.
91 Macdonald, *Gold Coast*, p. 40.
92 H. Tedlie, 'Materia Medica and Diseases', in *Mission from Cape Coast Castle to Ashantee: With a Statistical Account of That Kingdom and Geographical Notices of Other Parts of the Interior of Africa*, by T.E. Bowdich (London: John Murray, 1819), pp. 370–80 (p. 375).
93 Bowdich, *Teembo*, p. 18.
94 Austin, *Labour*, pp. 140–50.
95 Austin, *Labour*, pp. 73–7.
96 See, for instance, Wilks, Levtzion, and Haight, *Chronicles*.
97 *Salaga Papers*, ed. by Marion Johnson (Legon, Accra: University of Ghana, 1965).
98 Louis Tauxier, *Le Noir Du Soudan: Pays Mossi et Gourounsi, Documents et Analyses* (Paris: Emile Larose, 1912); A.W. Cardinall, *The Natives of the Northern Territories of the Gold Coast: Their Customs, Religion and Folklore* (London: George Routledge & Sons, 1920).
99 Benedict G. Der, *The Slave Trade in Northern Ghana* (Accra: Woeli, 1998), pp. 10–26.
100 R. la T. Lonsdale, 'Kumasi and Salaga, 1881', SAL/41/3. In Johnson (ed.), *Salaga Papers*.
101 V.S. Gouldsbury, 'Report of his Journey into the Interior of the Gold Coast, 1876', SAL/21/2. In Johnson (ed.), *Salaga Papers*.
102 Cardinall, *Northern Territories*, pp. 83–5.
103 PRAAD/A/ADM/56/1/128, Report on food supply in Frafra, 1911, Captain H. Wheeler, Acting Provincial Commissioner, North Eastern Province, Zuarungu, 'Food supply in Frafra,' 31/5/1911.
104 Cardinall, *Northern Territories*, p. 264.
105 Cardinall, *Northern Territories*, pp. 82–3.
106 More work deserves to be done to this end, as most of the recent histories of African foodways have focused on Atlantic Africa. A notable exception can be found in Simpson Miller, *Food and Identity*, pp. 179–219.
107 C.S. Kponkpogori, C.J. Natomah, and O. Rytz, *Gonja Proverbs* (Legon, Accra: University of Ghana, 1966), p. 10.
108 A.K. Awedoba, *An Introduction to Kasena Society and Culture through Their Proverbs* (Lanham, MA: University Press of America, 2000), p. 181.
109 Sebastian K. Bemille, *Dàgàrà Proverbs* (Berlin: Dietrich Reimer, 2010), p. 188.
110 Kponkpogori, Natomah, and Rytz, *Gonja Proverbs*, p. 40.
111 Samuel Akon et al., *Kusaas Siilima: Kusaasi Proverbs* (Tamale: Ghana Institute of Linguistics, 1980), p. 12.
112 Akon et al., *Kusaas Siilima*, p. 27.
113 Bemille, *Dàgàrà Proverbs*, p. 199.
114 Meyer Fortes, *The Dynamics of Clanship among the Tallensi: Being the First Part of an Analysis of the Social Structure of a Trans-Volta Tribe* (Oxford: Oxford University Press, 1945), p. x.

115 Meyer Fortes, 'The Political System of the Tallensi of the Northern Territories of the Gold Coast', in *African Political Systems*, ed. by Meyer Fortes and Edward Evan Evans-Pritchard (Oxford: Oxford University Press, 1940), pp. 239–71 (pp. 250–1).

116 C. Von Francois, 'Salaga in 1888', SAL/18/1. In Johnson (ed.), *Salaga Papers*.

117 J.G. Christaller, 'Recent Explorations in the Basin of the Volta (Gold Coast) by Missionaries of the Basel Missionary Society', *Proceedings of the Royal Geographical Society and Monthly Record of Geography*, 8.4 (1886), 246–56 (p. 254).

118 V.S. Gouldsbury, 'Report of his Journey into the Interior of the Gold Coast, 1876', SAL/11/1. In Johnson (ed.), *Salaga Papers*.

119 For Salaga, see Johnson (ed.), *Salaga Papers*; for earlier, albeit second-hand information on Yendi, see Bowdich, *Mission*, p. 178.

120 Allan, *African Husbandman*, p. 240.

121 Akon et al., *Kusaas Siilima*, p. 12.

122 Austin, Baten, and Van Leeuwen, 'Biological Standard of Living', pp. 1298–9.

123 R.S. Rattray, *The Tribes of the Ashanti Hinterland* (Oxford: Clarendon Press, 1932), p. 138.

124 Rattray, *Law*, p. 37.

125 PRAAD/A/ADM/56/1/128, 'Food supply in Frafra'; Cardinall, *Northern Territories*, p. 74.

126 Cardinall, *Northern Territories*, p. 74.

127 Cardinall, *Northern Territories*, p. 29.

128 Cardinall, *Northern Territories*, p. 28.

129 Gary Granzberg, 'Twin Infanticide: A Cross-Cultural Test of a Materialistic Explanation', *Ethos*, 1.4 (1973), 405–12.

130 Helen L. Ball and Catherine M. Hill, 'Reevaluating "Twin Infanticide"', *Current Anthropology*, 37.5 (1996), 856–63; Guang Guo and Laurence M. Grummer-Strawn, 'Child Mortality Among Twins in Less Developed Countries', *Population Studies*, 47.3 (1993), 495–510.

131 Erkki Haukioja, Risto Lemmetyinen, and Mirja Pikkola, 'Why Are Twins so Rare in Homo Sapiens?', *The American Naturalist*, 133.4 (1989), 572–7 (p. 576).

132 Tauxier, *Le Noir*, p. 329.

133 Cardinall, *Northern Territories*, p. 69.

134 RH/MSS.Afr.S.2003, Yvonne P. Fox, 'Three chapters of memoirs on life in the Northern Territories of the Gold Coast', c.1930s.

135 Field, *Religion and Medicine*, pp. 180–3.

136 Rattray, *Religion*, pp. 56, 66.

137 Fortes, 'Field Study', pp. 265–6.

138 Field, *Religion and Medicine*, p. 183.

139 Wolf Bleek, 'Did the Akan Resort to Abortion in Pre-Colonial Ghana? Some Conjectures', *Africa*, 60 (1990), 121–31.

140 Rattray, *Religion*, p. 67.

141 Wilks, *Asante*, p. 673.

142 Iliffe, *African Poor*, pp. 4, 6.

143 Goody, *Cooking*.

144 For instance, McCann, *Stirring the Pot*, p. 4. This is not an entirely inaccurate reading; Goody's account does not detail the range of foods produced, even among the LoDagaa (Dagaaba), or attest to the significant skill necessary to procure, produce, process, and refine the raw ingredients grown, hunted, or gathered in the savannah. Yet his central point – about class – is often overlooked in rejoinders to this debate.

145 Fran Osseo-Asare, *Food Culture in Sub-Saharan Africa* (Westport, CT: Greenwood Press, 2005); McCann, *Stirring the Pot*; La Fleur, *Fusion Foodways*; Logan, *The Scarcity Slot*; Simpson Miller, *Food and Identity*.

146 Watts, *Silent Violence*.

4
Feeding the cocoa boom, c.1896–1957

In 1955, in the rural Asante constituency of Atwima Nwabiagya, a new highlife was taking off. Sung through the streets of its villages by young people and school children, it went as follows:

> If you want to send your children to school, it is cocoa,
> If you want to build your house, it is cocoa,
> If you want to marry, it is cocoa,
> If you want to buy cloth, it is cocoa,
> Whatever you want to do in this world,
> It is with cocoa money that you do it.

Written by Fred Sarpong, a journalist, trader, politician, and sometime songwriter, it has been said that the original *Twi* lyrics 'goes with a much greater swing'.[1] With the end of British rule coming into sight, Sarpong's highlife voiced support for Asante nationalism and opposition to Kwame Nkrumah's Convention People's Party (CPP), then leading the charge towards self-rule.[2] This song worked as political propaganda because cocoa income was the primary vehicle for personal advancement in rural Asante, but also because rural Asante's cocoa industry was the primary source of foreign exchange for the entire colony. Nkrumah's aspirations for the entirety of an independent state relied heavily on the output of a relatively small number of Asante farmers. By the end of the colonial period, the health of the Gold Coast economy was largely dependent on the vagaries of the international cocoa market; so too was the health of the growing numbers of people whose livelihoods depended on the money which cocoa provided.

Between the late nineteenth century and the first rendition of Sarpong's song, Asante's economy had changed from one primarily oriented towards subsistence agriculture to one reliant upon the commercial cultivation of cocoa. Unlike in some other parts of Africa, the Gold Coast's shift to cash-cropping was spearheaded by indigenous entrepreneurship, rather than the efforts of European settlers. By 1910, perhaps only 30 years after its introduction, these 'rural capitalists' had transformed the Gold Coast into the biggest exporter of cocoa in the world.[3] In 1893, cocoa exports measured less than two tons, earning only £93 for the colony. By 1920, the 124,000 tons of cocoa shipped out were worth more than £10 million. The combined value of the seven next most important agricultural exports – the 17 million tons of kola nuts, guinea grains, palm kernels, palm oil, rubber, cotton, and copra – made only £830,000.[4] By the 1930s, cocoa exports averaged more than two hundred thousand tons and could represent as much as three-quarters of the colony's annual export earnings, propping up the transport and distributive sectors as well as an expanding urban world which depended on and was concentrated around the geography of the cocoa boom.[5]

Of course, as we have already seen, extra-subsistence production was common throughout Asante following the end of the Atlantic slave trade and before the introduction of cocoa. During these years there was 'a general readiness both to respond to the market opportunities and to use extra-economic means, from slavery and polygyny to market controls, to make those responses more effective'.[6] However, encouraged by colonial administrations and stimulated by the ever-growing supply of imported goods, greater integration with the global market drove the expansion of cocoa, sowing the influence of the cocoa trade throughout the fabric of Asante life. As the state and the individual cultivators became increasingly dependent on the cash which could be earned from cocoa, social conflict also spread. The draw of the cocoa economy was such that, as one observer recalled, 'everyone went "cocoa mad", lawyers threw down their briefs, clerks gave up their berths and all devoted their time to buying and shipping cocoa'.[7] 'Chaos' was the word Gwendolyn Mikell chose to describe the social and economic turmoil of the Gold Coast's cocoa revolution, as cocoa altered traditions of kinship and dominated independence politics throughout the colony.[8] Jean Allman also chose to describe the 'chaos' of Asante gender relations during this period, when the pursuit of cash and cocoa undermined the value of domestic reproduction and refigured the roles of wives and mothers across the kingdom. At the same time, cash and cocoa provided new avenues for women's economic emancipation, which in its own turn led to increasingly severe enactments of patriarchal control.[9]

At the intersection of these chaotic worlds – the commercial and domestic, the public and the private – is where the social epidemiology of good and bad nutrition often lies. In Asante, these are two worlds which are largely indivisible. As the Gold Coast's Director of Agriculture explained in 1918, unpaid 'family labour' and free access to 'tribal' land meant that 'cocoa can be more cheaply produced in this country than in any other country with which I am acquainted'.[10] The boom in commercial production was, therefore, facilitated by refiguring the domestic modes of production, the primary concern of which had previously been the health, happiness, and hungers of the household. These changes were only complicated by the nature of Asante domestic structure, or what has been described as the 'remarkable' paradox that, 'in spite of their matrilineal inheritance system, the Ashanti basic unit of labour in mining, trading and farming has always been the conjugal family'.[11] Cash and then cocoa tested this paradox by upsetting the relative importance of production and reproduction in Asante understandings of wealth.

As the main tenets of Asante production shifted further in response to the cocoa boom, local food cultures and patterns of childrearing changed as well. Forest agriculture moved to accommodate cash-crops and the production and relative worth of food crops changed in response. Expanded agricultural production drove an increased demand for familial labour, which impinged on the time available for childrearing, as well as for extra-familial labour, which fostered the growth of an immigrant labouring class. Huge increases in the value of extra-subsistence production promoted internal migration and propped up the expanding urban areas which were concentrated almost exclusively in the South – the Northern Territories' administrative centre in Tamale being the primary exception. In these growing cities, social reproduction and the domestic economy were largely removed from the nineteenth-century model and cast the nutrition environment of the rural forest into sharp relief. For some in rural Asante, these changes meant opportunities for employment within an expanded food market. For others, it meant dislocation from the subsistence economy and reliance on purchased food. Cocoa influenced nutrition and food security throughout the kingdom; however, these were not necessarily malign influences. Cash had the potential to fill any gaps in subsidence and the diversification of employment facilitated new routes into wealth. Sadly, the converse was now also true, and deficits in cash or employment could tie food insecurity and malnutrition to emergent forms of poverty. Massive shifts in the Gold Coast economy meant that the demography of malnutrition changed. The economy, and individual position within it, suddenly became relevant to the social aetiology of malnutrition.

Social reproduction in the colonial economy

Although the expansion of cocoa production in Asante should be considered the result of indigenous industry, it is important to remember that colonialism provided the backdrop against which these developments took place. Through a combination of free trade and indirect rule, Whitehall guided the development of British colonies, dependencies, and protectorates around the world. An important aspect of this, and one especially relevant for a study of malnutrition, is the way in which the colonial establishment attempted to refigure the African domestic environment, as well as the degree to which it succeeded.

Writing in the late 1960s, Ester Boserup noted that 'colonial administrators and technical advisers are largely responsible for the deterioration in the status of women in the agricultural sectors'.[12] In subsequent years, feminist economists have explained the degree to which female labour is ignored in the neoclassical tradition of economic thought fundamental to Western governments and colonial administrations alike.[13] One illustrative aspect of this is the common misrepresentation of the nature of family. In his 1820 *Essay on Government*, James Mill, one of the founders of classical economics, explained that:

> All those individuals whose interests are indisputably included in those of other individuals may be struck off without inconvenience. In this light ... women may be regarded, the interest of almost all of whom is involved in that of their fathers or in that of their husbands.[14]

Well into the twentieth century, the view still propagated by influential textbooks was that 'family affections generally are so pure a form of altruism, that their action might have shown little semblance of regularity, had it not been for the uniformity of the family relations themselves'.[15] This rationale assumes that the family operates as a single unit and, in doing so, denies the possibility of intra-family conflict and the inequitable allocation of resources. Yet in Asante, as was often the case elsewhere in Africa, 'the property of a wife was quite distinct from that of the husband'.[16] Such distinctions can cause significant divergences in health and wellbeing within a family unit. Regarding colonial Nyasaland, Megan Vaughan explained that 'the rights and duties of husbands and brothers were the subject of constant negotiation'. This was a particular problem in times of economic stress, such as the 1949 famine where 'the suffering of women ... was constructed as much around government famine relief policy as it was around marriage and kinship structure'.[17]

The suffering of women often also reflects in the suffering of their children. Conceptualising the family as a single economic unit obscures and undervalues those labours associated with the basic survival and expansion of the family, part of which includes the work necessary to secure the health and nutritional status of every dependent member. Ultimately the neoclassical approach to economics focuses on the 'productive economy', which makes money, and takes for granted the 'reproductive economy', which sustains human needs. The contribution provided by the reproduction and maintenance of the labour force through childbirth, childcare, and myriad domestic responsibilities is devalued as the accumulation of capital acquires a significantly greater value. As the family unit is appraised simply on its productive ability, reproductive labour is rendered invisible in any calculation of its worth.[18] Such erasure is usually gendered, as the subsistence activities omitted in production statistics are unevenly ascribed to women. The status, freedoms, and agency of women in any given society are, therefore, particularly relevant to the health and wellbeing of the children born into that society.

Built broadly on the back of these Euro- and andro-centric economic theories, the insidious influence of colonial capitalism was only amplified by the more active colonisation of the domestic, that which sought to reformulate African production and the African family along European lines.[19] By the late 1920s, the colonisation of motherhood through baby shows was widespread (see also Chapter 2); new mothers were also routinely encouraged to visit maternity clinics, with gifts of sugar, soap, and children's clothes.[20] However, Asante mothers were largely ambivalent to the mothercraft agenda and, through sheer demand, had converted the child welfare centre in Kumasi into the curative centre they wanted, rather than the education centre which the administration had envisaged. Indeed, by 1932, the Health Service was attempting to offload responsibility for child welfare to Medical and Sanitary Services 'in view of the fact that the various Infant Welfare Clinics in the Gold Coast are now about 99% curative and only about 1% preventive in scope'.[21] Where Asante mothers attended more transparent forms of domestic engineering, such as child bathing sessions and missionary lectures, it was often for specific, mundane reasons, such as for recipes or medicine and baby powder.[22] Even so, the reconstruction of the mundane pioneered the colonisation of the home, furthering social and cultural ties to a metropolitan model of social reproduction.

Domestic change in colonial Asante

The expansion of capitalist production in pre- and early-colonial Asante radically altered the domestic economy of the average Asante household. Indirect rule provided the backdrop for the tense domestic environment of the early twentieth century. Writing in the early 1920s, Rattray's elderly informants readily recognised this, noting that 'you have dealings with and recognise only the men; we supposed the European considered women of no account, and we know you do not recognise them as we have always done'.[23] Important tenets of colonialism – such as welfare, education, taxation, and the marketing of Western goods – combined in order to abet the economic reformulation of gender roles which, rooted in the conflicting traditions of matrilineality and capitalistic accumulation, was already underway across the kingdom. What emerged was, in many respects, at odds with the situation in the nineteenth century. As recorded in 1957 by the sociologist and later prime minister Kofi Busia, it was common understanding that 'cocoa ruins the family, divides blood relations'.[24]

This does not mean to say that women in nineteenth-century Asante enjoyed anything like gender parity. Women were the property of men and the sexual freedom and social mobility of young women was circumscribed by law, tradition, and taboo.[25] However, women, and particularly post-menopausal women who had returned to their matrikin, did find some power in a matrilineal gerontocracy which recognised age and lineage before gender. Here the male elder (*abusuapanin*) and the female elder (*obaapanin*) sat together in authority over the matrilineage (*abusua*). At the centre too, the queen mother (*Asantehemaa*) was considered the co-ruler of the kingdom and the primary counsel to the *Asantehene*. Although political centralisation and military expansion in the eighteenth century allowed for the development of chieftaincy, kingship, and a greater formal degree of patriarchy, the enduring presence of the matrikin granted women a considerable degree of influence into the twentieth century.[26] As Rattray explained, if women had been more involved in warfare and not been bound by taboos concerning menstruation, 'the Ashanti woman, under a matrilineal system, would, I believe, eclipse any male in importance'.[27]

In the nineteenth century, household duties were also defined with a greater degree of fairness than in later years. Women cultivated food crops and performed the great bulk of the domestic responsibilities – cleaning, cooking, and childcare, the drawing of water, and the collection of firewood. Men were expected to clear land for cultivation, help during the harvest, and build and maintain the houses. Still, in terms of general subsistence, women provided more than two-thirds of the labour required to farm. Men, however, also concerned themselves with extra-subsistence activities – panning for or mining gold, collecting kola and rubber, long-distance trade, weaving, metalworking, tapping palm wine, hunting and trapping.[28] Although a husband did have the legal right to 'profit by the fruits of … [her] labour and later that of her children', this did not 'entitle the husband to order about either wife or children like slaves'. Instead, the standard relationship was such that it 'amounts only to the mutual assistance that persons living together and sharing a common ménage would naturally accord to each other'.[29]

However, as cocoa, which initially belonged wholesale to men, was granted a higher station in the increasingly monetised economy than food crops, the continued rights of men to the labour of their wives allowed for gross inequalities within the traditional household. In previous years, female cultivation of food had allowed women a valuable return on their labour, that of the house's food. Cocoa farms, however, required much more labour, yet were considerably more valuable than food farms and, unlike food farms, which were left to fallow every few years, cocoa farms held their value for decades.[30] Women's work on their husband's cocoa farms massively increased their conjugal contribution to household wealth. Despite this, the labour of Asante women was, as Roberts has explained, only compensated by the 'continued obligation of her husband to provide part of her subsistence from his own earnings'.[31] As Allman and Tashjian explain, 'conjugal labour in the production of cocoa severely undermined the reciprocity that had previously been a defining element of Asante marriage'.[32]

As Asante commercialism grew through the nineteenth century, the abolition of slavery led to a greater demand for 'legitimate' labour, something which only increased with the emergence of the cocoa industry at the beginning of the twentieth century.[33] Familial labour attained a greater value, and women, as the potential producers of both children and cocoa, were particularly valuable. In Brong, a little north of Asante proper, Mikell found an increase in polygyny and recorded 'older Brong males ... [who] could remember the search for wives which occurred at the turn of the century when cocoa sank roots'.[34] As male elders cashed in on their female dependents, brideprice became artificially inflated and now often included payments not refundable on divorce. Meanwhile, and despite the British banning pawnship, female pawns and pawn wives also found a ready market.[35] Even in 1938, the Nowell Commission, the then most comprehensive study of the cocoa industry, explained that an individual 'could always hand over four or five of his nieces when he needed capital'.[36] Given the increasingly repressive domestic landscape, women began to utilise the space created by the British administration, increasingly contesting divorces or inheritances in colonial courts. Meanwhile, many others sought to escape the bounds of marriage altogether. As the costs of marriage grew, both for men looking for a wife and for men whose wives were looking for a divorce, Native Authorities and the colonial government attempted to restrict what was considered unbridled female emancipation and the emergence of a female petite bourgeoisie. Brideprices were forced down by Native State Councils, which also passed laws to regulate adultery and divorce.[37] In the most extreme cases, in the period between 1929 and 1932, unmarried women over the age of 15 were detained until they gave the name of a man whom they would agree to marry. These men were then summoned to court and obliged to pay a 'release fee' of five shillings in return for their newly betrothed.[38] As was the case elsewhere on the continent, constraints on female autonomy in Asante were codified as a crisis of morality and legitimised as part of a dialogue which concerned 'epidemics' of prostitution, adultery, and venereal disease.[39]

Abetted by indirect rule, the arbitration of marriage, divorce, adultery, and death became concentrated in the hands of Asante chiefs and allowed for the colonisation and commercialisation of the domestic under the apparently legitimate veneer of tradition. As with elsewhere on the continent, this spread to the realm of childrearing. Chiefs, for instance, served to propagate the use of Western education. In exchange for his cooperation, Tafohene Yaw Dabanka was allowed to educate six of his children for free at the Wesleyan Missionary School for girls.[40] As education became an increasingly important route into wealth and influence, its provision became a growing concern for Asante households. Since fathers were traditionally responsible for training their children in a profession – hunting, mining, fishing, or farming – the payment of school fees was understood as the responsibility of the father.[41]

Increasing the cost of childrearing and placing the responsibility for the payment of childrearing in the hands of Asante fathers also further undermined the economic authority of Asante mothers. As the *Asantehemaa* was given to praying for during the *adae* ceremony, the gendered objectives of the nineteenth-century economy were that 'the women bear children and the men gain riches'.[42] As we have already seen (see Chapter 2), children were absolutely central to Asante perceptions of affluence and, in many respects, acted as the female counterpart to male material wealth. However, under colonial capitalism, women found their position as the arbiters of biological wealth at least partially usurped by their husbands' cash-earning.

In the 1950s, and at the sharp end of a demographic transition which was particularly painful for Asante mothers, who had been stripped of some of their social value and economic potential, the anthropologist Meyer Fortes described the divergence between male and female perceptions of value. Fortes noted that, although they recognise that 'contraception is contrary to Ashanti ideals and sentiments', 'some educated men talk of the need for family limitation so as to enable better provision to be made for the education and standard of living of children'. He goes on to cite the story of 'an educated Ashanti friend' who 'decided to limit his family to three children' by sending 'his wife to stay with her parents after the birth of their third child':

> At the end of a year, he was obliged to yield to her protests and to allow her to come back to him. He then proposed that they should try to limit their family by practising continence. Outraged and in distress, his wife accused him of making this suggestion as a pretext for seeking to divorce her. She ran to her mother's brother, who called a meeting of the elders of his own and the husband's families. The husband was reprimanded at this meeting and was obliged to promise never to repeat his offence.[43]

As subsistence agriculture waned in importance, and as cocoa replaced childbearing as the primary route to wealth, the economic position of wife and mother within the family was devalued to what was clearly a distressing extent. The scale of Asante's domestic transformation has received much fuller and more nuanced discussion elsewhere – Allman and Tashjian's *'I Will Not Eat Stone'* providing something of a definitive account – but it is important to recognise the breadth of these changes, since diets and deficiencies are often the result of domestic structures. It is, in fact, precisely these changes which dictated child welfare, nutrition security, and the production of food across the Gold Coast's cocoa belt.

Nutrition and capitalist domesticity in rural Asante

The second, smaller section of F.M. Purcell's lengthy investigation into nutrition on the Gold Coast concerned a number of Akan 'forest villages' in Akim and Asante. Finding the Akans shorter and weaker on average than their neighbours in the savannah or on the coast, Purcell explained that they had 'adapted themselves to an inferior diet by economy in physique and in output of energy' and, although 'the standard of physique among Akans is low ... clinical signs of dietic deficiency are uncommon among adults, and gross deficiency diseases are rarely seen'.[44] Generally, 'the diet of adults in the forest villages is ample and well balanced', although deficiencies in animal produce meant that 'the diet lacks good quality protein'.[45]

This absence of protein was taken by Purcell to be the primary nutritional problem in the forest. Although thrifty physiologies were assumed to alleviate many of the ill-effects among the adult population, children were found to be particularly vulnerable in the Akan food environment, where a 'general oedema ... is common and believed to be caused by a chronic lack of good quality protein food during the years of greatest need'. Purcell tied this oedema to the ongoing debate between Stannus, Trowell, and Williams (see Chapter 2), explaining that it 'may be severe in the fatal infantile pellagroid syndrome, which prevails throughout the forest country'.[46] Later investigations supported these conclusions. Sybil Russell, working in Asante since 1924, first as part of the Scottish Mission and later as a government consultant, also found oedematous malnutrition to be widespread across Asante, where 'protein is in short supply, especially for the children, who are served after their elders; and carbohydrate, of poor quality ... forms the bulk of each meal'.[47]

In the 1930s, kwashiorkor played an important role in Akan infant mortality. In Akim, Purcell recorded that as many as 10 per cent of infant deaths were caused by *ahonhon*.[48] In the 1940s, 'cases of undernutrition and malnutrition were frequently seen' in Kumasi's hospitals.[49] Russell, however, was keen to clarify what Purcell had overlooked, explaining that, exacerbated by endemic malaria, ascaris, and enteritis, the 'marked lack of protein' in the local diet meant that, for the typical baby, 'only continued breast-feeding tides him over a critical period'.[50] As elsewhere in the Gold Coast, and elsewhere around the world, kwashiorkor in

Asante related first to the domestic environment and was only afterwards influenced by the state of the local food economy. Even by the 1930s, however, cash, cocoa, and colonialism had enacted significant changes to both Asante childrearing and Asante food production. Although the few investigations specifically regarding malnutrition in the Gold Coast grant useful glances into the nature of malnutrition in the forest, the insight they garner is fleeting, apolitical, and disinterested in giving nutrition any form of historical narrative. Instead, the changing state of nutrition in the colonial forest has to be constructed with reference to the changes seen across the Southern Gold Coast throughout this period.

At a macroeconomic level, even the League of Nations recognised that changing demands for labour across the continent were a drain on nutritional efficiency, with Burnet and Aykroyd noting that 'while intertribal strife has disappeared, porterage work, work on roads and railways, etc., have disturbed the easy traditional routines of the native and have often subjected him to unaccustomed physical strain'.[51] This increased burden, however, did not fall evenly on colonies, or even on households. The remodelling of Asante domestic responsibilities meant that mothers throughout the rainforest had to bear much of the burden, adapting traditional methods of social reproduction to the conjugal responsibilities demanded by an invigorated capitalist economy. The nutritional effects were, for Purcell at least, plain to see:

> Unless the general standard of living of the African housewife and her family improves, the diet can hardly improve either. It is an unbalanced social organisation which ordains that the woman shall draw water and prepare the food; shall work in the house and in the field.[52]

Despite this, Purcell still emphasised 'parental neglect and ignorance of child welfare' in the aetiology of malnutrition.[53] Even in the 1950s, Grant noted that 'where care is inadequate in terms of western standards, it appears to be related to ignorance rather than to indifference'.[54]

These conclusions complemented the broader colonial articulation of nutrition epidemiology across Britain's African territories (see Chapter 2). This tendency to blame indigenous social structures, rather than to consider recent transformations of indigenous societies, can be seen in Uganda too, where the state mantra was that malnutrition is 'not due so much to absolute poverty as to ignorance, conservatism and superstition'.[55] It would later fall to African doctors to explore the interaction between malnutrition and poverty.[56] In view of the tendency to bring children to hospital too late, Mulago Hospital's Latimer Musoke did not blame maternal ignorance but explained that:

> The life of the mothers of most of our patients is very arduous. She had the responsibility of growing food for the family, assisting the husband in cultivating fields of cash-crops, providing water and firewood for the family and looking after her own four to eight children ... It is with these problems that the mother had to forsake her home and other children to bring her sick infant to hospital.[57]

Similarly, Kenyan medical pioneer Bernard Omondi concluded that 'the far too common picture of kwashiorkor ... was rare in the old days'. However, 'the desire to get employment and earn money, to build good houses and to educate ones children is detrimental to child life in the present stage of economic struggle particularly in the low-income class of people who value money more than food'.[58] While Omondi may be guilty of nostalgia, both Omondi's Kenya and Musoke's Uganda can probably be compared with the situation seen across the Southern Gold Coast.

Throughout the early twentieth century, money gained a greater importance in the daily lives and social standing of the average Asante family. Over the course of the colonial period, access to money determined access to land, to labour, to Western commodities, to education, and even to salvation, as memberships to Christian churches could only be met with cash.[59] The vast majority of Asante cultivators were caught in a divergent economy. To stay in the self- or semi-self-sufficient economy of the recent past would cut them off from the cash economy, the draws of the expanding commodities and education markets and, by way of the relative nature of poverty, make them poor in comparison with their neighbours. Cash-cropping, by comparison, impinged upon individual economic agency, undermining self-sufficiency in favour of the market or the diminishing capacity of their neighbours to produce food.[60] However, the culturally prevalent desire for wealth – something which had ensured the chaos of the cocoa revolution and the kingdom's epidemic of indebtedness – was reflected in what McCaskie calls a 'powerful drive to demonstrate status as a consumer'.[61] Of course, the switch to cash-cropping was rarely wholesale and the wealth of the forest ecology generally prevented food insecurity, at least for those with ready access to land. Despite this, reduced direct investments in social reproduction – for instance, food production, hunting, trapping, or even breastfeeding – had the potential to upset individual and household nutrition security, if not nutritional status.

This switch, as with much in Asante's colonial history, is muddled by matrilineality. According to the historian and prominent pan-Africanist politician J.B. Danquah, in nineteenth-century Asante the burden of childrearing was such that 'a father has right of use over his children, but the true ownership is vested in their maternal family. The tie between mother and child can scarcely be broken; but the relationship between father and child can be destroyed by a customary process.'[62] Since the maternal line was the cornerstone of Asante society, children could be removed from a father's protection by a male relative on the mother's side if the father's duty of care fell below what was expected, including if the father were 'too poor to bring up the child properly'.[63] However, by the mid-1930s, the *abusua*'s authority over its children only existed in a vestigial form and had largely been forgotten. Instead, reformulated by colonial economics and Westernised ideas of family, the process of fathering became conflated with a status of 'fatherhood' which granted men 'inalienable' rights of ownership over their children without any corresponding duty of care.[64] In this respect, the formal growth of an Akan patriarchy undercut the support previously granted by the strength of ties to the matrilineal kin. According to Allman and Tashjian, the burden of domestic reproduction which had been 'shared via a complex web of fluid social relationships between matrilineal kin and conjugal units [now] fell squarely on the shoulders of Asante's colonial mothers'.[65] This progressively bound infant welfare to the wealth of individuals, rather than to that of the wider kin group.

The cocoa economy also accompanied significant and often gendered changes in food supply and diet. Within Akan marriages or in the relationship between lovers in Asante, the provision of food from man to woman is absolutely central. In fact, the Akan-Twi verb stem *di* (to consume or enjoy) refers to eating as well as to sex. To some extent, traditional Asante unions were centred on this reciprocal exchange of food for cooking and sex. Prior to colonisation, the male provision of food was presented in the form of land for food farming and, more directly, in the form of additional food, often animal products caught or purchased with extra-subsistence income. In fact, supplying one's wife with relish-food contributed to the construction of Asante masculinity, since 'if the man lives with the matrikin, thin soup sent by the wife could be a source of embarrassment to him'.[66] Indeed, when men went to their farms, Purcell recorded that 'much of this time may be passed merely in setting steel foot traps in the forest for game'. In the late 1940s, these exertions meant that 'the total amount of meat obtained by trapping the several species of small antelope is much higher than we had earlier expected; the consumption is much higher than in the Northern Territories'.[67] However, even as Purcell was writing, this arrangement was beginning to change. Cash-earning gained greater importance across the South and cash-for-food increased relative to the physical provision of food or land. Into the postcolonial period, the anthropologist Katherine Abu explained that:

> 'Chop money', the Ghanaian English phrase for 'money for food', is the subject of much marital strife ... Sisters living together and in a position to observe the contents of each other's cooking pot are easily aware of how well each is supported by her husband or lover ... Comparing the 'chop money' is considered to be a prevalent feminine vice.[68]

Although the provision of chop money was subject to some social scrutiny, as a means of spousal support it was particularly problematic. When men physically brought the food they were to contribute to that day's meal, it was clear when it was not enough. However, in the form of chop money, this form of familial support 'placed the burden of making it sufficient on the wife and her resourcefulness'.[69]

Since male involvement in food growing was traditionally fairly limited, men's movement out of the food economy did little to disrupt the food security of the average Akan family. However, as men moved away from the provision or acquisition of supplementary foodstuffs, nutrition security was increasingly equated with one's standing in the emergent cash economy. Increasingly, dietary supplementation was defined by cash wealth and Purcell found that 'many are too poor to buy meat from the market or obtain it from a trapper'.[70] By the late 1940s, Marjorie Brown, the Gold Coast's first nutrition officer, described the general pattern of the forest diet:

> The main meals consist, almost invariably, of a mass of starchy food served with a soup or stew. The soups and stews always contain pepper, tomatoes and onions and there is usually at least one other vegetable, more commonly there is some each of okros, garden eggs and spinach and there may be a few beans. Meat and fish are used when they are available and can be afforded. This basic recipe gives a plain soup.[71]

The difference between this recipe and those socially stratified but still meat-heavy diets given by Bowdich for the early nineteenth century (see Chapter 3) suggests a remarkable decline in supplementary relish-foods for the average family.[72] This is also attested to in the archaeological record, with significantly fewer animal bones found in Banda's early-colonial middens.[73] Bound as it was to sexuality and an idealised masculinity, the provision of chop money or extra-subsistence food was particularly sensitive, and the norms of conjugal interaction made it difficult for wives to address their husbands when their chop money fell short.[74] Any such reduction in individual circumstances could impinge on the health and nutrition of dependent children. In the past, women were more able to remove themselves and their children from a poorly supported domestic environment, leaving behind only their rights over the food crops that would only be productive for a few more years. However, as kin relationships changed in favour of the father, and as women's contributions to the cultivation of cocoa grew, any such relocation necessitated abandoning long-term investments in this new, dominant form of wealth, as well as rights over their children.[75] Into independence, most women were said to add to their chop money, meaning dietary supplementation was increasingly reliant on female cash-earning.[76] Even in the nineteenth century, it was said that 'by way of a hard life', 'a strong, healthy middle aged looking woman is a rarity'.[77] Given the increasingly strained livelihoods of Asante women in the twentieth century, it may be little surprise that one 1940s survey noted that 'below the age of 16 years equal proportions of both sexes showed stigmata of malnutrition, but above that age deficiency signs were noted in 17 out of 76 females examined but in only three out of 50 males'.[78]

Spurred on by the need for cash as economic security, Asante women turned to the internal food markets, the colonial courts, and the Gold Coast's emerging urban spaces in an attempt to secure the economic agency necessary to provide an adequate diet for themselves and their dependents in this new environment. Economic agency came, of course, through land – Asante women wrested land from their husbands, had it donated by their kin, or bought it with the profits of their entrepreneurship, ultimately becoming exploiters of employable labour themselves.[79] By the 1950s, nearly half of the sedentary cocoa farmers in Akim were women.[80] However, increasing demands on maternal time and energy outside of the household can significantly affect the nutritional status of their infant children. The European experience suggests that maternal employment closely correlates with child survival. For instance, in Lancashire during the economic crisis of 1868 and in German-occupied Lille during the First World War, the rise in maternal unemployment actually led to a decline in infant mortality, as mothers were able to stay close and care for their young children, despite the harsh local economic conditions.[81] The inverse was probably true for a growing number of women in the colonial Gold Coast, since, 'with farming and selling occupying the attention of many women, the daily care of young children may be partly in the hands of girls who are only a little older than those in their care'.[82]

Although Asante mothers were well aware that 'the children often become seriously ill at the time of weaning, or soon after, recognising as well many of the symptoms of kwashiorkor', most were prone to forego the social insurances of the past in order to deal with the increasingly demanding positions of mother and wife.[83] This was a particular problem for younger mothers, who, in the early 1950s, reported an earlier age for weaning than those aged over 35 years. For younger women, pregnancy was the reason most frequently given for the cessation of breastfeeding, while older women generally weaned their babies due to farm work.[84] Although age-related declines in fertility will have played a part in this, it is also likely that the economic security eked out by older women allowed them a greater degree of agency over their childbearing and the care of their children. Older women were more likely to have access to their own cocoa farms, to have capital accumulated through the longer-term sale of foodstuffs, or, at least, to have the support of their older children. Younger women were more likely to need the social insurances afforded by large numbers of children. The relationship between infant nutrition and maternal employment outside of the home is complex and generally relates to whether the loss of maternal care is made up for by additional income or food production.[85] Of course, this trade-off is highly individualised and depends on personal economic status, rather than localised levels of food or nutrition security. In this environment, if household demands for cash exceed the earning power or productive capacity of a mother, exertions outside of the home, especially in terms of time, may well be detrimental to the nutritional status of a young child.

Increasing demands on household labour did not stop with married parties either. While education preceded fertility limitation for some families, the earning power of children was more easily realised and more readily exploited for others.[86] In the more sparsely populated Brong area, an Akan cocoa farmer with 5 wives and 27 children told researchers, 'I wish I had even double the number of children I have at present ... there would be no need to engage labourers to weed my cocoa farm and to help in the plucking and in carrying the dried beans to the nearest weighing station if I had more children.'[87] This fits with findings which saw that children – and especially female children who were less likely to have money spent on their education – were frequently incorporated into the growing business of porterage throughout the Gold Coast well into the 1940s.[88] In 1911, one Medical Department officer described

> the distressed appearance of the cocoa carriers along the road ... all day long a procession of them passed to the south, old men and women, children of all ages, each staggering under a too heavy burden ... their condition of profuse perspiration and laboured breathing recalling the appearance of an athlete after some supreme effort.[89]

Relative to the nineteenth century, the ubiquitous production of cocoa and the diversifying commodities market encouraged a rather different perception of subsistence and a more concerted focus on extra-subsistence pursuits. In practice, this meant that the burdens and rewards of the cocoa economy were shared inequitably across households and across the kingdom. As Austin has explained, the cocoa boom was not built on the substitution of leisure for labour. Instead, cocoa encouraged a reallocation of resources from the less-productive cash-earning activities of the nineteenth century to the more productive ones offered by an exotic new crop. This surge of productivity ameliorated the loss of unfree labour and facilitated the employment of free labour.[90] However, it seems likely that, emboldened by an overtly patriarchal colonial administration, the exploitation of familial labour was an important bridge in this broader transition.

This gendered division of labour and food distribution may well have contributed to maternal malnutrition and likely contributed to a stillbirth rate which was consistently higher than any other region in the colony (see Table 4.1). In Gambia, Ceesay et al. found that high-protein and high-energy prenatal dietary supplementation 'reduced retardation in intrauterine growth' and 'was associated with a substantial reduction in the prevalence of stillbirths and early neonatal mortality'.[91] Of course, the frequent incidence of stillborn babies will interact with the rainforest's specific disease burden, especially the hyperendemicity of malaria. However, the fact that Ashanti had a notably higher incidence of stillbirths than the Eastern and Western regions or the Trans-Volta – all areas with similar levels and forms of endemic disease – points to socio-economic differences.

Asante's fertile ecology and the lack of time needed to cultivate usually reliable crops like plantain meant that the Asante could enter a part-subsistence economic model without compromising their calorific intake to any great extent.[92] In fact, into the 1920s, food farming

Table 4.1 Regional stillbirth rates for hospital deliveries, 1954.[93]

Region	Total births		Percentage stillborn
	Live	Still	
Accra	2,114	339	13.82
Eastern	924	160	14.76
Western	1,312	253	16.17
Trans-Volta/ Togoland	480	90	15.79
Ashanti	1,247	349	21.73
Northern Territories	1,176	112	8.70
Total	7,253	1,303	15.21

complemented the production of cocoa, since young cocoa plants were shaded by taller food crops such as plantain and cocoyam.[94] The forest's general abundance also meant that, throughout the colonial period, 'the bulk foods, plantain, cocoyams, etc., are over-produced and much is left to rot in the farms ... it is concluded that more is wasted than used'.[95] However, as early as the 1930s, the then Director of Agriculture recognised that the pursuit of cocoa had the potential to undermine individual nutritional status within the forest, since 'the tendency is strong towards neglecting the production of food and using imported supplies instead'. He also recognised the potential for this to become a cyclical problem, since, 'in some areas ... the supply of land for shifting-cultivation is lessening fairly rapidly and the income from cocoa is likely to continue to decrease'.[96] In Nigeria, colonial administrators had also noted the perilous period of transition from subsistence to cash-crop agriculture, explaining that 'some farmers appear to sell enough cocoa to be able to buy reasonable quantities of food for their families, but other families have much younger cocoa which has to be cared for with cash from the sale of their food crops. Hence they have a lower food intake.'[97] It is probably reasonable to assume that, in some cases, dietary deficiency in Asante had similar causes. As cash and cocoa assumed greater significance in the kingdom's economy, food could be sold to foster cocoa production, and land previously dedicated to the growth of food crops could be redistributed under cocoa. In short, the food economy was increasingly neglected in favour of the cocoa economy, leading to what was described in 1943 as 'the anomaly of a rich (economically) area being qualitatively the worst fed'.[98]

When cocoa began to mature, the complementary relationship between food and cash-cropping reversed, as the cocoa trees grew to form a shade canopy, denying light to shorter food plants. Progressively, and especially in densely populated districts, the land utilised for food-cropping diminished, requiring modifications to modes of food production and acquisition.[99] Declining access to land, as well as newly diversified demands on household labour, promoted dietary changes. As early as the 1940s, 'the Medical Department ... sounded a note of warning on the undeserved popularity which cassava ... attained', stating that 'harmful effects on growth and health will result if it replaces whole grain food such as millet, maize or rice'.[100] Within 10 years, only plantain and yam outstripped cassava in terms of Asante's gross production.[101] Cassava was already prominent in food cultures across the region, especially among the Ewe-speakers of the lower Volta plain, where unreliable rainfall earned cassava the name *agbeli*, 'there is life'.[102] Introduced during the Columbian Exchange, and initially the food of slaves or pigs, cassava grew in popularity as a reliable, high-yielding staple which could be grown on marginal land. By the 1930s, cassava began making inroads into Asante diets, sometimes replacing plantain in *fufu* and displacing other, more nutritious foodstuffs around the farm.[103] By the time Grant undertook her fieldwork in 1952, she found that in Mampong, as in Ayeduase, 'the women of the area plant less legumes now than formerly, preferring to plant cassava because it grows prolifically and with little cultivation.'[104] As in earlier years, the usual method of weaning was such that 'as the child grows he begins to eat bits of starchy food thrust into his hand. He may or may not be given maize porridge, but whenever he cries he is always offered something to eat.'[105] However, combined with already short periods of child spacing and a tradition of early weaning – two aspects of Asante childrearing also influenced by the kingdom's cash-crop transition – this meant that the substitution of maize for cassava in weaning foods will have had some impact on the nutritional status of infants consuming this staple. Although the income effect of cocoa production may well have outweighed the effect of this substitution for most, it probably played into a general decline of nutrition security, if not of nutritional status per se.[106]

In fact, across the Gold Coast, average nutritional status only improved during these years. Historical anthropometric data have found that the cohort of Second World War recruits born between 1905 and 1920 outgrew the cohort of First World War recruits born between 1880 and 1893 by an astonishing 2 cm on average, implying a considerable improvement in health and nutrition during childhood.[107] Moradi et al. suggest that, in Asante, these increases were driven by the income derived from cocoa production. However, they also likely reflect the liberation of unfree labour and the democratisation of access to subsistence, as well as improved healthcare and reductions in nutrition–disease interactions.[108] Of some thirteen thousand children under six months of age seen at child welfare centres around Asante in 1956/7, only 69 (0.53 per cent) were considered malnourished. Nutritional deficiencies were far more common among older children and were clearly associated with weaning (see Table 4.2). However, improvements in average nutritional status cannot necessarily speak to changes in nutrition security. Moreover, such statistics can only partially address the details in the historical epidemiology of malnutrition, particularly the way in which food and nutrition related to space as well as to poverty, ethnicity, and class. For instance, throughout the colonial period, only relatively wealthy agriculturalists had the time to invest in preventive care or regular infant welfare attendances, whereas urban Asante had regular access to these facilities. In Kumasi, in 1935, Cicely Williams found that around three-quarters of paediatric outpatients or admissions into city hospitals were from outside of the city. The welfare centre, on the other hand, was patronised mainly by those from around the town, leaving carers better informed and children less susceptible to severe deficiencies later on.[109] Since maternal time was increasingly fraught, committing to the long commute to and from the hospital was often untenable for rural parents. It is, therefore, unsurprising that when these children were eventually brought to Kumasi their nutritional status had declined beyond that of their urban counterparts.

The majority of expatriate observers in the Gold Coast forest recognised that, although severe deficiency may have been rare, sub-clinical malnutrition was absolutely ubiquitous. In rural Ayeduase, Grant found that, as late as the 1950s, 'most showed some signs of protein deficiency'.[110] In 1953, Brown also noted that, although 'there are fortunately not many children who suffer from this severe form of kwashiorkor ... there are many who suffer from kwashiorkor in a mild form'.[111] For Williams, who arrived in the Gold Coast around twenty years before Brown or Grant, malnutrition was an

Table 4.2 Incidence of malnutrition in Child Welfare Clinics by age, Ashanti Region, 1956–7.[112]

Age	n. Cases	n. Malnourished	% Malnourished
<1 mo.	2,610	10	0.38
1–6 mo.	10,467	59	0.56
6 mo.–2.5 yrs	8,429	569	6.75
>2.5 yrs	3,066	123	4.01

apparently normal part of childhood, explaining that 'the average child of 18 months weighs no more than he did at 9 months ... he is pot-bellied and spindle-legged, peevish, helminthic, and in constant abdominal discomfort'.[113] At two years, children 'are nearly all thin, pot-bellied, unhappy, and suffering from all manner of diseases such as malaria, worms, yaws, scabies and ulcers'.[114] Ultimately, the narrative of nutritional *illness* was one of continuity in the face of economic growth. In 1958, the director of the Kumasi Central Hospital recognised that 'there were many cases [of kwashiorkor] seen at this hospital' and came to the conclusion 'that there is little improvement, if any, over the past 10 years in the nutrition of children'.[115] As colonial officials were often prone to do, Williams insisted that kwashiorkor related to maternal ignorance, explaining that, when she arrived in the Gold Coast in 1929, 'it was soon evident that malnutrition was a big problem, though poverty was not. There was little real shortage of money or food, but there was deep ignorance of how a child should be fed.'[116] It was also Williams's contention that malnutrition was broadly endemic and resulted from 'the usual diet in this country'.[117] However, the conclusions forwarded by Williams – as well as those insights proffered by Purcell, Grant, and Brown – fail to countenance nutrition with historical perspective. Over the previous 30 years, the 'usual diet' in the country had changed. Money, too, only recently assumed real relevance with regard to diet and nutrition security and, where cash-earning did assume such relevance, it had to be integrated into the process of food acquisition. These factors all had an impact on the increasingly capitalistic economics of social reproduction, changing the methods by which Asante children were fed.

Throughout the colonial period, it seems likely that the kingdom's nutrition security was in decline, even if nutritional status was generally improving. The material benefits of Asante's integration into the global economy were felt by children born into the colonised kingdom, but failures to succeed in this economic environment could result in clinical malnutrition much more readily than in the immediate precolonial past, where food and nutrition security had been bound together in a complex system of familial responsibility. However, as the sanctity of such responsibilities began to erode, malnutrition was largely determined by individual position in the modern economy. This, as we will see, was something felt much more acutely by particular sections of society.

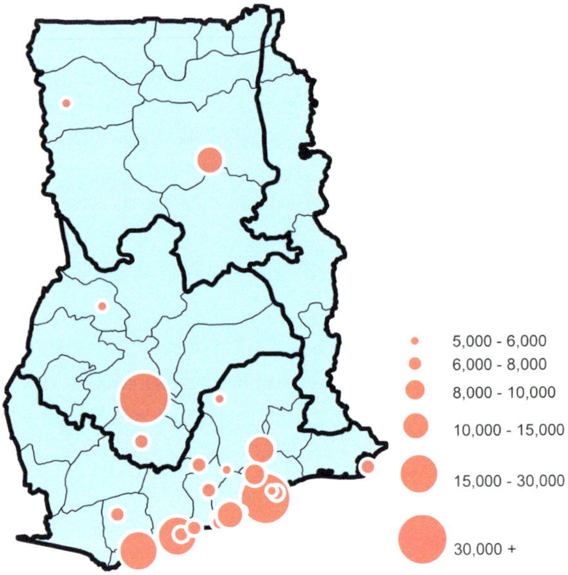

Figure 4.1 Towns with populations of 5,000 or more people, 1931.[118]

Nutrition and gendered poverty in Southern cities

The cocoa boom did not only affect childrearing in Southern forests. Increasing output and mounting profits had also allowed for the development of a form of urbanism across the South which was largely impossible in the Northern savannah (see Figure 4.1). Coastal towns, in particular, swelled in order to ship forest produce and mediate the trade between indigenous inland producers and overseas buyers. Forest towns

Table 4.3 Population living in urban areas, 1960.[119]

	Total population	Population in towns >5,000 people	Population in towns >10,000 people	Percentage population in towns >5,000	Percentage pop. in towns >10,000
Accra	491,817	393,383	372,588	80.0	75.8
Ashanti	1,109,133	276,772	235,496	25.0	21.2
Brong-Ahafo	587,920	91,491	33,980	15.6	5.8
Eastern	1,094,196	220,765	140,449	20.2	12.8
Northern	1,288,917	101,639	83,600	7.9	6.5
Volta	777,285	102,101	42,276	13.1	5.4
Western	1,377,547	365,023	236,405	26.5	17.2
All regions	6,726,815	1,551,174	1,144,794	23.1	17.0

also grew, cash-crop agriculture and the concentration of gold deposits supporting a more diversified employment structure as well as a more profitable trading sector. By the time of the 1960 census a full quarter of those living in the Ashanti Region lived in towns with populations of five thousand people or more, with the vast majority residing in Kumasi. In the savannah only 7.9 per cent lived in such large conurbations, nearly all of whom were in Tamale, the colonial government's distributive centre and administrative capital for the Northern Territories (see Table 4.3).

Where social reproduction was devalued in the traditional, agrarian economy of rural Asante, it gained greater worth in the rapidly expanding urban world. In the pre- and early colonial periods, the Gold Coast's established towns were small, largely homogeneous communities with balanced gender ratios and traditional domestic structures. In 1891, Accra recorded 6,467 men and 6,362 women, whereas Cape Coast was made up of 3,526 men and 3,603 women. However, by 1931, there were 20 per cent more men in Accra than women.[120] In the new industrial towns, the pattern was more immediate and much more dramatic. The establishment of a railhead and a deep water harbour in 1898 and 1928 respectively transformed Sekondi-Takoradi from a collection of Ahanta villages into a bustling, multi-ethnic urban city. Here, in 1901, men outnumbered women by five to one.[121] In Sekondi-Takoradi, as in other industrial towns, such as the mining centres of Obuasi or Tarkwa, men usually arrived alone, driven by the growing need for cash income or by a lack of opportunity in their rural homelands. The women that followed were similarly drawn to the economic possibilities provided by this pattern of development. Since the colonial government was loath to provide its labour force with housing or food, the value of domestic and conjugal services became heavily inflated across the urban colony and the sale of cooked food, the provision of boarding houses, and the sale of sex provided urban women with new and highly lucrative avenues for capital accumulation.[122] As the historian Emmanuel Akyeampong has explained, 'women found more spaces within the emerging social order to assert their autonomy, to accumulate wealth on their own, and to define marriage and what they expected of it'.[123]

As in the rural world, marriages and other conjugal relationships in the city were rarely the meetings of equals. In fact, the profitability of domestic and conjugal services, and the surplus of male industrial labour, meant that women were often better off than men in the urban economy. Initially, urban workers suffered through low but rising wages and enjoyed a stable cost of living, with any increase in wages providing commensurate improvements in the standard of living. However, during the 1930s, food prices rose sharply as real wages plummeted, leaving those dependent on wages particularly vulnerable throughout the rest of the colonial period.[124] By the late 1940s, Kofi Busia's social survey of Sekondi-Takoradi noted that 'men were seen at nights weaving mats or handbags in order to supplement their wages … the little extra they earned from weaving in the evenings enabled them to pay their rent which they could not otherwise pay, as their wages barely sufficed for their food.'[125] Conversely, the 1953 Accra Expenditure Survey decided to sample only households with wage-earning heads, explaining that 'for other families, where occupations consist largely of trading and other activities, family income tends to move with prices, so that price changes have a less important effect'.[126] Akyeampong suggests that, during this period, it was men who really needed women, since 'urban life was a disappointment … dissolution was reflected in an intensification in gender conflict, mirrored in court cases, and a male elaboration of "romance" or "love"'.[127] In this environment, women had a lower impetus to marry and a greater risk of exploitation if they did. Highlife songs like '*Wo Pe Tam Won Pe Ba*' ('You Like Cloth but You Don't Want Children') and 'Give Me the Bush Girl' speak to the conflict produced when romance was not forthcoming.[128]

Female economic security was, in part, achieved through their domination of the marketplace. In the nineteenth century, the production of and trade in foodstuffs was understood as women's work and, with the urban expansion of these markets, women in town and county were culturally and practically primed to expand such enterprises. By 1948, women made up 73 per cent of those employed in commerce in Accra and nearly 90 per cent of women working in Accra were employed as traders.[129] Ioné Acquah's social survey of late-colonial Accra found that female traders were 'in many cases … the mainstay in the home and … generally speaking, more economically independent than … their counterparts in western countries'.[130]

Urban women in the Gold Coast also enjoyed markedly more independence than rural women in the Southern colony.[131] In the same way that conjugal relationships in rural Asante were increasingly defined by economic individualism, urban women collectively defended these gendered economic interests in view of patriarchal social structures and the male bias in salaried employment.[132] Originating in the freedoms of the colonial period, these trends seeped over into the independence era. By the early 1970s, the vast majority (well over 90 per cent) of women in Accra lived with their matrilineal relatives rather than their husbands, largely in order to secure their standing and authority within the household.[133] These women put considerable effort into circumventing traditional systems of inheritance in order to provide specifically for their daughters' future security.[134] Even those women without extensive kin networks could find extra-entitlement support through the sale of sex or through flexible, informal relationships. When Margaret Field asked about the perception of sex workers in Accra in the mid-1950s, she was told: 'it is her work. When a man has to stay in a town like Kumasi one of the things he may need is a woman. Also travellers need somewhere to stay the night.'[135] In both Accra and Sekondi-Takoradi, sex workers were almost exclusively from ethnic groups foreign to the immediate area.[136] Sex work was, simply, one of several ways in which migrant women could profit from their urban advantage and benefit from the inflated cost of social reproduction in the early-colonial city.

Since informal earnings did not rely directly upon the saturated and often erratic labour market, female income in the city was often more stable than men's. Although trade unions and mutual assistance funds grew in popularity, labour movements and urban dissent were slow to develop and the colonial period saw the development of a disenfranchised and often desperately poor male proletariat.[137] Calls for wage increases throughout the early 1940s were compounded by the 1945 Department of Labour finding that 'the labourer in Government service earns on average ten shillings a month less than domestic servants, and very much less that the average earnings admitted by earners in trade'.[138] This postwar cost of living crisis was so great that it fomented the conditions for the 1948 Accra Riots which led, indirectly, to Kwame Nkrumah's 1951 election victory and the formal process of decolonisation in Africa.[139]

Throughout this period, unemployment, destitution, itinerancy, homelessness and hunger were growing yet uniquely male concerns.[140] These were particular problems for Northern migrants who, without the support of established kin, existed at the furthest fringes and, in Accra, made up most of the 'hard core of persons who habitually sleep out'.[141] These men were also the most likely to resort to crime, whereas, between October 1946 and March 1948, only 3.2 per cent of those convicted in Sekondi-Takoradi were women. Few of those men convicted were indigenous Ahanta and the vast majority were from outside of the Southern colony.[142] In Sekondi-Takoradi, social marginality and economic insecurity meant that the poor were 'habitually underfed' and the destitute 'were all in a poor state of health and appeared to be suffering

Table 4.4 Regional distribution of deficiency diseases reported in hospitals, 1951–3.[143]

	Beriberi	Pellagra	Scurvy	Other deficiency states	Total nutrition-related
Accra	229	0	9	93	331
Ashanti	26	72	21	1,799	1,918
Eastern	41	47	11	2,239	2,338
N.T.s	25	289	11	1,655	1,980
Trans-Volta	0	0	2	193	195
Western	68	187	155	2,042	2,452
Total	389	595	209	8,021	9,214

from nutrition deficiencies'.[144] For the very poorest in Sekondi-Takoradi, Busia found that diets consisted 'of little else besides disproportionate quantities of cheap starchy foods'.[145] In this environment, malnutrition was tied to poverty and food insecurity, to kinlessness and unemployment, all particular problems for single male migrants. According to Medical Department returns (see Table 4.4), between 1951 and 1953 Accra's greatest nutritional problem was beriberi, a disease which, across the colony, affected perhaps twice as many men as women.[146] Although these figures will be complicated by frequent misdiagnoses, beriberi, a thiamine deficiency, was relatively well understood by the 1950s. It was usually seen to accompany diets composed of polished white rice or, perhaps, cassava – economical alternatives to traditional staples but substitutions which were nutritionally deficient.[147] The pioneering Ghanaian epidemiologist Fred Sai found that beriberi was an 'almost unknown disease among the local inhabitants' and instead concentrated among 'Liberian immigrants working as beach boys ... living on a diet largely consisting of polished rice'.[148] In the Gold Coast, beriberi reflected a particularly urban form of poverty where diet and food acquisition intersected with ethnicity, employment, and social insecurity.

Children, on the other hand, appear to have been better off in the cities than in the countryside across the South. The economic agency and group security exercised by urban women combined with greater access to healthcare and the flexible care provision allowed by informal employment in order to grant considerably lower levels of nutritional illness in the city than in surrounding rural areas (see Table 4.4).[149] Concerted efforts to combat high rates of infectious disease in politically and economically sensitive areas also assuaged the threat of disease–nutrition interactions in the city. Public works addressed water supply and sewerage at the same time as healthcare was made free and much more accessible.[150] Child welfare clinics emerged first in the cities too: in Accra in 1921 and, by the end of the decade, in Sekondi, Kumasi, Cape Coast, Koforidua, and Ho. In 1926, the colony's first paediatric hospital, the Princess Marie Louise Children's Hospital also opened in Accra. Between 1925 and 1930, attendances at infant welfare centres grew six-fold, from 20,000 to 130,000.[151] By 1932, infant mortality in Accra had fallen to 95 per thousand, down from 368 per thousand in 1916.[152] Maternal mortality and crude death rates also declined along similar lines.[153] By 1955, more than thirteen thousand children were on the registers of Infant Welfare Clinics around Accra and, according to Acquah, 'it would appear that all children are taken to the clinic during the first year of their lives'. The expanding cadre of midwives and allied health professionals which concentrated in the cities paid 'special attention to all premature babies, infants suffering from malnutrition and foster-children' and were said to 'endeavour to visit every new-born baby'.[154] In per capita terms, Accra had more doctors, more nurses, and more beds, and saw more patients than any other region.[155] In 1954, deliveries in Accra's hospitals accounted for nearly 30 per cent of the entire colony's institutional deliveries.[156] However, between 1951 and 1953, Accra's hospitals reported, on average, only 3.6 per cent of the colony's nutrition cases. The mechanism here is surely the same as that reported by Williams in 1935 Kumasi, with pervasive preventive medicine and the uptake of best practice offsetting the need for curative hospital care.[157]

Apparently the social and medical advantages of life in the city also outweighed the pervasive decline of the traditional, family-based systems of social support which were especially apparent in the city.[158] Having become 'consuming units' and 'a burdensome charge on income', 'the children of dead relatives were, in some instances, being neglected' by their adoptive families.[159] However, this appeared to present in the form of troubling numbers of juvenile delinquents, unschooled and unruly, rather than in any epidemic of poorly nourished waifs and strays.[160] In fact, children born around Kumasi and the Accra plains achieved a greater adult stature than their rural counterparts across the South.[161] Accra's indigenous Ga outgrew the rest of the Southern colony and presented in the Gold Coast Regiment's personnel files with a higher BMI and a greater average chest circumference.[162] Additional data show that Accra schoolchildren were generally taller and weightier than Northern children of the same age.[163] This may also have had something to do with the greater prevalence of expensive, supplementary foods like meat and fish in the cities – much of which was now imported, tinned produce – especially given its relative decline in the countryside. As Cardinall noted in 1931, 'per capita consumption of meat is infinitely greater in the larger centres than in the rural districts where the people cannot be classified in any sense as meat-eaters'.[164] In the 1930s, Williams saw 'in every village' 'children, especially those of the toddler stage, so unhealthy as to be conspicuously unshapely'. She recognised the same pattern in 'many towns' but apparently saw infant ill-health as a particular problem of village life.[165]

Nutrition and entitlement in the cocoa economy

As in the nineteenth century, the social epidemiology of malnutrition in the colonial Asante village was largely dictated by wealth. It related to access to capital and to spare time, to the availability of land to grow cocoa, and to the availability of labour to work that land. Wealth largely dictated the quality and quantity of food available in the household. Likewise, the amount of time a family was able to spend on childcare generally depended upon the position of the mother within the household, as well as her individual position within the wider economy. If a mother had the support of her husband, her older children, or her matrikin, she would have had more time for her nursing child and better food for herself and her at-risk children. Similarly, if she was able to benefit from the degree of land or capital necessary to employ extra-familial labour, then the burdens of production reduced and allowed her to address social reproduction instead. If she could not enjoy these advantages, if she were poor, then her children's nutrition would likely have been in question.

However, the colonial period saw a significant change in the demographics of wealth and the nature of poverty. The prevalence of unfree labour declined under colonial rule, meaning that poverty and nutrition insecurity was no longer the reserve of the unfree but was, instead, tied to an expanded notion of social status. Although conceptualising class is problematic in Africa, economic standing in colonial Asante was largely defined by individual distance from the diversifying means of production. Following the emergence of the cottage cocoa industry, the 'second stage of the capitalistic process' in Asante was the 'systematic large-scale employment of farm labourers'.[166] By 1938, the Nowell Commission explained that the cocoa industry was 'dependent on migrant labour which comes in from the Northern Territories, where money crops are inadequate ... who tramp down to the cocoa districts from the north for the cocoa season and return by lorry to their homes and families in the food planting season'.[167] Following the initial expansion of cocoa, the industry relied on hired labour working either as sharecroppers under the *abusa* or *nkotokuan* systems (one-third of the crop was received by *abusa* farmers, while the *nkotokuan* earned a fixed number of loads) or as casual wage labourers, whose efforts were mainly used to establish new farms. In many respects, the development of cocoa in Asante followed a process of class formation and exploitation which was common in other parts of Africa. In Uganda, for instance, the growth of rural capitalism and the establishment of a landlord–tenant relationship allowed for the formation of a group which Mahmood Mamdani has described as 'kulaks', members of a 'petty bourgeoisie' who supplemented familial labour with undervalued and politically unorganised migrant labour.[168] In colonial Asante, the intensified production of cocoa promoted similar forms of class formation and necessitated the exploitation of such labour.

Although the colonial environment was particularly trying for Asante mothers, whose precarious position could undermine the health of their young children, the inalienable rights of Asante women over the use of communally owned, stool lands assuaged the threat of hunger for those individuals able to capitalise on this advantage. The potential benefits of the new economy were not, however, open to everyone. While outside labour was welcome in the kingdom, both the colonial state and the Asante chieftaincy committed themselves to preventing the purchase of land by non-Asante Africans. In 1936, for instance, following the sale of land in the southern reaches of Asante to individuals from the Eastern Province, Chief Commissioner F.W. Applegate explained to the *Asantehene* that 'such procedure I think you will agree is bound to work deleteriously and against the common good of Ashanti'. The *Asantehene* agreed, subsequently warning chiefs, 'I should be glad if you and your Elders would take every possible precaution against the outright sale of Stool lands to strangers.'[169] Supported by the colonial government, Asante's hereditary rulers continued the monopolistic defence of Asante's 'broad forest rent'.[170] For non-Asante labourers, 'lacking both capital and rights over forest lands, it was a remarkable achievement to become a cocoa farmer (farmowner) at all'.[171]

These exclusionary processes established a class of rural labourers disconnected from the subsistence economy and reliant on the market for both their food and nutrition security. In the precolonial nineteenth century there was no real value to the bulk foods which grew so prolifically across the kingdom. However, the cocoa boom dislocated the food economy from the wider economy and the number of immigrants and labourers without access to land increased just as food crops were being neglected. Likewise, cocoa brought more money into Asante and the rest of the South at the same time as demands for food outstripped its supply. The increasingly unstable food market and the threat of inflation meant that, by the late 1940s, price controls had to be implemented across the region. By the 1950s, the lack of locally grown foodstuffs drove demand for imported food, encouraged a flourishing black market, and led to heavy inflation.[172] The Watson Commission, brought in to explain the social conditions behind the 1948 Accra riots, found that 'the prices of staple foods on a number of urban and country markets [were] probably about 2½ times the pre-war level'.[173] Despite stresses in the rural food economy, the cocoa belt ran an impressive surplus in terms of food production. In Akim-Abuakwa, for instance, between June 1952 and May 1953 the difference between production and consumption amounted to 15,000 tons of food crops.[174] However, this surplus production largely bypassed the rural market in favour of the greater purchasing power of the Gold Coast's urban areas. This movement was promoted by an Africanising state bureaucracy which, following the 1948 Accra Riots over the spiralling cost of living, recognised urban food security as an important tool for political dissent. Despite significant and mounting shortcomings in the rural food economy, the Akim-Abuakwa survey plainly acknowledged that, as far as Nkrumah's incoming CPP government was concerned, 'the main agricultural problem in the Gold Coast at the present time is the supply of foodstuffs to growing urban communities'.[175]

Such conclusions pave over the weaknesses of a rural food economy which had facilitated the production of malnutrition as a failure of entitlement. Later twentieth-century research in Ghana concluded that variations in food prices 'explain a significant proportion of the variance of the conditional probability of child survival'. Simply increasing the prices of three staple foods (maize, cassava, and plantain) by 10 per cent decreased median child survival time by almost 12 per cent.[176] Modified conclusions are probably applicable for the colonial Gold Coast, where fewer children were entirely dependent on a less expansive market economy. Where they were, though, they were particularly vulnerable in times of familial or local economic crisis. The nutritional impact of one such crisis, the 1937–8 cocoa 'hold-up' – a widespread refusal of farmers, chiefs, and brokers to sell cocoa to expatriate trading firms – was obvious to Purcell:

> On being stationed for a few months in 1938 in Koforidua, on the fringe of the forest, I have observed some ten cases of severe malnutrition, of which six were pellagrous; nearly all were children of Kotokoli parents, indigenous northern immigrants, dependent on uncertain employment by the local cocoa farmers. The hold-up of cocoa in the year 1937 caused much economic hardship: labourers were not paid. As a class the local Kotokolis were underfed; infantile pellagra [kwashiorkor] among them in 1938 was probably associated.[177]

It is reasonable to assume that any real decline in the purchasing power of a market-dependent farmer or labourer meant simultaneous reductions in individual entitlement as well as in the nutritional status of the individual and their dependants. Here the occupational makeup of rural Asante is important. If an individual produces food as a smallholder or a sharecropper they get their return in food, do not have to endure the vagaries of the market, and are less likely to suffer significantly through those food shortages accompanied by price increases. Wage labourers, on the other hand, have to deal with erratic price increases in a highly imperfect capital market. Even if smallholders do not produce food, in the wake of drought or in harsh market conditions they will not be incomeless – they will just endure a lower income, which may not facilitate the employment of labourers. By contrast, those who sell services, labour, or handicrafts are more exposed to price fluctuations, as not only is their income less in relative terms, but their clients or employers are less likely to be able or inclined to buy their services or products.[178] It is for this reason that – to take a famous example of Amartya Sen's – Bengali barbers starved during the 1943 famine.[179] It is for largely the same reasons that the 1937 cocoa hold-up resulted in kwashiorkor for Kotokoli children.

For some, food insecurity as a result of economic exclusion will have been compounded by social marginality. In Uganda, the nutritionists Bennett and Stanfield summarised the mechanism behind migrant susceptibility to total-calorie deficiencies, explaining that marasmus

> is more likely to occur in the children of poorly nourished mothers with recurrent untreated fevers who do not receive ante-natal care, who deliver at home and whose lactation fails. This group of factors might have occurred more in poor immigrant women who had not yet mastered the local language or learnt how to use medical services.[180]

Twenty years after Purcell's investigations in Koforidua, the director of the Kumasi Central Hospital still recognised an ethnic dimension in the epidemiology of nutritional disease, noting that there are 'many patients from Northern Ghana. Most of the paupers come from this area.'[181]

If insufficient household income is taken as the root socioeconomic cause of severe malnutrition, the income of an indigenous Asante, even if it was equal to that of a migrant labourer, was often buoyed by land ownership, kinship, and familial support. In general, the movement away from slavery and pawnship preceded a historic improvement in the bargaining power of migrants in the forest.[182] However, due to their limited 'entitlement package', and their lack of entitlement to socialised sources of food, it was the landless and rootless parts of the population that felt the highs and lows of the food market most acutely. Here labourers could not access the domestic security afforded by the 'broad forest rent' as 'principals' but only as 'agents'.[183] This growing demographic was required to succeed continuously in order to avoid conjunctural crises which, brought about by any relative decline in their economic fortunes, represent a new type of structural poverty.[184] For this emergent precariat, sporadic bouts of nutritional stress were a very real possibility, dependent on individual ability to weather economic change. As Purcell explained in the 1930s, 'plantain is eaten by all; it is abundant and cheap, but the price may rise 100% from 25 for 1d to 12 for 1d, in times of relative scarcity. (Such an increase should embarrass only the very poorest).'[185] Progressively, though, any such price increases had the potential to embarrass more and more people. The trajectory of Asante class formation during these decades meant that more people fell into the category of the 'very poorest'. For perhaps the first time in Asante history, a significant part of the population was at real risk of food and nutrition insecurity, a result of new, structural flaws in the internal food economy.

Notes

1 Quoted in Dennis Austin, *Politics in Ghana, 1946–1960* (London: Oxford University Press, 1964), p. 275. This is Austin's own verdict on the song's specific swing.

2 For the history of Asante nationalism, see Jean Allman, *The Quills of the Porcupine: Asante Nationalism in an Emergent Ghana* (Madison, WI: University of Wisconsin Press, 1993); Austin, *Politics*, pp. 250–315.

3 Polly Hill, *The Gold Coast Cocoa Farmer: A Preliminary Survey* (Oxford: Oxford University Press, 1956); Polly Hill, *The Migrant Cocoa-Farmers of Southern Ghana: A Study in Rural Capitalism* (Cambridge: Cambridge University Press, 1963).

4 Gold Coast Government, *Agricultural Department Annual Report* [*ADAR*], 1900 (Accra: Government Printer, 1901); *ADAR*, 1920, p. 62.

5 *ADAR*, 1955/6, p. 30.
6 Gareth Austin, '"No Elders Were Present": Commoners and Private Ownership in Asante, 1807–96', *The Journal of African History*, 37.1 (1996), 1–30 (p. 29).
7 Quoted in Roger J. Southall, 'Farmers, Traders and Brokers in the Gold Coast Cocoa Economy', *Canadian Journal of African Studies*, 12.2 (1978), 185–211 (p. 196).
8 Gwendolyn Mikell, *Cocoa and Chaos in Ghana* (New York: Paragon House, 1989).
9 Allman, 'Rounding up Spinsters'.
10 W.S. Tudhope, *Enquiry into the Gold Coast Cocoa Industry: Final Report, 1918–1919* (Accra: Government Printer, 1919), p. 12.
11 Kwame Arhin, 'Succession and Gold Mining at Mansu Nkwanta', *Research Review, University of Ghana*, 6.3 (1970), 101–9 (p. 107).
12 Ester Boserup, *Women's Role in Economic Development* (London: George Allen & Unwin, 1971).
13 For feminist critiques of neoclassical economics, see, among many others, Paula England, 'The Separative Self: Androcentric Bias in Neoclassical Assumptions', in *Beyond Economic Man: Feminist Theory and Economics*, ed. by Marianne A. Ferber and Julie A. Nelson (Chicago, IL: University of Chicago Press, 1993), pp. 37–53; Lourdes Benería, 'Toward a Greater Integration of Gender in Economics', *World Development*, 23.11 (1995), 1839–50.
14 James Mill, *An Essay on Government*, ed. by Currin V. Shields (Indianapolis, IN: Bobbs-Merrill, 1955), pp. 73–4.
15 Alfred Marshall, *Principles of Economics* (London: Macmillan & Co., 1920), p. 20.
16 Macdonald, *Gold Coast*, p. 290.
17 Vaughan, *Story of an African Famine*, p. 147.
18 A similar point is made at more length in Michelle Murphy, *The Economization of Life* (Durham, NC: Duke University Press, 2017), pp. 17–34.
19 See Meillassoux, *Maidens, Meal and Money*; Comaroff and Comaroff, 'Home-Made Hegemony'.
20 Allman, 'Making Mothers', p. 29; see also Nancy Rose Hunt, '"Le Bebe En Brousse": European Women, African Birth Spacing and Colonial Intervention in Breast Feeding in the Belgian Congo', *The International Journal of African Historical Studies*, 21.3 (1988), 401–32 (p. 418).
21 PRAAD/A/CSO/11/6/4, Infant welfare centres – Principles, 1931–2, H. O'Hara May, Deputy Director of the Health Service to Director of Medical and Sanitary Services, 1932.
22 Allman, 'Making Mothers', pp. 41–2.
23 R.S. Rattray, *Ashanti* (Oxford: Clarendon Press, 1923), p. 84.
24 K.A. Busia, *The Position of the Chief in the Modern Political System of Ashanti: A Study of the Influence of Contemporary Social Changes on Ashanti Political Institutions* (London: Published for the International African Institute by Oxford University Press, 1951), p. 127.
25 See, for instance, T.C. McCaskie, 'State and Society, Marriage and Adultery: Some Considerations Towards a Social History of Pre-Colonial Asante', *Journal of African History*, 22.4 (1981), 477–94.
26 Emmanuel Akyeampong and Pashington Obeng, 'Spirituality, Gender, and Power in Asante History', *The International Journal of African Historical Studies*, 28.3 (1995), 481–508.
27 Rattray, *Ashanti*, pp. 81–2.
28 Austin, *Labour*, pp. 107–10.
29 Rattray, *Law*, p. 25.
30 Allman and Tashjian, *'I Will Not Eat Stone'*, p. 62.
31 Penelope Roberts, 'The State and the Regulation of Marriage: Sefwi Wiawso (Ghana), 1900–40', in *Women, State, and Ideology: Studies from Africa and Asia*, ed. by Haleh Afshar (Albany, NY: SUNY Press, 1987), pp. 48–69 (p. 54).
32 Allman and Tashjian, *'I Will Not Eat Stone'*, p. 65.
33 Gareth Austin, 'Between'.
34 Mikell, *Cocoa and Chaos*, p. 201.
35 Beverly Grier, 'Pawns, Porters, and Petty Traders: Women in the Transition to Cash Crop Agriculture in Colonial Ghana', *Signs*, 17.2 (1992), 304–28; Roberts, 'The State'; Gareth Austin, 'Human Pawning in Asante 1800–1950: Markets and Coercion, Gender and Cocoa', in *Pawnship, Slavery and Colonialism in Africa*, ed. by Paul E. Lovejoy and Toyin Falola

(Trenton, NJ: Africa World Press, 2003), pp. 187–224; Kwame Arhin, 'Monetisation and the Asante State', in *Money Matters: Instability, Values and Social Payments in the Modern History of West Africa Communities*, ed. by Jane I. Guyer (Portsmouth, NH: Heinemann, 1995), pp. 188–201.

36 Quoted in Grier, 'Pawns, Porters, and Petty Traders', p. 319.

37 Roberts, 'The State', pp. 61–7; Arhin, 'Monetisation'.

38 Allman, 'Rounding up Spinsters'.

39 Jean Allman, 'Of "Spinsters", "Concubines" and "Wicked Women": Reflections on Gender and Social Change in Colonial Asante', *Gender & History*, 3.2 (1991), 176–89. This 'gender chaos' is part of a continent-wide pattern; see, for instance, Silberschmidt, *'Women Forget'*; Amadiume, *Male Daughters*.

40 Allman, 'Making Mothers', p. 29.

41 Jean Allman, 'Fathering, Mothering and Making Sense of Ntamoba: Reflections on the Economy of Child-Rearing in Colonial Asante', *Africa*, 67.2 (1997), 296–321 (p. 308).

42 Rattray, *Ashanti*, p. 105.

43 Fortes, 'Field Study', p. 265.

44 PRAAD/A/ADM/11/1/1294, Purcell, 'Report', p. 109.

45 PRAAD/A/ADM/11/1/1294, Purcell, 'Report', p. 4.

46 PRAAD/A/ADM/11/1/1294, Purcell, 'Report', pp. 109–10.

47 E.H. Jellinek, 'The Russells of Edinburgh: A Medical Dynasty', *Proceedings of the Royal College of Physicians of Edinburgh*, 31.4 (2001), 342–51; Russell, 'Malnutrition', p. 110.

48 PRAAD/A/ADM/11/1/1294, Purcell, 'Report', p. 113.

49 Russell, 'Malnutrition', p. 110.

50 Russell, 'Malnutrition', p. 110.

51 Burnet and Aykroyd, 'Nutrition and Public Health', pp. 448–9.

52 PRAAD/A/ADM/11/1/1294, Purcell, 'Report', p. 117.

53 Purcell, *Diet and Ill-Health*, p. 66.

54 Faye Woodard Grant, *The Nutrition and Health of Children in the Gold Coast* (Chicago, IL: University of Chicago, 1955), p. 7.

55 Uganda Government, *Review of Nutrition in Uganda: A Summary of Previous Work and An Appreciation of the Present Position* (Entebbe: Government Printer, 1945), p. 1.

56 John Iliffe, *East African Doctors: A History of the Modern Profession* (Cambridge: Cambridge University Press, 2002), p. 141.

57 Latimer K. Musoke, 'An Analysis of Admissions to the Paediatric Division, Mulago Hospital in 1959', *Archives of Disease in Childhood*, 36.187 (1961), 305–15 (p. 305).

58 Quoted in Iliffe, *East African Doctors*, p. 108.

59 Arhin, 'Monetisation'.

60 This is very similar to the pattern seen in southern Uganda. See Nott, 'Malnutrition in a Modernising Economy', p. 244.

61 T.C. McCaskie, 'Accumulation: Wealth and Belief in Asante History: II the Twentieth Century', *Africa*, 56.1 (1986), 3–23 (p. 13); see also Wilks, *Asante*, p. 673; Austin, *Labour*, pp. 140–50.

62 J.B. Danquah, *Gold Coast: Akan Laws and Customs and the Akim Abuakwa Constitution* (London: G. Routledge & Sons, 1928), p. 189.

63 Rattray, *Law*, pp. 8–10; see also Allman and Tashjian, *'I Will Not Eat Stone'*, p. 86.

64 Allman, 'Fathering, Mothering', pp. 312–13; see also Dorothy Dee Vellenga, 'Who Is a Wife? Legal Expressions of Heterosexual Conflicts in Ghana', in *Female and Male in West Africa*, ed. by Christine Oppong (London: George Allen & Unwin, 1983), pp. 144–55.

65 Allman and Tashjian, *'I Will Not Eat Stone'*, p. 125.

66 Katherine Abu, 'The Separateness of Spouses: Conjugal Resources in an Ashanti Town', in *Female and Male in West Africa*, ed. by Christine Oppong (London: George Allen & Unwin, 1983), pp. 156–68 (p. 161); for an insight into the relationship between food and masculinity, see Stephan Miescher, *Making Men in Ghana* (Bloomington, IN: Indiana University Press, 2005), pp. 121, 131–2.

67 PRAAD/A/ADM/11/1/1294, Purcell, 'Report', pp. 96, 99.

68 Abu, 'Separateness of Spouses', pp. 160–1.

69 Allman and Tashjian, *'I Will Not Eat Stone'*, p. 66.

70 PRAAD/A/ADM/11/1/1294, Purcell, 'Report', p. 4.

71 Marjorie Brown, 'Nutrition in the Gold Coast: A Summary of Information Relating to the Present Position of Nutrition in the Gold Coast', in *Conférence interafricaine sur l'alimentation et la nutrition. Dschang, Cameroun, 3–9 Octobre 1949* (Paris: La Documentation Française, 1949), pp. 96–103 (p. 98).
72 Bowdich, *Mission*, p. 319.
73 Logan, *The Scarcity Slot*, p. 109
74 Abu, 'Separateness of Spouses', p. 161.
75 Allman and Tashjian, *'I Will Not Eat Stone'*, p. 65.
76 Abu, 'Separateness of Spouses', pp. 160–1; Christine Oppong, *Middle Class African Marriage: A Family Study of Ghanaian Senior Civil Servants* (London: George Allen & Unwin, 1981), pp. 87, 95.
77 W. Terry Coppin, 1884. Quoted in Austin, *Labour*, p. 172.
78 M.J. Colbourne et al., 'A Medical Survey in a Gold Coast Village', *Transactions of the Royal Society of Tropical Medicine and Hygiene*, 44.3 (1950), 271–90 (p. 282).
79 Dorothy Dee Vellenga, 'Matriliny, Patriliny, and Class Formation Among Women Cocoa Farmers in Two Rural Areas of Ghana', in *Women and Class in Africa*, ed. by Claire Robertson and Iris Berger (New York: Africana Publishing Company, 1986), pp. 62–77.
80 Polly Hill, 'Women Cocoa Farmers', *Economic Bulletin of Ghana*, 2.6 (1958), 70–6.
81 Marco Breschi and Massimo Livi Bacci, 'Month of Birth as a Factor in Children's Survival', in *Infant and Child Mortality in the Past*, ed. by Alain Bideau, Bertrand Desjardins, and Héctor Pérez Brignoli (Oxford: Oxford University Press, 1997), pp. 157–73 (pp. 161–2).
82 Grant, *Nutrition and Health*, p. 7.
83 Grant, 'II', p. 697.
84 Grant, 'II', p. 697.
85 For more on this complicated relationship, albeit with limited relevance for the historian, see, for instance, Joanne Leslie, 'Women's Work and Child Nutrition in the Third World', *World Development*, 16.11 (1988), 1341–62; Patricia L. Engle, 'The Effect of Maternal Employment on Children's Welfare in Rural Guatemala', *New Directions for Child and Adolescent Development*, 20 (1983), 57–75; Marie T. Ruel et al., *Urban Challenges to Food and Nutrition Security: A Review of Food Security, Health, and Caregiving in the Cities* (Washington, D.C.: IFPRI FCND Discussion Paper No. 51, 1998), p. 40.
86 Allman and Tashjian, *'I Will Not Eat Stone'*, pp. 94–6.
87 Quoted in Kaye, *Bringing up Children*, p. 23.
88 Kwabena O. Akurang-Parry, '"The Loads Are Heavier than Usual": Forced Labor by Women and Children in the Central Province, Gold Coast (Colonial Ghana), c.1900–1940', *African Economic History*, 30, 2002, 31–51.
89 Gold Coast Government, *Medical and Sanitary Department Report* [*MDAR*], 1911 (Accra: Government Printer, 1912).
90 Gareth Austin, 'Vent for Surplus or Productivity Breakthrough? The Ghanaian Cocoa Take-off, c. 1890–1936', *The Economic History Review*, 67.4 (2014), 1035–64.
91 S.M. Ceesay et al., 'Effects on Birth Weight and Perinatal Mortality of Maternal Dietary Supplements in Rural Gambia: 5 Year Randomised Controlled Trial', *BMJ*, 315.7111 (1997), 786–90 (p. 786).
92 In Buganda, a similar rainforest economy in southern Uganda, plantain attained near-mythic status. Plantain could yield 10 times the produce of a yam garden and be cultivated all year round, but it provided only one-tenth of the protein and a little under a quarter of the energy of a maize-based diet. See C.C. Wrigley, *Crops and Wealth in Uganda: A Short Agrarian History* (Kampala: East African Institute of Social Research, 1959), pp. 7–8.
93 *MDAR*, 1954, p. 141.
94 Austin, *Labour*, pp. 54–5.
95 Beckett, *Akokoaso*, p. 76.
96 TNA/CO/323/1570/7, Committee on Nutrition in the Colonial Empire, Economic Advisory Council: papers circulated, 1938. Memorandum by the Gold Coast Director of Agriculture, 'Agriculture in relation to Human Nutrition', 29/6/1938.
97 W.R.F. Collis, J. Dema, and A. Omololu, 'On the Ecology of Child Health and Nutrition in Nigerian Villages, Parts I and II', *Tropical and Geographical Medicine*, 14 (1962), 140–63, 201–29.

98 TNA/CO/859/68/1, Nutrition research survey: Gold Coast, 1941–3. Minutes by S. Culwick on a follow-up report on nutrition in the Gold Coast, 5/11/1943.
99 Austin, *Labour*, p. 66.
100 TNA/CO/859/68/1, Nutrition research survey: Gold Coast, 1941–1943. E. Norton Jones, Secretary for Social Services, to the Colonial Secretary, 'Nutrition', 17/11/1943.
101 *ADAR*, 1950/1, p. 23.
102 See E.V. Doku, *Cassava in Ghana* (Accra: Ghana Universities Press, 1969); La Fleur, *Fusion Foodways*, p. 167.
103 La Fleur, *Fusion Foodways*, pp. 155–81; McCaskie, *Identities*, p. 48; Austin, *Labour*, p. 66.
104 Grant, *Nutrition and Health*, p. 61.
105 Russell, 'Malnutrition', p. 110.
106 Moradi, Austin, and Baten, *Heights and Development*, p. 28.
107 Alexander Moradi, 'Confronting Colonial Legacies – Lessons from Human Development in Ghana and Kenya, 1880–2000', *Journal of International Development*, 20.8 (2008), 1107–21 (p. 1113).
108 Moradi, Austin, and Baten, *Heights and Development*, pp. 27–8.
109 Cicely D. Williams, 'Maternal and Child Health in Kumasi in 1935', *Journal of Tropical Pediatrics*, 2.3 (1956), 141–6 (p. 142).
110 Grant, 'II', p. 701.
111 Marjorie Brown du Sautoy, *Some Gold Coast Foods or What to Eat for a Balanced Diet* (Accra: Government Printing Department, 1953), 20.
112 PRAAD/K/ARG/13/4/37, Child Welfare Clinics (Midwives' Returns). These are incomplete returns from various clinics for September 1956 to April 1957.
113 Williams, 'Child Health', p. 99.
114 WL/PP/CDW/B.1/3. 'Gold Coast Handbook of Nursing. Children's Section, Accra'.
115 PRAAD/K/ARG/13/3/12, Annual Report MOH, 1957–8, Kumasi Central Hospital Report, 1957, p. 23.
116 Cicely D. Williams, 'Council on Foods and Nutrition', *Journal of the American Medical Association*, 153.14 (1953), 1280–5 (p. 1281).
117 WL/PP/CDW/B.1/3, Cicely Williams's Papers, 'Gold Coast Handbook of Nursing. Children's Section, Accra'.
118 A.W. Cardinall, *The Gold Coast, 1931: A Review of Conditions in the Gold Coast in 1931 as Compared with Those of 1921 Based on Figures and Facts Collected by the Chief Census Officer of 1931, Together with a Historical, Ethnographical and Sociological Survey of the People of That Country* (Accra: Government Printer, 1932).
119 Ghana Government, *1960 Population Census of Ghana* (Accra: Census Office, 1962).
120 Gold Coast Government, *Report on the Census of the Gold Coast Colony for the Year 1891* (Accra: Census Committee, 1892); Gold Coast Government, *The Gold Coast Appendices, Containing Comparative Returns and General Statistics of the 1931 Census* (Accra: Government Printer, 1932).
121 Gold Coast Government, *Report on the Census for the Year 1901* (Accra: Census Committee, 1902).
122 The gender history of Gold Coast urbanisation is thoroughly illustrated in Emmanuel Akyeampong, '"Wo Pe Tam Won Pe Ba" ("You like Cloth but You Don't Want Children"): Urbanization, Individualism & Gender Relations in Colonial Ghana, c.1900–39', in *Africa's Urban Past*, ed. by David M. Anderson and Richard Rathbone (Oxford: James Currey, 2000), pp. 222–34.
123 Emmanuel Akyeampong, 'Sexuality and Prostitution among the Akan of the Gold Coast c. 1650–1950', *Past & Present*, 156, 1997, 144–73 (p. 157).
124 Robertson, *Sharing*, p. 30.
125 K.A. Busia, *Report on a Social Survey of Sekondi-Takoradi* (London: Crown Agents for the Colonies on behalf of the Govt of the Gold Coast, 1950), p. 23.
126 Gold Coast Government, *1953 Accra Survey of Household Budgets* (Accra: Office of the Government Statistician, 1953), p. 2.
127 Akyeampong, 'Urbanization', p. 227.
128 Akyeampong, 'Urbanization', p. 228.
129 Gold Coast Government, *Census of Population 1948, Report and Tables* (Accra: Government Printer, 1950).

130 Ioné Acquah, *Accra Survey: A Social Survey of the Capital of Ghana, Formerly Called the Gold Coast, Undertaken for the West Africa Institute of Social and Economic Research, 1953–1956* (London: University of London Press, 1958), p. 72.
131 Busia, *Report*, pp. 29–46.
132 For economic individualism within the household, see, for instance, Abu, 'Separateness of Spouses'; Allman and Tashjian, *'I Will Not Eat Stone'*, pp. 45–78.
133 Robertson, *Sharing*, pp. 64–7.
134 Robertson, *Sharing*, pp. 48–56.
135 M.J. Field, *Search for Security: An Ethno-Psychiatric Study of Rural Ghana* (London: Faber and Faber, 1960), p. 123.
136 Acquah, *Accra Survey*, p. 73; Busia, *Report*, pp. 107–8.
137 The origin of trade unionism in the Gold Coast's mines is detailed in Jeff Crisp, *The Story of an African Working Class: Ghanaian Miners' Struggles, 1870–1980* (London: ZED Books, 1984), pp. 56–93.
138 TNA/CO/927/2/3, Series of reports by Miss P. Ady relating to wages and standards of living in Accra, 1945–6. 'Wages and Standards of Living in Accra', p. 12.
139 An official accounting of the riots can be found in Andrew Aiken Watson, *Statement by His Majesty's Government on the Report of the Commission of Enquiry into Disturbances in the Gold Coast, 1948* (London: HMSO, 1948); for more context and analysis, see Austin, *Politics*, pp. 66–8.
140 Acquah, *Accra Survey*, pp. 80–1. See also Adame Labi and B. Selormey, *Report on the Enquiry into Begging and Destitution in the Gold Coast, 1954* (Accra: Government Printer, 1955); Busia, *Report*, p. 24.
141 Acquah, *Accra Survey*, pp. 53–4; Busia, *Report*, pp. 110–11.
142 Busia, *Report*, pp. 106–7.
143 *MDAR*, 1953, p. 83.
144 Busia, *Report*, pp. 24, 110–11.
145 Busia, *Report*, p. 23; Field, *Security*, p. 33f.
146 *MDAR*, 1942–55.
147 For a comprehensive history of beriberi, see Kenneth J. Carpenter, *Beriberi, White Rice, and Vitamin B: A Disease, a Cause, and a Cure* (Berkeley, CA: University of California Press, 2000). For Purcell's account of beriberi in the Gold Coast, see F.M. Purcell, 'Beri-Beri or Epidemic Dropsy', *West African Medical Journal*, 7.4 (1934), 143–5.
148 Fred T. Sai, 'The Impact of Urban Life on the Diets of Rural Immigrants and Its Repercussions on the Nutritional Status of the Community', *Ghana Medical Journal*, 6.4 (1967), 134–9 (p. 137).
149 Female agency has been seen to reflect in infant mortality decline across the world. See, for instance, John C. Caldwell, 'Routes to Low Mortality in Poor Countries', *Population and Development Review*, 12.2 (1986), 171–220 (p. 184).
150 Quoted in K. David Patterson, 'Health in Urban Ghana: The Case of Accra 1900–1940', *Social Science & Medicine. Medical Anthropology*, 13B.4 (1979), 251–68 (pp. 253–4).
151 *MDAR*, 1925; *MDAR*, 1930–1.
152 Stephen Addae, *The Evolution of Modern Medicine in a Developing Country: Ghana 1880–1960* (Bishop Auckland: Durham Academic Press, 1996), pp. 227–39.
153 PRAAD/A/CSO/11/5/1, Maternal mortality and morbidity in the Gold Coast, 1932; Patterson, 'Urban Ghana', p. 265.
154 Acquah, *Accra Survey*, p. 135; *MDAR*, 1955, p. 49.
155 Gold Coast Government, *Report of the Commission of Enquiry into the Health Needs of the Gold Coast* (Accra: Government Printer, 1952), pp. 5, 31.
156 *MDAR*, 1954, p. 141.
157 Williams, 'Maternal and Child Health in Kumasi in 1935', p. 142.
158 PRAAD/A/ADM/5/4/62, Welfare and mass education in the Gold Coast, 1946–51, 'Report of the Department of Social Welfare and Community Development 1946–1951'.
159 Busia, *Report*, p. 94.
160 Geoffrey Tooth, *A Survey of Juvenile Delinquency in the Gold Coast* (Accra: Government Printer, 1946).
161 Moradi, 'Confronting Colonial Legacies', p. 1114.

162 Gold Coast Regiment personnel records, enlisted 1938–60. Alexander Moradi, 'Men under Arms in Colonial Africa: Gold Coast Regiment', anthropometric data provided by author, 2009.

163 Compare *MDAR*, 1948, p. 16, with B.B. Waddy, 'Heights and Weights of Children in the Northern Territories of the Gold Coast', *Journal of Tropical Medicine and Hygiene*, 59.1 (1956), 1–4.

164 Cardinall, *The Gold Coast, 1931*, p. 104. It is interesting to note that urban access to imported animal produce was seen, by some, as a pernicious threat to adult health, as well as to the colony's food sovereignty – see Robins, '"Food Comes First"', p. 172.

165 Williams, 'Child Health', p. 97.

166 Hill, *Migrant*, p. 187.

167 Metcalfe, *Great Britain and Ghana*, p. 653.

168 Mahmood Mamdani, *Politics and Class Formation in Uganda* (London: Heinemann, 1976), pp. 151–3.

169 Both quoted in Austin, *Labour*, pp. 257–8.

170 Austin, *Labour*, p. 258.

171 Austin, *Labour*, p. 260.

172 PRAAD/K/ARG/2/1/9, 'Price controls, general, 1948–53'.

173 Watson, *Statement*, p. 38.

174 Gold Coast Government, *Agricultural Statistical Survey of South-East Akim Abuakwa 1952–3* (Accra: Office of the Government Statistician, 1953), p. 10.

175 Gold Coast Government, *Akim Abuakwa Survey*; see also Gerardo Serra, 'Towards a Political Economy of Statistics: A Study of Household Budget Surveys in the Gold Coast, 1945–1957' (presented at the African Economic Development: Measuring Success and Failure conference, Simon Fraser University, Vancouver, 2013).

176 Victor Lavy et al., *The Impact of the Quality of Health Care on Children's Nutrition and Survival in Ghana*, Living Standards Measurement Study (Washington, D.C.: World Bank, 1995), pp. 1–68 (p. 16).

177 Purcell, *Diet and Ill-Health*, p. 43. For the specifics of the hold-up, see Rod Alence, 'The 1937–1938 Gold Coast Cocoa Crisis: The Political Economy of Commercial Stalemate', *African Economic History*, 19 (1990), 77–104.

178 Sen, *Poverty*, pp. 5–6.

179 Sen, *Poverty*, pp. 67, 154–5.

180 F.J. Bennett and J.P. Stanfield, 'The Pattern of Malnutrition in Uganda', *Journal of Tropical Pediatrics*, 17 (1971), S5–10 (p. S7).

181 PRAAD/K/ARG/13/3/12, Kumasi Central Hospital Report, 1957, p. 25.

182 Austin, *Labour*, pp. 424–30.

183 Austin, *Labour*, p. 429.

184 This pattern can also be seen in southern Uganda; see Nott, 'Malnutrition in a Modernising Economy'.

185 PRAAD/A/ADM/11/1/1294, Purcell, 'Report', p. 96.

5
Hunger in the 'labour reservoir', c.1896–1957

In 1899, in a now infamous statement of imperial indifference, Sir Frederick Hodgson, then Governor of the Gold Coast, opined on the future of the Northern Territories in a despatch to Joseph Chamberlain, then Secretary of State for the Colonies. After noting the relative paucity of marketable products found or grown in the recently colonised North, Sir Frederick explained:

> For the present I, therefore, cannot too strongly urge the employment of all available resources of the Government upon the development of the country to the South of Kintampo leaving the Northern Territories to be dealt with in future years ... I would not at present spend upon the Northern Territories – upon in fact the hinterland of the Colony – a single penny more than is absolutely necessary for their suitable administration and the encouragement of the transit trade.[1]

Unlike in other parts of the Empire, in the Northern Territories the encouragement of the transit trade – and the more general promotion of colonial capitalism – was somewhat dependent on this considered lack of state investment.

Further south, the rapid development of the gold and cocoa industries was demanding massive inputs of waged labour. The Northern Territories served as the most obvious source of manpower for the growing mines and sprawling plantations of Asante and the Colony. The most persistent argument relating to the origins and effects of this mass migration takes that the colonial government led the purposeful 'underdevelopment' of the North in order to feed the needs of Southern industry. As an agent of metropolitan capital primarily concerned with the extraction of gold and cocoa, the colonial state exploited the human resources of the savannah by treating the Northern Territories as a labour reservoir.[2] This line of thinking leads neatly to a 'dependency theory' framework of economic development which sees the wealth of the metropole built upon the underdevelopment of a colonised periphery, the wealth of which, in turn, depends upon the underdevelopment of its own peripheries.[3] Or, as Samir Amin has generalised with regard to Africa, 'the necessary corollary of the "wealth" of the coast was the impoverishment of the hinterland ... the culmination of the colonial trade was balkanisation, in which the "recipient" micro-regions had no "interest" in "sharing" the crumbs of the colonial cake with their labour reserves'.[4] Here migration into the centre was actively detrimental to the development of productive agricultural advances in outlying regions.[5]

The problem with dependency theory is, as Jean-François Bayart has most famously explained, that its 'woolly universalism' overlooks the depth and variance of the African past in favour of an ahistorical and explicitly political reading of the world.[6] By assuming that colonialisation and globalisation have charted universal patterns of peripheral poverty, dependency theorists are commonly seen to ignore the influence of diverse precolonial histories; the novelty and variability of localised economies; and the import of African agency within these historical processes. As we have already seen in Asante, insights drawn from demography and anthropology offer a means to more nuanced histories of capitalist development and attendant changes in food, poverty, health, and nutrition. However, this should not be taken to deny the value of a centre–periphery model. The health inequalities and infrastructural disparities which can be seen in modern Ghana undoubtedly reflect the priorities of an extractive colonial system. Attendance first to the health needs of the colonists and then Southern producers – all the while overlooking the greater demands of Northern health – speaks to the relative worth of human capital within the colonial economy. The erosion of nineteenth-century polities and market integration with the rest of the Gold Coast and the rest of the British Empire also preceded a general decline in purchasing power for Northern subsistence farmers. Although southward migration was stimulated by the growing demands of this changing economic landscape, labour migrancy was a considered reaction to both new and long-standing pressures. Negotiated between migrants and their families remaining at home, increasing southward migration was nonetheless responsible for significant disruptions to the social and familial structures around which food production and childcare had previously been oriented. As we have also seen in Asante, new forms of nutrition insecurity derived as much from the pervasive devaluation of domestic reproduction as from the enduring struggle for food. Unlike in Asante and the Colony, however, the Northern Territories received little state support to mediate the worst effects of their capitalist transition.

Health disparities and colonial infrastructure

At a fundamental level, nutrition is determined by the provision of adequate care and the provision of adequate food. The adequacy of any household or community's childcare and food supply is greatly influenced by localised patterns of infrastructure and state organisation. The provisioning of clean water, sanitation, and power; the span and efficacy of public health campaigns and famine relief programmes; regulations regarding land management and working conditions; and a great number of factors besides these are all critically important in determining nutritional status. Particularly pertinent, however, is the general provision of healthcare and education. In an influential survey article, the demographer Jack Caldwell – who had previously cut his teeth at the University of Ghana – outlined 'the routes to low mortality in poor countries'.[7] Explaining how poorer nations such as Costa Rica, Vietnam, Cuba, and Sri Lanka could outperform rich nations like Oman, Saudi Arabia, or Libya, Caldwell highlighted the various interactions between mortality decline and state and social organisation. In part, national successes resulted from per capita expenditure on health and social care, improved staff numbers vis-à-vis total population, and a greater proximity to modern healthcare. However, as in oil-rich Saudi Arabia or Libya, the proliferation of modern medical services did not translate into lower child mortality until a cohort of educated young mothers grew up to recognise its worth.[8] The social orientation of individual communities was also found to be important. Female autonomy, a regard for education, and a history of egalitarianism, radicalism, and political activity create an environment where health facilities and schools are demanded and utilised, but are not accepted uncritically.[9] Although these determinants are wrought over the course of centuries, the state still determines whether its citizens have the means to address such traditions. The state determines access to healthcare and education but also to political franchise and, in that, governments can mediate our understandings of health and our demands for greater wellbeing.

For decades, access to health, education, and even politics in colonised spaces was mediated by colonial administrations. For colonial governments and Christian missionaries, these were, in part, tools to control and coerce; informed at least initially by racist ideologies, hospitals and schools were often viewed with suspicion by their intended public.[10] On a more fundamental level, the scientific perception of health often did not fit with indigenous understandings of illnesses caused by 'immutable and supernatural laws'.[11] Here, Medical Officers lamented that their patients:

> Failed to take proper advantage of the medical facilities available to them … not a single one of the people we advised to come to hospital for treatment actually came, for like so many people in the Gold Coast they regarded the hospital as the last resort of the sick when all traditional medicines had failed.[12]

Although later campaigns against trypanosomiasis and yaws made use of powerful and effective curatives, a cautious approach to Western medicine is not entirely surprising.[13] In 1932, for instance, a two-year-old boy died at the Princess Marie Louise Children's Hospital in Accra after being injected for yaws; in 1937, 19 people died across Bawku and Navrongo following tryps injections; in 1942, 3 more people died in Wa, again following tryps injections.[14] Surgery and anaesthesia were more readily respected but many people preferred traditional medicines for the treatment of leprosy, blindness, and infertility.[15] The uptake of Western medicine in the Gold Coast was, therefore, rather haphazard, informed by the successes and failures of colonial healthcare, as well as by traditional epistemes. As late as the 1980s, one study in Northern Ghana suggested that children's ambivalence to Western medicine could not be disentangled from its original introduction as part of an invasive foreign regime.[16] As Caldwell explains, access to 'services clearly play a role, although the message is that health cannot simply be bought'.[17] In the colonial world, the manner and the historical context in which these services were provided must also be borne in mind.

In the Gold Coast, the provision of public services was closely linked to imperial interests and the generation of capital. In the extractive colonial economy, public-service provision was usually oriented towards the protection and advancement of its most valuable and immediate sources of human capital. In the earliest instances, Western medicine in West Africa concerned itself specifically with European health. With the ascendency of British rule, ill-health was understood as an explicit threat to colonial power in the new colony. For instance, British defeat and withdrawal from the 1864 Anglo-Ashanti war was largely due to mass morbidity during the march into the forest. The successful 1874 campaign, on the other hand, was extensively planned to preserve troop health through the advanced establishment of hospital and quarantine huts, pre-planned camp sites, and the provision of raised beds.[18] Still, European mortality remained high into the twentieth century. In the first years of the colony, morbidity was so severe that there were two governors at any one time, so that one could always be on sick leave.[19] Medical officers accompanied the later extension of colonial administration and health services began with the distribution of anti-malarial drugs to colonists in commercial and mining centres. Preventive healthcare was likewise created primarily for the benefit of government officials, with sanitary water and sewerage concentrated in a few areas. The state only granted the African population access to these new forms of healthcare when 'cultural isolation was found to be an ineffective preventive measure'.[20]

The steady if piecemeal expansion of medicine and education was largely arranged around the vagaries of capital formation. Spending was dependent upon development policy and determined by the globalising market, concentrating on the productive centre of Asante and the commercial centres which were growing up around the coastal ports. By 1921, there were six medical officers in Asante, two of whom were assigned to industrial projects.[21] However, the Northern Territories received far less attention than either Asante or the Colony. Following his 1929 tour of the North, Governor Alexander Ransford Slater called the medical provision in the Territories 'nothing short of scandal', going on to explain that:

> There is only one hospital worth the name, viz at Tamale. At Wa there is a so-called hospital full of people sleeping on the floor, but the building is an ancient ramshackle one badly situated next to the noisy centre of town … at Lawra … a totally illiterate but faithful old retainer … attends regularly every morning with lint to give a little elementary aid to persons suffering from sores etc. This is the sum total of the hospital facilities in a district with nearly 100,000 inhabitants, for at Tumu there is nothing.[22]

Although Slater ordered immediate improvements, and medical services did begin to expand throughout the North, the North/South disparity in healthcare provision was formed during colonial government (see Figure 5.1) but endured well into independence. Extant Northern

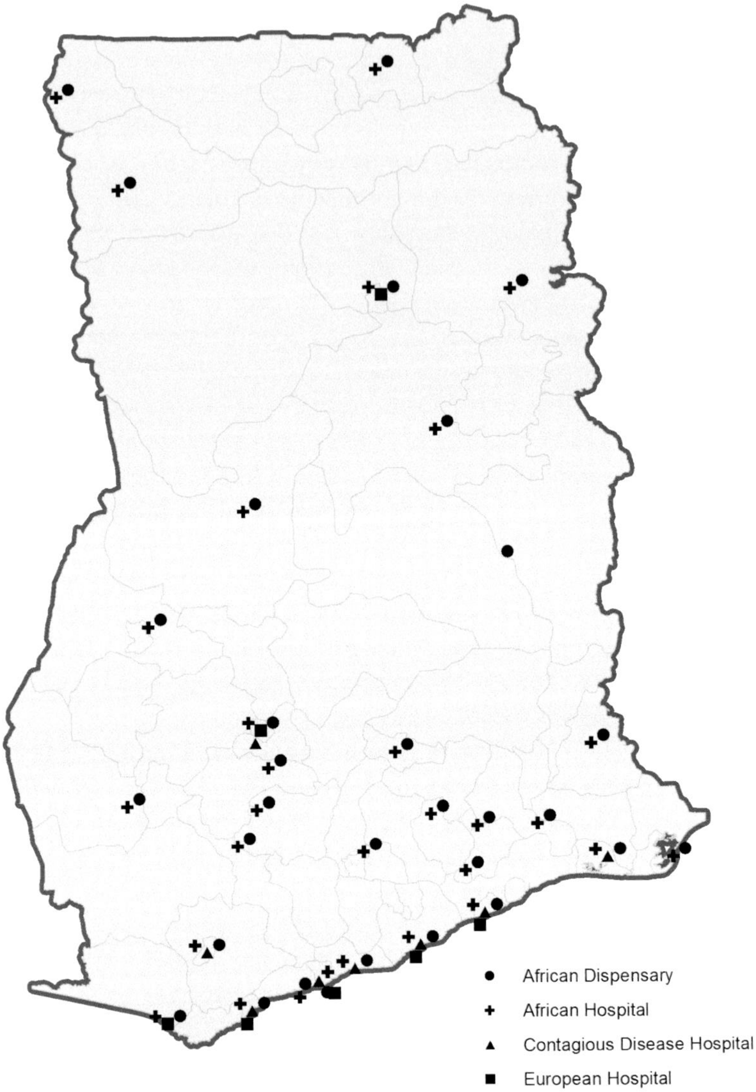

Figure 5.1 Healthcare provisioning, 1929/30.[23]

hospitals were available but were also habitually understaffed, as the country's few doctors gravitated towards the profitable urban centres of the South.[24] Large towns only received the attention of an itinerant medical officer, if at all, and there were rarely more than four doctors throughout the Northern Territories. In 1951, there was one doctor for every 120,000 people in the Northern Territories, 1:27,000 in Asante, and

1:24,000 in the coastal colony. The population to bed ratio was similarly skewed at 1:1,500 in the Ashanti Region and 1:4,300 for the North.[25]

Similar disparities were seen in the provision of nutrition and child welfare services. In the early 1930s, child welfare clinics operated in every major conurbation in Asante and the Colony. By contrast, in 1932, enquiries into the establishment of Tamale's first child welfare clinic were met with a telegrammed reply from Accra: 'old power house Tamale may be used for Infant Welfare work but no expenditure on alteration or improvement should be incurred.'[26] These were years of retrenchment which threatened the colony's child welfare project in general. Still, this trend of hesitant and inequitable spending left an enduring legacy of infrastructural inequality, devaluing infant health in the North and allowing for fundamental misunderstandings of Northern nutrition. Indeed, by 1955, there were 15 child welfare clinics in Kumasi alone, and 33 in the rest of the Ashanti Region.[27] The year before, the Medical Department had reported that, apart from Bimbilla Health Centre, 'in the Northern Territories there was only a hospital clinic service' providing child welfare services.[28] Attendances at these two centres amounted to 7,040, compared with 49,787 in the Ashanti Region.[29]

Ultimately, the colonial state did not invest in health infrastructure in the North because it saw limited value in the local economy. Unlike Asante, the North housed little exploitable agriculture, and few valuable mineral deposits. Unlike the coast, the North was not well positioned to act as a centre of colonial commerce. When the Northern Territories were appended to the Gold Coast, they were never expected to turn a profit but were instead annexed to defend against inroads from the French or German empires. Indeed, between 1892 and 1906, the administration of Protectorate of the Northern Territories ended in a deficit of £112,125, despite £318,307 in imperial grants.[30] Given the expense of simply administering the North, the government was loath to provide any additional health or social care, especially considering the scale of the North's disease burden, much of which was tied to the unique demands of life in the Territories.[31] For instance, epidemics of cerebrospinal meningitis often occurred at the beginning of each year, when harmattan winds drove residents into housing which was often overcrowded and poorly ventilated.[32] Onchocerciasis, or river blindness, was also particularly prevalent in the North, draining labour from communities with already marginal levels of productive human capital.[33] By the 1950s, perhaps 3 per cent of the North's total population was clinically blind. However, it was only following a 1951 publication which showed onchocerciasis to be endemic among riverside populations along the *lower* (i.e. southern) Volta that the nature of river blindness in the North was also addressed.[34] As with many of the North's other diseases, blindness went 'unnoticed, or if noticed, disregarded'.[35] Louse-borne relapsing fever and trypanosomiasis also appeared as epidemics particular to the North throughout the colonial period. Alongside epidemic illness, less dramatic, endemic concerns took an even higher toll on the health of Northern populations.[36] In general if dispassionate terms, B.B. Waddy, a medical officer in the north-west, explained the area had 'the misfortune to be a hyperendemic focus of yaws and onchocerciasis, and a hypersusceptible epidemic focus of sleeping sickness and cerebro-spinal meningitis', in addition to 'the usual holoendemic malaria and some lively foci of schistosomiasis'.[37]

Generally, health and nutrition in the Southern colony was considerably better than that seen in the Northern Territories. In the late 1930s, Purcell calculated that as many as 27 per cent of the children born in the savannah would die within their first year. In the forest, infant mortality was estimated at around 10 per cent.[38] The 1948 census found similar if less extreme variations in child survival.[39] With regard to nutrition, schoolchildren in 1940s Accra were markedly taller and heavier than children measured in Northern schools nearly a decade later.[40] However, the breakdown of microenvironments through improving transport links and increased trade did cause the incidence of epidemic illness in the South to increase during the early twentieth century, although to a lesser extent that in the North (perhaps due to some partial immunity garnered by early interaction with Europeans).[41] There were a number of limited smallpox outbreaks, the ferocity of which was eroded by increasingly widespread vaccinations, but the real exception is the 1918 epidemic of Spanish influenza, which caused a major loss of life throughout the South.

The influenza epidemic also provides a useful example of the politics of healthcare provisioning in the Gold Coast. Throughout 1918, many people were highly critical of the performance of the Medical Department. In Keta, one resident 'publicly accused the government of callousness; others were bitter about the shortage of physicians. The government was denounced for its failure to train African doctors, its lack of interest in the health of non-White populations, and discriminatory practices which protected a "trade union" of British physicians.'[42] One district commissioner, seeking to blunt African accusations of favouritism, was left to explain that in Accra a higher proportion of sick Europeans died (8 out of 77, or 10.4 per cent) than inmates of the capital's jails (18 out of 220, or 8.2 per cent).[43] The influenza epidemic received such attention from the administration largely because it affected the Southern colony. Northern epidemics, with a far greater combined effect than the influenza crisis, continued relatively unabated. Even the influenza death rate was higher in the North than elsewhere in the Gold Coast.[44] However, ill-health in the North rarely intersected with political dissent. Instead – for instance, in the north-western Lawra District, where the British appointed and propped up a system of ruling chiefs which often exploited their subjects apparently to the point of 'slavery' – the population sought political, spiritual, *and* medical protection from the local missions, the only visible form of White-colonial authority.[45] In the 1940s the colonial government finally attempted to address ill-health in the north-west, but only managed to do so with mission help.[46]

The Southern response to the 1918 epidemic was facilitated by a form of civil society made up of vocal, educated, and effective organisations and individuals agitating for the interests of a wider citizenry – something which was largely absent from the Northern Territories. A more obvious example of this can be found in the cocoa 'hold-ups' of the 1930s, where, in a longer protest against low prices, Asante farmers refused to sell to the expatriate firms that held a monopoly over cocoa buying.[47] As Mahmood Mamdani has explained, indirect rule was envisaged as a means to avoid such disruptions. Here, the employment of customary law and land tenure sought to maintain the peasantry as 'subjects' answerable to 'custom', rather than as 'citizens' with inalienable 'rights'. Across Africa, colonial governments refigured tradition and community into modes of domination which would facilitate the expansion of extractive economics.[48] However, in the cocoa belt, in mining towns, and in coastal areas, class formation and the growth of civil society undermined that mode of domination, threatening the profitability of the whole imperial exercise. Engineered development in the North sought to avoid such pitfalls and, instead, 'responded to the threat of civil society by designing development projects with an eye towards preserving African community'.[49] For instance, in 1950 the Gonja Development Scheme was given its mandate to redevelop 30,000 acres of marginal land for the semi-mechanised, commercial production of groundnuts. This was to be realised through the planned resettlement of tens of thousands of 'Frafra' peasants from the 'overpopulated' Zuarungu District, preserving 'tribal groups' and community order.[50] The Gonja scheme went into liquidation in 1957, but it was perhaps the grandest example of the sort of community-based development which, in 1926, Governor Frederick Gordon Guggisberg had envisioned as a 'bulwark' against the 'disintegrating waves of western civilisation'.[51]

As part of the subjugation of Northern civil society, the North was starved of education and denied the formation of the broad-based, politically expedient educated class which had been in development throughout the Southern colony since the end of the nineteenth century.[52] In 1914, C.H. Armitage, now the Chief Commissioner of the Northern Territories, requested funding for a number of local schools across the North, arguing that:

> With the Colony enjoying, in addition to the Education Department, the education services of the Church Mission Society, the Roman Catholic, Wesleyan, Basel and Bremen Missions ... a few crumbs from this feast of instruction might well be spared for the children of this Dependency.[53]

'Crumbs', however, proved to be an apt description and, throughout the first decades of the twentieth century, only a handful of schools were haltingly established across the Territories.[54] In 1925, Guggisberg explained to the governors of the school in Wa that, after Standard VII, 'the strictest care should be taken not to promote any but a very exceptional boy to a higher standard', a policy which endured into the 1940s.[55] Those missions which actively sought to educate Northern children found a hostile reception, since they were 'likely to disrupt the cherished political tranquillity of the Northern Territories'.[56] Education also threatened to undermine the value of Northern labour. As one district commissioner explained, 'in the near future there is a danger of the Protectorate being overrun by an excess of half-educated natives without a means of livelihood as they would consider manual labour beneath their dignity'.[57] Due in large part to such reservations, in 1925 there were only 356 boys and 21 girls in Northern schools, making up just 1.3 and 0.4 per cent of the colony's schoolchildren respectively. By 1954, the figures had grown significantly, with 8,011 boys and 2,140 girls in primary education in Northern schools, yet this still equated to just 2.9 and 1.6 per cent of primary enrolment across the colony. Underrepresentation was also seen at the higher levels: the first university graduate of Northern extraction passed out from a British university in 1953. The third Northern graduate, and the first to actually graduate in Ghana, came in 1960, three years after independence.[58]

The general absence of education infrastructure combined with the marginal nature of the savannah subsistence economy to restrain the development of Northern education. Educative childhoods were an expensive proposition which delayed children's transformation into productive assets; a 13-year-old in the cash economy could perhaps increase cash income by a third, or undertake labour to the same value.[59] Although competition for white-collar work was intense, and unemployment was a problem for the literate and illiterate alike, education was starting to become the surest route into influence and affluence in the South. In the North, however, productive human capital related more directly to family survival and any loss of child labour was felt much more acutely. Indeed, in the 1960s, one survey found that nearly half of all Northern respondents claimed that children aged five to nine years were 'earning their keep'. Of children between 10 and 14 years old, 74 per cent were considered productive members of the household. By contrast, in the region made up by Ashanti and Brong-Ahafo, only 17 and 56 per cent of respondents respectively considered their five-to-nine-year-olds and 10-to-14-year-olds 'productive'.[60] The patrilocal nature of Northern marriage devalued expensive investments in female children in particular and, even into independence, girls were underrepresented in Northern schools in particular (see Figures 5.2 and 5.3). Recalling the 1930s, Yvonne Fox explained that:

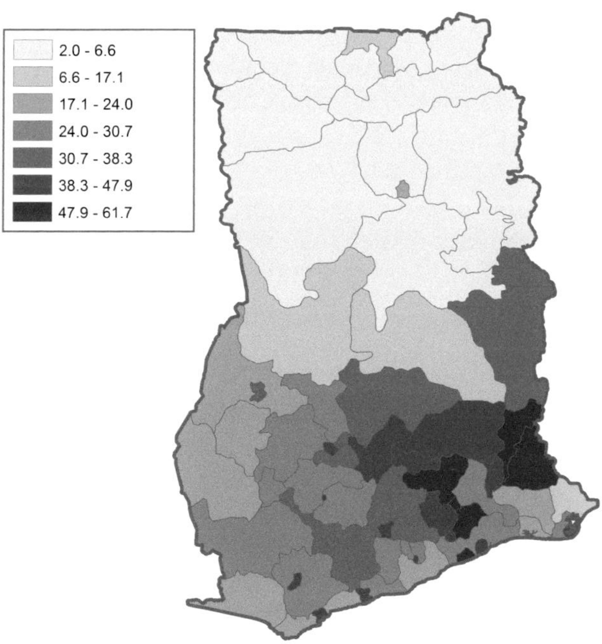

Figure 5.2 Percentage of girls aged 6–14 in regular education, 1960.[61]

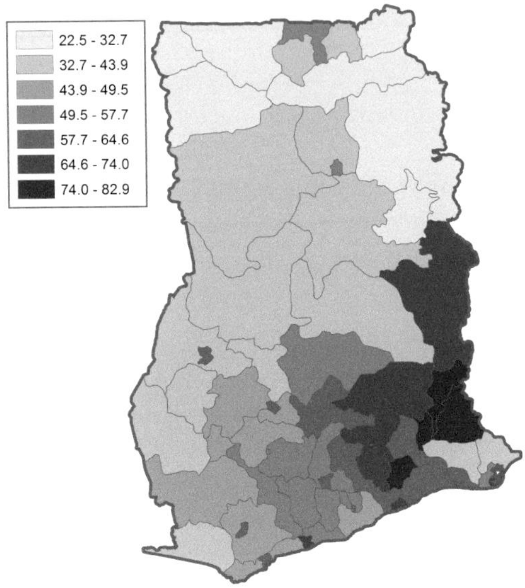

Figure 5.3 Gender disparity (girls as a percentage of boys) in regular education, 1960.[62]

> female education was none too popular. When parents sent their girls to school, they thought they should receive a payment or dowry of cows to compensate them for the loss of their daughters' services ... The chief of Sapelliga who had sent a daughter to school told R. that, before sending any other girl, he was waiting to see how this one turned out.[63]

The health advantages derived from female education were especially absent from the North, the lack of infrastructure and the socioeconomic environment of the savannah acting in conjunction to constrict education in general and female education in particular.

At the community level, the general dearth of education translated into widespread and disproportionate levels of illiteracy, and to a corresponding absence of political franchise.[64] At independence, this meant that Nkrumah's CPP struggled to integrate Southern Ghana with a recalcitrant hinterland disconnected from the rest of the emerging nation. Long denied purchase in the colony's politics, and wary of an independent political system 'which might result in the domination of the people of the north by those of the south', Northern voters turned out poorly for the CPP in the 1954 election.[65] Northern politicians feared that colonial retreat would simply mean the growth of 'black imperialism from the South' and actively fought for the continuation of British protection until levels of development – specifically in the form of infrastructure and educational standards – were broadly equitable. Eventually instead arguing for a federal Ghana, the Northern Peoples' Party (NPP) became the first in a tradition of parties espousing a monolithic Northern political voice, preferring 'being poor or living in poor conditions under their own government to feeling neglected under a rich government'.[66]

By the 1950s, as independence loomed, the state of health and nutrition across the country had, probably, never been better. Epidemic diseases had been successfully countered and nutritional status improved quickly. Children born in the later-colonial period significantly outgrew their parents, who had, in turn, outgrown their own parents.[67] International recognition of nutritional science had led to a greater recognition of the health effects of diet, and educationalists in the colony were taking notice too.[68] More and more girls were going to school and earning an education which had begun to include scientific theories of health and nutrition. By 1954, over 130,000 girls were enrolled in primary education, a 1,000 per cent increase on the 1934 figure.[69] As they grew, these children would imbibe the ubiquitous printed health education and diffuse its message among their neighbours and friends. All the while, with the success of vaccination campaigns and falling mortality rates, younger people became enamoured with the benefits of modern medicine; hospital admissions increased by 235 per cent between 1929 and 1955, as inpatient death rates almost halved. Over the same period, the number of outpatients seen rose by 74 per cent.[70] Despite this, the 'routes to low mortality' which were paved by these improvements were not evenly accessible across the emergent nation. Through underdeveloped infrastructure and the repression of civil society, the trajectory of colonial development entrenched the social and ecological bases of Northern ill-health. Inequities in health, education, and wellbeing are still very apparent in modern Ghana and, although these disparities may partly derive from the specific environmental and social determinants of disease in the savannah, their persistence was permitted by colonial policies which actively encouraged unequal development. As we will see in the next section, the considered underdevelopment of social services in the Northern Territories was complemented by a similar disinterest in developing the capacity and resilience of Northern agriculture.

Nutrition as coercion: migration and food insecurity in the colonial economy

Although rarely official strategy, the coercive potential of food deprivation was well understood by European colonists. In the most extreme manifestations, the suppression of food production was central to the broader suppression of indigenous resistance. Writing at the end of the nineteenth century, Charles Callwell's influential military textbook on the fighting of 'small wars' explained that when

> there is no king to conquer, no capital to seize, no organised army to overthrow ... it is then that the regular troops are forced to resort to cattle lifting and village burning and the war assumes an aspect which may shock the humanitarian.[71]

In 1896, the South Africa Company destroyed grain stocks in Rhodesia in order to force the surrender of the Ndebele.[72] During the following two decades, the colonial government in British-controlled Sudan curbed the independence of southern pastoralists through an 'administration by raids', the confiscation of cattle, and the destruction of villages.[73] In the Gold Coast's Northern Territories, where British militarism was subdued relative to other parts of the continent, early efforts to subdue the stateless, rebellious 'Frafra' repeated these trends, and military incursions left burned crops, razed villages, and epidemic disease in their wake.[74] Even as late as 1955, as part of their brutal repression of the Mau Mau revolt, the colonial government in Kenya allowed the growth of famine conditions in the ghettoised villages of Kikuyuland.[75] The mechanics of postcolonial famine has also been explained as a political construction; during the crisis in Darfur, food deprivation was manipulated by and to the advantage of powerful local actors.[76]

Food insecurity and endemic undernutrition should also be viewed in the same way – as a process which had artificial antagonisms as well as natural causes, and which produced beneficiaries as readily as victims. Even if hunger in the Gold Coast was rarely engineered by the state, its persistence in the savannah certainly benefited European concerns. Over the course of the colonial period, the Northern Territories began to look southwards, to Asante, the coast, and the export economy. Migrant labour became ever more important in the gold and cocoa industries growing across the South, a trend which was at least partly facilitated by Northern food insecurity. As we have seen in both the Asante domestic economy and the spatial inequities of infrastructural development, capitalist development often eschews the social reproduction of a given community while simultaneously promoting its capacity to produce at a level beyond subsistence. Prior to the concerted development agendas of the later-colonial period, these fundamental economic processes worked against the advancement of Northern subsistence and outmigration grew up at least in part to mitigate food insecurity at home.

As a result of this, successive colonial governments showed little interest in engaging with the structural causes of food insecurity, instead addressing its symptoms through the expansion of famine relief and the facilitation of migration. Although famine relief had been in place in the Anglo-Egyptian Sudan, Uganda, Tanganyika, and Southern Rhodesia throughout the 1910s, it was not until the 1930s that famine relief began in the Northern Territories, and this despite recurrent food shortages and an earlier general acknowledgement of structural shortfalls in food security. By 1933, every headman was required to send workers to a communal farm to expand reserves. Drought-resistant crops like cassava were promoted, as were locust-resistant root crops. Generally, though, these policies proved ineffective and most relief came in the form of trade embargos and food-for-work schemes.[77] In the late 1940s, Chief Commissioner W.H. Ingrams moved to reorient famine relief around a system of communal granaries and early warning systems. Although the compulsory requisition of grain was widely unpopular, it was at least partially successful, with communal reserves and early warning systems averting serious famine in 1953–4 and again in 1958–9.[78]

However, even these concessions were hard-won, and administrators in the North had to exhort the central state for famine relief well into the 1940s. Following the furore brought about by Purcell's public discussion of Northern nutrition (see Chapter 2), the Commissioner of the Northern Territories, G.H. Gibbs, was left to wring food aid from the Colonial Secretary, explaining that it is 'impossible to divine now if the people I have referred to would starve if given no assistance later in the year, but I am sure that starvation is not the means test that the Government would wish to apply'.[79] Even though he was said to recognise that 'there was always a danger of serious food shortage' in the Northern Territories, then Gold Coast Governor, Alan Burns, was hesitant to undercut the forces of free trade in order to bolster subsistence in the savannah. According to S. Culwick, a medical officer reporting on African nutrition security for the Colonial Office, Burns 'had been greatly impressed by the improvement seen in villages receiving palm oil and was in favour of subsidising its transport from the south, but there were difficulties in doing so because sending it north on any scale would interfere with exports to the UK'.[80]

During the horrific nineteenth-century famines in Ireland and then India, colonial adherence to the doctrines of Smith, Mill, and Malthus justified famine as an antidote to overpopulation and viewed any attempt to mitigate such crises through market manipulation as only accentuating the problem.[81] Such beliefs underpinned colonial food economies in Africa too, influencing famine relief and even non-crisis nutrition through similar if subtler mechanisms. In the Northern Territories, freedom of movement and the Southern economic advantage allowed valuable produce, in terms of both its economic and nutritional value, to be taken from the North and sold in markets where it would have a greater value. In the late 1930s, Purcell explained that 'there are the various species of antelope, and buffalo, but the amount of meat obtained from this sources is negligible in the more populous districts ... Much of the bush meat shot in the north, in Gonja, is by Ashanti hunters who take the kills down to Kumasi for sale.'[82] Fish, too, were subject to 'a somewhat predatory trade', where 'the Black Volta is fished by coast fishermen from Ada who establish camps alongside the river throughout its course, even far up beyond Lawra, during the dry season. A very small proportion, if any, of these catches is sold locally.'[83] Although interregional trade had the potential to improve wellbeing in impoverished areas such as northern Mamprusi (where 'the export of fowls to Kumasi is the main source of income'), it could also undermine the purchasing power of neighbouring people and drive valuable foodstuffs out of the North.[84]

Driven by population growth, urbanisation, and the cash-crop revolution, the colonial integration of Northern production with the expanding Southern food markets stimulated the southbound movement of staple foodstuffs too.[85] As early as the 1920s, the view of the North as a potential breadbasket of the Gold Coast meant that food insecurity increasingly related to market failure. Demand for food from buyers from Asante and from government departments in Tamale regularly outstripped supply, leading to rising prices which, throughout the 1920s, were complained about almost annually.[86] Although a small cohort of traders certainly benefited from these developments, the great mass of Northern subsistence farmers experienced broad declines in terms of purchasing power. This was a particular problem for perennially hungry, densely populated areas in the far north-east and north-west (see Figures 5.4 and 5.5) and served to accentuate a pattern where, in lean

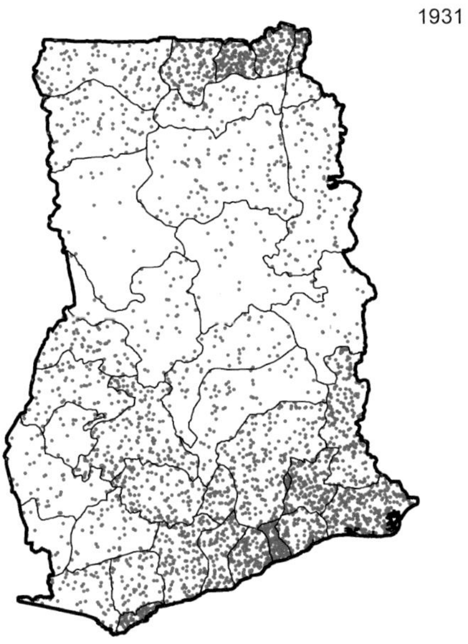

Figure 5.4 Population density, 1931.[87]

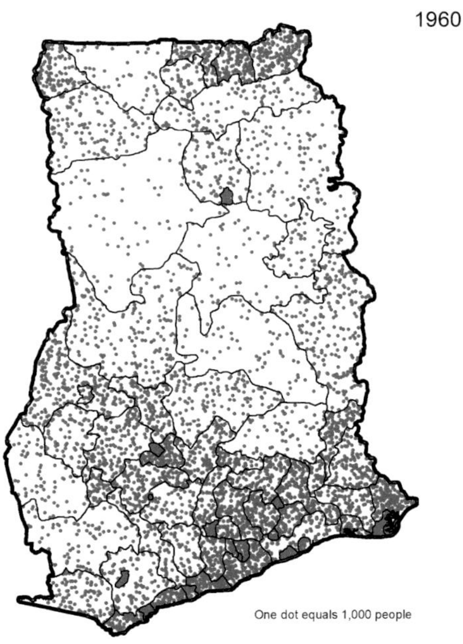

Figure 5.5 Population density, 1960.[88]

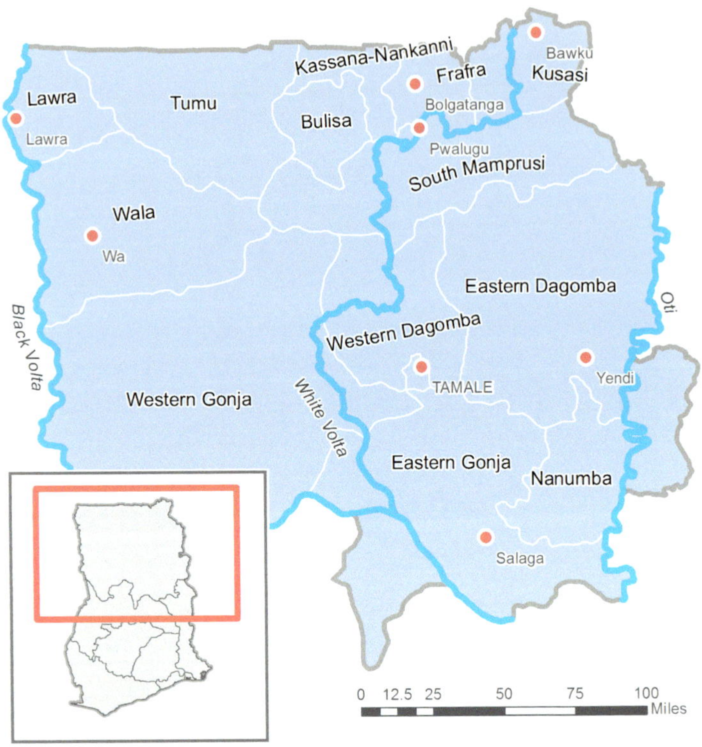

Figure 5.6 Districts, rivers, and settlements of note in the North, 1960.[89]

years, 'prices obtained for cattle sold under these circumstances are low and the prices that the Frafra have to pay for grain are extremely high'.[90] Although speculative trading pre-dated colonial rule, market integration under imperial administration encouraged the wider adoption (both spatially and quantitatively) of such practices, as well as the centralisation of even fairly small regional food economies. This was, in part, due to the fact that hunger in the Gold Coast's savannah was highly localised. In 1940, in the north-eastern community of Gawri, for instance, 'an eight week drought occurred which ruined the early millet. The poorer folk were chewing baobab fruit, a famine food in June; an abnormal misfortune; yet, at Zuarungu, eight miles to the south, there was a fair harvest.'[91]

As a main locus of the country's food insecurity, the movement of food into and out of the north-east was recorded at the Pwalagu ferry over the White Volta – the most direct route into and out of the 'hungry area' (see Figure 5.6). By the early 1950s, administrators could and did enact export bans on food crossing the river.[92] However, the growth of regional centres, such as Bolgatanga, alongside the emergence of local capitalists, undermined any such actions, allowing instead for the accumulation of food away from hungry rural areas.[93] Throughout the 1950s, prices in Tamale were consistently higher than those in Bolgatanga which were, in turn, consistently higher than those in Bawku.[94] In times of shortage, as in 1958, this became a particular problem for anyone reliant on backcountry markets:

> The bulk of the purchasing power for food is with those in Trade and Industry and the Profession [sic.]. These groups generally reside in the towns; hence the effective demand in the towns is better, and the rising level of prices, which is reflected in the villages, is initiated from the urban markets ... While the rural markets are short of supplies, the urban centres seem to be adequately supplied in the present time.[95]

These patterns of peripheral food insecurity remained consistent throughout much of the twentieth century (see also Chapter 6).[96]

This, again, fits into Amartya Sen's entitlement theory, this time at the macroeconomic level. Using the example of the 1972–4 Wollo famine in Ethiopia, Sen suggests that there does not need to be any widespread decline in food production to induce famine in individual villages or starvation in individual households. Across Ethiopia perhaps only 5–7 per cent of districts reported a fall in food availability against normal years, yet starvation and associated diseases brought the death toll to at least one hundred thousand. Hunger was concentrated in Wollo because a regional decline in purchasing power undermined local ability to command food imports from elsewhere.[97] In areas already compromised by highly localised Malthusian shortcomings, like the Gold Coast's north-east, these mechanisms can operate even at the district level, where the marketing of any excess foodstuffs is readily purchased by individuals with a greater 'entitlement package'. As with crises defined by a widespread reduction in food availability, market failures affect the poor most readily. Those least able to modify their entitlement packages, through access to livestock, land, or labour, are the most reliant on statist forms of famine relief and the most likely to starve when such relief is inadequate or unforthcoming. The growth of an integrated, colony-wide food market prompted these processes in lean years at the same time as food aid and facilitated outmigration in a colony-wide labour market provided new forms of relief.

The deterioration of peripheral food markets, macroeconomic entitlement failures, and a growing inability to remedy food insecurity through interaction with the local economy underwrote an enduring colonial labour policy which expressly championed Northern proletarianisation through southward migration. Over the course of the early twentieth century, the considered underinvestment championed by early-colonial administrators had begun to soften and, on his assumption of governorship in 1919, Guggisberg hoped 'within the next few years to see trains heavily loaded with groundnuts, shea-butter, corn, and cattle steaming south across the Volta'.[98] However, development in the North still had to fit within the demands of the colonial market; a year later, Guggisberg was to concede that 'every man of the Northern Territories is worth his weight in gold – for the mines, for private enterprise and for the development of those schemes the completion of which are necessary to secure progress and development'.[99] By 1937, the deleterious effects of emigration led the District Commissioner of Yendi to explain in a letter to Accra 'that the Protectorate [of the Northern Territories] has its own economic destiny to work out, and that that destiny is not solely to provide a reservoir of labour for the commerce and industry of the Colony and Ashanti'.[100] Progressively, over the course of the colonial period, labour migration became a more permanent transfer of people from North to South. By the time of the 1960 census, long-term rural migrants and expanding *zongo* communities in the city had left a million Northerners living across the South.[101]

However, it is wrong to assume that this process was actively arranged from Accra. For instance, and despite pressure from mining concerns, the government refused to implement policies of forced recruitment, instead only assisting in the mass recruitment campaigns of 1906–9 and 1920–3.[102] Similarly, aside from monopolies over the purchase and export of cocoa, expatriate enterprises had very little sway over the actual means of production.[103] At times, when officers did attempt to press men into mining or public works, they found an absence of young men, since many had already left for the South of their own accord.[104] As Guggisberg recognised in 1920, 'during the last two or three years, the NTs [Northern Territories] native has not rushed blindly into work in the South. He wants to know where he is going and what he is going to do. In fact, he has learnt to pick and choose, and to know his own value in the labour world.'[105] Cocoa farmers could usually afford to pay higher wages, and government work was seen to be much more agreeable than mining – mainly since it did not take place underground – and so labour diverted itself accordingly.

Rather than directly interfering with the processes of production, colonial governments concentrated on facilitating free trade. To these ends, the administration did provide infrastructure. Following Chief Commissioner Watherston's extensive road network plans, which established Tamale as the centre of the North, by 1910 the North had a 'well developed road network, superior in extent and construction to the roads in the South'.[106] Roads were established cheaply – often through unpaid labour working at the behest of chiefs and in lieu of taxation – and facilitated the growth of marketplaces, the penetration of marketable goods, and the flow of goods and people. Yet, unlike schools, roads did not necessarily allow the formation of a subversive civil society. Unlike hospitals and healthcare, roads were not built to assuage civil dissent. Although more direct involvement in development accompanied the beginnings of indirect rule in the 1930s, the Gold Coast was largely built on the ideals of market-driven growth in an integrated colonial market.[107] It was these considered investments in the development of the Northern Territories which corralled the Northern poor into a state of 'dependency'. As Inez Sutton has argued, 'the vision of the north as a supplier of labour conditioned colonial investment, or the lack of it, in Northern agriculture and especially infrastructure, so that little was done to create alternatives to labour migration when cash was demanded'.[108] As the colonial period progressed, demands for cash only increased. Market integration restrained the development of a more productive form of local capitalism at the same time as more regular interactions with the Southern colony and Western goods drove relativist understandings of poverty and brought new signifiers of social status, such as cloth and clothing.[109] Forced by both a particular development agenda and the weight of market forces, colonial capitalism provided the background against which the labour reservoir emerged. However, it was varied and often-changing interactions with savannah survival that actively shaped the adoption of migration.

Hunger, migration, and the limits of environmental determinism

The social shortcomings of capitalist development underline the history of colonialism in the Gold Coast, and the history of hunger in the Northern Territories cannot be entirely divorced from the political economy of colonial rule. However, the explanatory power of externalist economic histories of poverty, those which emphasise the top-down effects of policy, should be questioned in view of a savannah ecology which proscribes the ready escape from hunger. This was at least the thinking which prevailed among colonial staff. For instance, in the late 1950s, Waddy explained the cyclical and seasonal interactions of nutrition, disease, and labour across the savannah. His wearied account seems characteristic of a fatalism common to many medical officers posted across the North, and it is worth quoting at length:

> Throughout the dry season it is not possible to do any farming work, the ground is too hard. The heaviest work of the year takes place during the six weeks following the first rain, when the ground must be broken up for the season's planting. On the area of ground broken up and planted, depends the size of the harvest. At this period, last season's food stocks and therefore diet are at their lowest. The season's guinea worms emerge, sometimes almost immobilizing whole villages. Exacerbations of yaws "rheumatics" cripple many adults. In hyperendemic onchocerciasis areas, children lead out the blind men, perhaps 20 per cent of the adult males, to hoe pathetically. Mosquitoes breed afresh and this moment is the likeliest for adult malaria in a semi-immune community. Everything in fact conspires to make the community physically inefficient at this all-important time. If all the adverse factors operate together, famine results – as I have often seen. At best, farming effort is confined to the area round houses right up to the walls, where human excreta preserve some fertility in the overworked soil. There is never any excess food to sell, therefore there are no bought clothes or blankets for warmth. Inevitably, cold night air is abhorred and houses are unventilated. If any of the adverse factors cease to operate or are weakened, one improved harvest results in more food and energy next season. The cycle is broken and progress may be uninterrupted. This, too, can be seen in part of the Northern Territories where one may walk from a village five miles into the bush before leaving the last farm. In such a place crops are no longer grown close to the houses. With food to sell, the standard of living rises quite obviously: clothes, kerosene lamps and bicycles being the outward and visible signs.[110]

Later, Waddy would go on to clarify the relationship between disease and hunger in the north-west, explaining that 'any further adverse factor, such as the death of one or two active men, an extra crop of guineaworms, or a raid on the farm by game animals, could and did bring villages to starvation'.[111]

Patterns of malnutrition fit into this formulation and can also be explained as a bio-ecological phenomenon, linked with cycles of infection and seasonal demands on labour and food supply. In preindustrial Europe, children born in the winter were more susceptible to respiratory infections, while children being weaned in the summer lost the protective influence of breastfeeding during the time of year when infectious disease is more common.[112] In The Gambia, malnutrition peaked immediately following the annual rainy season epidemics of bacterial gastroenteritis.[113] In the Northern Territories too, a common cause of the high infant mortality was given as *bwinne*, 'a form of enteritis, infantile diarrhoea, which prevails each year in epidemic forms'.[114] In the densely populated Nangodi polity of north-eastern Ghana, it was later explained that the period of maximum physical activity (planting and weeding) coincided with the peak of the hungry season (between April and June), contributing to a cyclical pattern of food insecurity and malnutrition.[115] Even in the less pressured areas further south, the stresses of a single rainy season influenced nutritional status and the same mechanisms – disease, labour demands, and declining food supplies – acted against infant health despite the richer food environment. In Dagomba areas, for instance, low population densities allowed for a more profitable form of shifting cultivation and longer fallow periods, with at least some land, labour, and capital left over to grow cash-crops and diversify the local employment structure.[116] Nevertheless, one medical officer still came to conclude that 'there is always undernutrition because the calories value of the diet is insufficient for the needs of the body. It is probably only in the months of September, October, November and December that a diet of adequate calorie value is achieved.'[117]

Although environmental frailties cannot be ignored, neo-Malthusian approaches to poverty should only be cautiously accepted by historians. By denying individuals any understanding of their own poverty, or any agency over their own survival, neo-Malthusian approaches to hunger suffer some of the same shortcomings as dependency theory. Though reflective of external forces, Northern demography was also actively shaped by an entrenched understanding of the relationship between famine and family in unstable and highly variable savannah environments. Although death and disease were essentially unknowable, the survival of the family was known to rely on its ready modification in the face of constant threats; outmigration has to be fitted into this pragmatic pattern of household manipulation.

Labourers entering into mine work, for instance, commonly began their journeys in poor health, and some communities may have even sent men producing a net deficit in terms of household food production.[118] In the early 1920s, death from hunger or thirst on the long road to or from the South necessitated the establishment of refuges in Kumasi in 1929 and Tamale in 1933.[119] By 1942, the Labour Department had established 37 camps along the main migration routes.[120] Conditions at the end of the journey were not much better either. Poor nutrition, parasites, and pre-existing diseases meant that, in 1923, death rates among migrant miners from the Northern Territories were around four times as high as the benchmark set by miners in the South African Transvaal. Out of the 711 Northern labourers recruited between October 1923 and February 1924, there were 43 deaths, only 3 of which were due to accidents. Moreover, 317 of these men spent an average of 31 days each in the mine hospital.[121] For many, the march southwards was undertaken probably not because of the bright prospects at the end of the road, but because of the dire prospects at its start.

Although migration was generally voluntary, it was still structured within pre-existing, family-based systems of social security. In this sense, we should question Iliffe's speculation that 'the weak household, bereft of able-bodied male labour, has probably been the most common source of poverty throughout Africa's recoverable history'.[122] Elsewhere, outmigration has had a positive effect on familial survival. During Ireland's Great Famine, mass migration probably saved a great many lives by readjusting the ratio between food supply and population.[123] If it was women primarily left behind, the households they headed were not necessarily hungry either. In Zambia, cooperation in the distribution of food and labour across complex exchange networks made up for male absence in even decidedly poor households.[124] In another famous case study, Tiffen et al. show that outmigration from the densely populated Machakos area of eastern Kenya effectively mitigated the problems of soil desiccation and erosion. Located close to Nairobi, high levels of off-farm income could be readily earned in the burgeoning city and then invested in land improvements back home. Coinciding with high global coffee prices and low levels of taxation, productivity and living standards rapidly improved in the later colonial period.[125]

Positive interactions between migration and food security have historical precedents in West Africa too. As the historian Philip Curtin has explained, food insecurity led communities to actively address the limitations of their environments. The pastoral Fulani, for instance, adapted to the climatic instability of their original home, the middle valley of the Senegal River, to drift across sub-Sahelian West Africa, eventually assuming the position of cattle keepers for sedentary farmers – Curtin's main point being that nutrition is a 'mediating element in man's relationship with his environment'.[126] This is a relationship embedded in the culture of the savannah, where one Gonja proverb advises,

> The tortoise says that where there is food, there he turns his neck and goes (to eat).[127]

In fact, simply enabling migration may have provided citizens of the colonial North with a greater degree of agency over their own food security. According to Cardinall, 'several people, commenting on the famine early in 1919, said that had it not been for the White man's presence, which provided safety in travelling to more favoured parts, they would have had to sell their own offspring'.[128]

Neither climate nor ecology is particularly stable in the savannah – in fact, significant and largely unpredictable variations in rainfall are the norm.[129] In the same way that successful later-colonial famine relief systems relied upon early warnings regarding failed rains, facilitating outmigration worked to alleviate food insecurity by allowing a flexible and responsive means to modify household food security upon the recognition that a crop was likely to fail.[130] Of course, this is something which actual farmers are infinitely more able to deduce than any administrator. The first large-scale famine relief project, undertaken in 1931, proved to be a costly failure largely because of this. By the time that imported food relief reached Kumasi, much of it had spoiled and, by the time it reached the North, there was no famine in any case. Such accounts prove the difficulties encountered in monitoring food availability and funnelling relief into the Territories, as well as the ability of the Northern poor to quickly adapt to approaching shortfalls in production.[131] Hunger in the savannah was rarely consistent but was, instead, dependent on highly localised conditions which could vary significantly from year to year. In view of this, Purcell found a symbiosis in the seasonal pattern of migration which saw 'the men leave after harvest in December [and] return for the April sowing; which suits everybody'.[132]

As a considered response to the realities of distinct spatial and temporal pressures, migration was especially valuable for the heavily populated and perennially hungry Kassena-Nankani, Frafra, and Kusasi districts which, together with Builsa District, make up the 'hungry area' in the far north-east, which is occasionally and inaccurately referred to as North Mamprusi (see Figure 5.6). It was here that Purcell and other colonial officers focused their energies. Taking average consumption for a number of compounds in each area (10 in Zuarungu, for instance) over the course of between 7 and 10 days, Purcell's data show the degree to which basic consumption varied by locality, season, and household wealth (see Table 5.1).[133]

Hunger in Ghana's north-east is unique and its deep history is difficult to speak to. It seems likely that more viable communities operating under a tradition of shifting cultivation were sedentarised in the eighteenth or nineteenth century by warfare, slaving, disease, and, latterly, vying European empires.[134] As the recently 'fossilised' populations grew in size, fallow periods were shortened and eventually abandoned in some areas, with little compensatory improvement to farming practice. By the early 1900s, Cardinall noted that 'there is, comparatively speaking, very little uncultivated land, and that lies chiefly along the valleys of the larger rivers and is what is commonly called orchard bush'.[135] In this bush, 'everywhere one comes across ancient middens of which the origin is unknown and which are situated at a distance one from the other as are the dwelling places of the people today'.[136] Though the relationship between overpopulation and depopulation could not be entirely attributed to the colonial *causes célèbres* of trypanosomiasis or soil erosion, the cyclical nature of disease, death, and depopulation was recognised by the first concerted investigations undertaken during the early 1940s.[137] By 1944, it was concluded that 'extinction has already overtaken 8 villages within ten miles of Kwapong, 5 within the last decade'.[138]

It was not until the 1960s that a plausible cause was forwarded. In a landmark investigation, John Hunter explained that a history of endemic onchocerciasis had long made life untenable in the river valleys and that communities were instead forced to concentrate on non-infected watersheds (see Figures 5.7 and 5.8). Traversed by a dense network of seasonal streams and larger tributaries of the White Volta, the Gold Coast's north-east provided a great deal of fast-flowing water for blackfly vectors of onchocerciasis to breed in. However, on higher ground, less fertile land and high population densities preceded soil erosion and a general decline in food security. Riverside populations suffered and starved under the demands of endemic blindness until they were partially restored by new waves of settlement, pushed towards the river by the hunger forming on the watersheds. Hunter suggests that this cyclical process of advance (driven by famine) and retreat (driven by disease) had been evident in certain areas since at least the nineteenth century.[139]

Table 5.1 Average daily calorie intakes for compounds in communities across the Northern Territories, 1940–1.

Location	Date	Lowest compound average^	Highest compound average^	Average across compounds^	Yearly average across compounds^	Inequality ratio (1 = absolute equality)	Point on Figures 5.7 and 5.8*
Lawra	Oct-40	788	1,099	923	2,064	0.72	~
	Dec-40	2,222	4,180	2,831		0.53	
	Mar-41	1,704	2,940	2,431		0.58	
Sandema	Sep-40	1,235	4,567	1,908	1,787	0.27	1
	Dec-40	1,400	3,500	2,105		0.40	
	Feb-41	1,025	1,717	1,348		0.60	
Chaana+	Sep-40	519	1,990	930	1,532	0.26	2
	Dec-40	908	2,177	1,351		0.42	
	Feb-41	709	[Unreadable]				
Zuarungu	Jul-40	1,165	2,408	1,597	1,419	0.48	3
	Nov-40	1,198	2,059	1,572		0.58	
	Dec-40	866	1,768	1,388		0.49	
	Feb-41	805	1,498	1,118		0.54	
Tongo	Sep-40	1,225	2,065	1,677	1,408	0.59	4
	Dec-40	1,155	2,060	1,546		0.56	
	Feb-41	674	1,671	1,001		0.40	
Nangodi	Oct-40	965	2,124	1,388	1,385	0.45	5
	Feb-41	906	2,054	1,382		0.44	
Sekote	Dec-40	854	1,969	1,484	1,346	0.43	6
	Feb-41	820	1,623	1,207		0.51	
Kokgo	Oct-40	875	2,036	1,436	1,306	0.43	7
	Dec-40	630	1,680	1,155		0.38	
Navrongo	Aug-40	1,085	1,939	1,415	1,221	0.56	8
	Dec-40	1,050	2,100	1,399		0.50	
	Jan-41	475	1,210	850		0.39	
Nakon	Sep-40	690	1,616	999	808	0.43	9
	Dec-40	485	1,717	1,193		0.28	
	Feb-41	230	649	327		0.35	

^Averages are in terms of consumption units, which are weighted at 1.2 for adult men, 1 for adult women, 0.8 for male children, and 0.6 for female children.
*These points are only rough estimates based on the centre of the recorded survey location.
~Off map, in Upper West. See Figure 5.6.
+It is unlikely that the averages are fairly representative of Chaana, 'the families surveyed were very poor.'

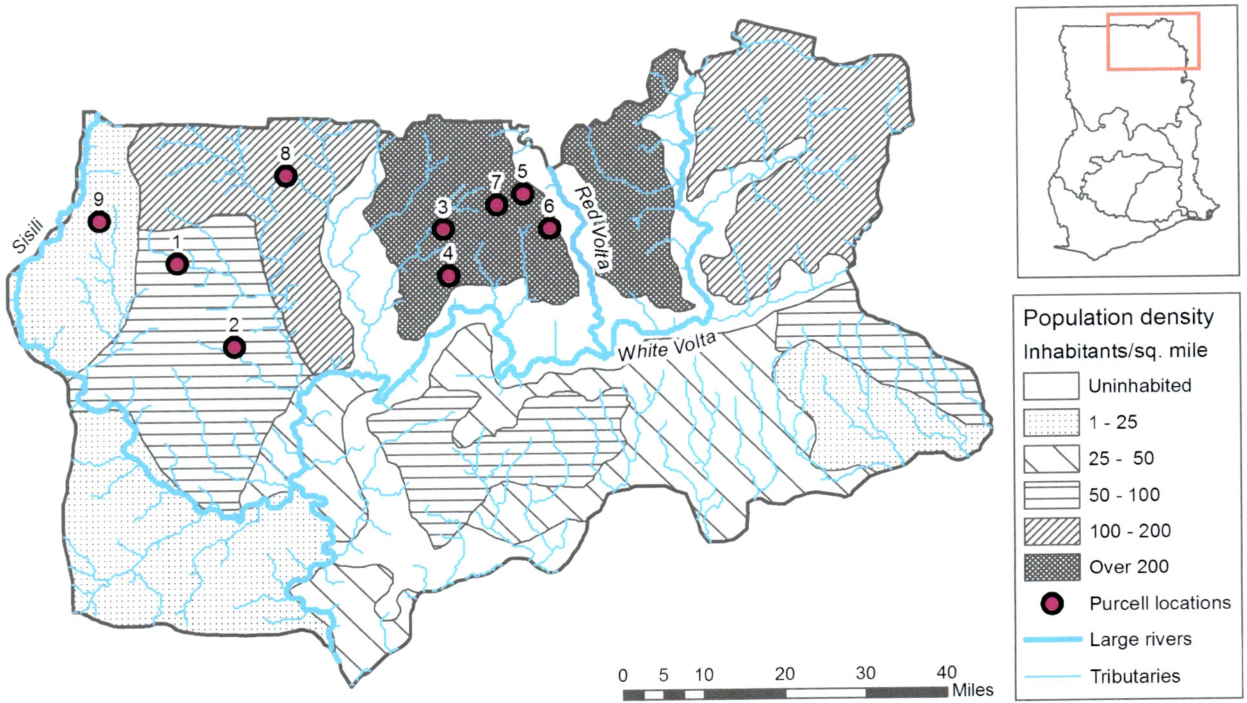

Figure 5.7 Watercourses and population distribution in north-eastern Ghana, 1960.[141]

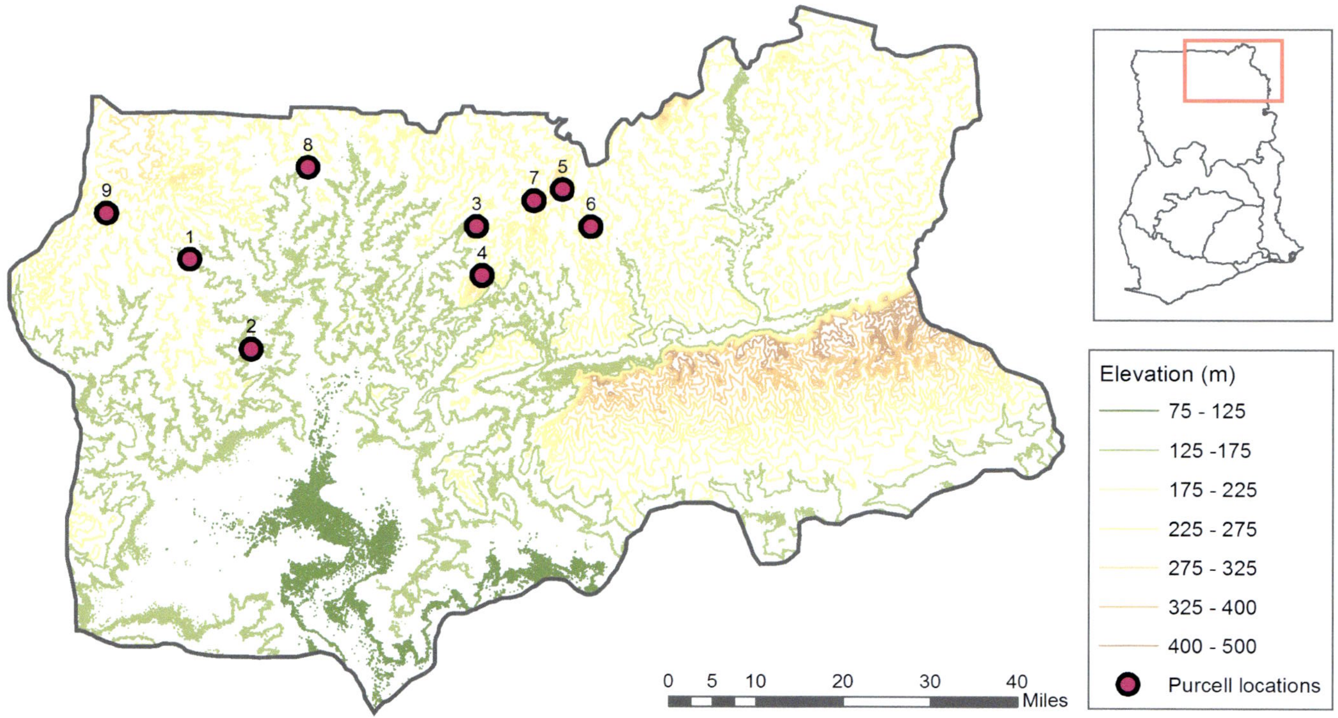

Figure 5.8 Topography of north-eastern Ghana.[142]

As a locus of disease and demographic intrigue, the focus of numerous important ethnographies, and a meeting point of the British and French empires, a cross-border economic history of this part of the West African savannah deserves to be written. What we do know about poverty and hunger here has been best described by Jérôme Destombes as a pattern of 'hungry watersheds' and 'famished valleys'.[143] Although we might question this simplistic topographical metaphor, poverty and food insecurity do seem to have followed the contours of savannah geography. The depopulation of the riverine and lowland areas most likely to harbour onchocerciasis and other waterborne disease vectors undoubtedly affected nutrition. Removed from the social insurances and more dynamic marketplaces of the more populous areas, and bearing the greatest disease burden, Purcell found Nakon (see marker no. 9 on Figures 5.7 and 5.8) to be especially hungry. Sitting in a broad, shallow valley alongside the Sisili River, Nakon presented, according to Purcell, 'several cases of extreme stunting' and an 'obvious correlation between the poor physique of the people and the prevalence of starvation'.[144] In the 1960s, one investigator estimated that child mortality in Nakon may have been around 50 per cent.[145]

In Nakon, Purcell found a community slowly dying. This was a process eminently more visible to those living around it and, as was the case with many aspects of ill-health, the geography of disease fitted into a socio-spiritual epistemology. In the same way that infanticide was born from communal understanding of infant viability, land made untenable by disease was readily recognised by those living alongside it. In 1940s Sekoti (marker no. 6), the agriculturalist C.W. Lynn was told that sickness, blindness, and 'bad fairies' causing the death of children were the primary reasons for leaving an area:

> The Chief and his followers asserted however, that the soil was excellent for farming, and only the presence of 'bad fairies' prevented the extensive farming which had obviously been followed there not many years before … Questioned more about the 'bad fairies' it was said that they did not interfere until a flourishing compound had been established with many children, then they came from the riverside and hum-bugged the people.[146]

In the village of Zorse, in Kusasi District, a late 1980s study found that a family head may still uproot their family on account of frequent sickness and on the advice of indigenous religious practitioners 'who may advise him that the place is not healthy for his family, that there are spirits who cannot be appeased'. However, strong attachments to ancestral land meant that migrations were not undertaken lightly. Most ultimately moved only short distances, 'within Kusaok [the Kusasi homeland], where a man may have maternal relatives'.[147]

Densely populated areas were communally and spiritually reinforced as islands of relative safety. On these watersheds, in places like Zuarungu (marker no. 3), hunger was less severe. Here, in contrast to Nakon, Purcell found that 'many who are in poor general condition show no specific signs of malnutrition; they are merely weak from hunger' (see Table 5.1 for the difference in consumption between Zuarungu and Nakon).[148] Although places like Zuarungu were affected by a seasonally deficient diet, they avoided the chronic deprivation caused by the riverine disease burden and the attendant deficit of labour. Instead, in Zuarungu, C.W. Lynn's 1931–2 investigation suggests that it was access to scant land which played the decisive role in determining the depth of hunger (see Table 5.2). Reduced population pressures facilitated investments in human and animal capital, helping also ensure food security. Indeed, further from the largest rivers and with more access to land, it was Lawra in the north-west, Sandema (marker no. 1), and Chaana (marker no. 2) which enjoyed the greatest average consumption (see Table 5.1). However, for congested compounds or for congested districts, the facilitation of outmigration provided an important and flexible means to relieve the pressures of overpopulation, especially in times of crisis.

By the 1960s, 38 per cent (or 22.6 square miles) of the Nangodi polity beside the Red Volta had been abandoned. Retreating since at least 1918, riverine settlements in areas particularly prone to onchocerciasis had shrunk by as much as 75 per cent between 1948 and 1960 alone.[149] Situated close to a major tributary of the Sisili River, similar patterns of environmental pressure and labour shortages in Tumu preceded 'a gradual exodus of the younger people', leaving 'those remaining [to] wage a gradually losing fight with what is aptly described as the "bush"'.[150] Such conclusions highlight the interaction between external influences and the natural environment, yet also stress the element of choice apparent in the Northern fight against poverty. The 'fight' with the bush was a decision informed by collective experience, as was the 'exodus' to the South. Where once the flight would be to the overburdened watershed, it was now mines and plantations which offered more attractive respite from want.

In the 1930s, Fortes put 'absenteeism' of Tallensi men at between 7 and 15 per cent, depending on the time of year.[151] Between the 1948 and

Table 5.2 Comparative statistics for compounds with and without food shortages, Zuarungu, 1931–2.[152]

	Means from 10 compounds with no food shortage	Means from 19 compounds short of food
Acres of farmed land per compound	8.16	5.66
Men farming	3.4	3.4
Acres farmed per man	2.4	1.6
Persons living in compound	14.7	11.5
Units of livestock (Fowl = 1 unit)	399	136
Persons per acre	1.8	2.03

1960 census, the population of the Tallensi homeland, the Frafra District, had actually declined, as 23 per cent of 'Frafras' were now accounted for elsewhere, the vast majority employed as 'general labour' on cocoa farms or gold mines.[153] Comparisons between Fortes' 1930s survey and Keith Hart's late 1960s one suggest that demographic and health pressures in the far north-east worked in conjunction with increasing external opportunities in order to promote outmigration. In Tongo, where the adult male population per compound averaged 2.6 men in 1934, by 1967 this had doubled to 6.0. However, of these six men, only half were working on farms at home. In an era of falling child mortality and swelling families, only outmigration mitigated what could have been calamitous demographic and environmental pressures.[154] Despite a continuing element of uncertainty, by the 1960s cash income from the South was important for hungry families and could bring in far more than local extra-subsistence earnings.[155] As in Machakos, such income may have played a role in the partial adoption of innovative, capital-dependent agricultural techniques promoted by colonial agricultural officers during the 1940s and 1950s. However, the deeply peripheral position of the Gold Coast's north-east precluded the investments afforded in Machakos, and developments were never really sustainable or productive.[156] Still, the expanded labour market broadened the 'opportunity structure' of even these poor and peripheral areas. Over the course of the colonial period, increased mobility, the growth of regional urban centres like Tamale and Bolgatanga, the reduced cost of transport, and the social security provided by *zongo* communities in Southern towns bolstered the viability and profitability of the migrant economy at home and in the urban world elsewhere. This allowed previously insular communities to expand and operate within and across regions, promoting the movement from short- to long-term migration.[157]

Of course, the viability and profitability of migration was not universal. It was, perhaps, not even the norm. In Kusasi, for instance, David Cleveland presents a particularly dismal view of long-term migration, where the colonial pursuit of proletarianisation undermined traditional demographic controls and perhaps heightened insecurity at home. No longer dependent upon lineage or land for bridewealth, outmigration may have preceded fertility increases and actively furthered population pressures.[158] The labour market was also notoriously unreliable throughout this period, and men from the Northern Territories were particularly liable to suffer destitution or death in Tamale or in the towns of the South.[159] Moreover, profits made away from home did not necessarily filter back to those left at home. In the 1930s, remittances from Tallensi migrants were rare and long-term migrants were sorely missed during the harvest.[160] Long-term economic migration was understandably 'a source of considerable concern to their elders', largely because it threatened the family-oriented social security which supported the dependent poor in particular.[161] By the mid-1950s, it was said that 'in Tamale and the North beggars beg for food and the problem there is one of poverty, lack of sufficient food during the months before the harvest is ripe, old age and sickness'.[162] North–south migration was also seen to accentuate the Northern disease burden, facilitating the spread of trypanosomiasis and, later, sexually transmitted disease. Throughout the Northern Territories, syphilis was known as the 'Kumasi Sickness'.[163]

Although southward migration shaped Northern fortunes throughout this period, the relative value of outmigration varied significantly between households. For instance, where migration relieved pressure on the supply of food in one household, in another the loss of labour undermined the basic tenets of food production. However, as the most important expression of economic agency available in the 'dependent' colonial economy, migration was approached with the same pragmatic flexibility that had long ensured Northern survival. Its uptake should be taken as proof of Hart's suggestion that, even in the furthest reaches of the Gold Coast, those opportunities that were offered by the colonial economy were readily recognised and regularly taken.[164] These were, on average, years in which nutritional status improved across the North. Heights increased for those born in the savannah as bargaining power grew for – and remittances grew from – Northern migrants working cocoa farms in the forest.[165] The opportunities offered by migration were only valuable as long as the opportunities remained viable.

In this respect, the benefits granted by market integration also obscure the structural vulnerabilities which came alongside it. In Machakos, Tiffen et al.'s story ended in 1989, just as the Kenyan economy began to contract; a 1999 restudy presented a dour picture of the following years, a period in which reduced off-farm income meant fewer people could afford the expensive agricultural inputs which had previously ensured productivity. Poor families continued to invest their labour in physical improvements to the land, such as terracing, but the consequent increase in productivity was not enough to match the increase in population. In 2000 drought hit Machakos, with some people ultimately succumbing to starvation.[166] We can, perhaps, trace a similar story through the history of Northern Ghana, where the erosion of demographic insurances during periods of economic growth preceded the return of hunger in later episodes of market contraction.

Perhaps more importantly, the use and value of outmigration was also responding to the quickly changing and spatially dependent demands of the globalising Gold Coast economy. Into the 1950s, migration began to drain areas less prone to endemic food insecurity, such as the far north-west or the sparcely populated areas, like Gonja and Dagomba areas a little further south. Here, migration was not simply dictated by survival but also by adventure and the desire for new forms of status and wealth.[167] Dagaaba migrants saw travel to 'Kumasi' as a way of seeing the world, acquiring status goods and perhaps also a wife on their return; one interviewee remarked that '"if you did not go to 'Kumasi,' the girls will not even mind you when you talk to them"'.[168] For some time, at least in the north-west, cash was only a minor motivator behind migration. In 1937, after counting the district's tax revenue, the commissioner of Lawra-Tumu was 'surprised to see that most of the takings were ... old coins, and a large proportion showing signs of having been buried.'[169] Into the later colonial period, however, the need for cash, to purchase bicycles or cloth, motivated more sojourns south. By 1952 it was

> generally accepted that the reasons why the men leave the North for work in the Colony and Ashanti are as follows: to make money to take home either as savings or as goods ... [and] because there is little to keep them in the North during the dry season when there is no farming to be done and food and water are short.[170]

The motivations behind migration were never static but changed according to various temporal and spatial demands.[171] At first, outmigration was rooted in structural, absolutist understandings of poverty, bound up in famine, endemic hunger, and Malthusian crisis. Later, migration was encouraged by new, relativist acknowledgements of poverty, driven by personal aspiration and formed from increasing interactions with both the South and West.

Social reproduction and gender conflict in the migrant economy

Changes to food security are only part of the story of nutrition during these years. As elsewhere, nutritional status was also partially defined by the construction of the family, by childrearing practices, and by gender roles, all things which changed significantly as young men moved south for work. Since migration was initially seasonal and short-term, and since urban employment discriminated against women, wives and children were usually left behind. The Gold Coast's censuses speak to the scale of migration. By 1931, adult sex ratios for the North showed 92 men for every 100 women, highlighting the gendered nature of outmigration and the increasingly gendered burdens of everyday social reproduction. Most of the missing men seem to have been absorbed by the Colony and especially by Asante, where, in 1931, there were 112 men for each 100 women. By 1960, the figures for the North were even starker, with only 86 adult men recorded for every 100 women.[172] With a growing dearth of male labour, Northern subsistence was increasingly reliant on the labours of women forced into riskier modes of social reproduction.[173] Of course, women were never the passive victims of colonisation but, as in Asante (see Chapter 4), worked to actively ensure their security against the gendered hardships of the migrant economy.

Son preference and gender inequality was deeply entrenched in Northern communities. As we have already seen (see Figure 5.3), gender disparities in education were especially obvious in the North and similar patterns were also seen in health-seeking. In 1953, only 36 per cent of inpatients in the Northern Territories were women. For the same year, women in Asante made up 49 per cent of inpatients.[174] Gendered patterns of consumption also led to gendered nutritional indicators. Purcell, for instance, found that 'any and every kind of animal flesh may be eaten but most is usually consumed by male adults as part of a sacrificial rite'.[175] Richards found similar dietary patterns in Northern Rhodesia during the 1930s.[176] Much higher rates of adult female malnutrition were also found around this time in the Gold Coast's cocoa belt, but with little evidence for gender disparities in infancy.[177] Still, in comparison to men in Purcell's respective samples, women in the North were markedly shorter and lighter than their neighbours in the forest.[178] In Nangodi, during Hunter's 1963–4 survey, women suffered a greater degree of seasonal weight loss than men.[179] During one postcolonial food shortage, girls in hungry Upper Region villages presented with significantly lower BMIs than the men, boys, and adult women surveyed (see Table 6.3).[180] Elsewhere, such as during Nyasaland's 1949 famine, greater levels of female mortality have been explained in terms of lost direct entitlements to food from gardens and dwindling indirect entitlements, such as beer brewing, due to lack of demand.[181] Although the gendered nature of household labour requirements, food allocation, and health-seeking goes some way to explain anthropometric disparities, failures of entitlement better explain a mechanism of gendered neglect.

In the Northern Territories, female entitlement was probably lowest during the decade or so spent away from the constant care of mothers or grandmothers and before the relative safety of marriage, when, in the traditional economy, women's value was more readily recognised. In the patrilocal North, unlike in Asante, boys had traditionally contributed more to the food security and long-term maintenance of the family. The value of female children was, conversely, relatively short-lived. Before marriage, girls were a useful source of household labour but, after marriage, new wives would generally move into their husband's compound. Brideprice, usually in the form of cattle, went some way to make up for the family's loss of labour. However, at least in the 1930s, such livestock 'will as likely as not be used immediately to pay a debt or, more rarely, to make a special and urgent sacrifice'.[182] Even if they were not sold immediately, for many people livestock numbers would dwindle away over time, 'during the three or four hungry months, from April until June [when] the farmer is obliged to sell some, or all of his modest reserve of livestock … in order to buy essential food'.[183] On the other hand, resident, adult kin actively worked to avert such crises.[184]

In the marginal savannah environment, family structures were actively shaped by entitlements. As Fortes explained of the Tallensi, 'while taking a bride may be an affair of individuals, making a valid marriage is a cooperative concern'.[185] The family orientation of savannah food security left 'the head of the unit of food economy' heavily involved in each brideprice transaction of his dependent kin.[186] Marital food security worked the other way too, and a 'shortage of food' or a failure to support one's wife was considered a 'genuine grievance' and good grounds for a Tallensi woman to abandon her husband.[187] Food, and especially supplementary, famine foods were central to the making of a marriage. 'In congested Mamprusi', where groundnuts were

> the principal famine season food … every man seems to have a groundnut patch, and every woman has one also. The husband makes it for her; and is the first big thing a young man does for his betrothed. The crop belongs solely to the woman, to dispose of how she chooses.[188]

With the status and relative autonomy afforded by marriage, and more so by motherhood, rural women played a central role in extra-subsistence production and, by extension, food security. According to Purcell, women's supplementary income (pito brewing, shea butter manufacture, weaving, or the sale of firewood) 'may earn enough money to buy essential food in times of scarcity'.[189]

Women's position as the arbiters of valuable human capital afforded them a greater degree of autonomy outside of their parents' compound. Indeed, women's agency within conjugal relationships was common across the Northern Territories but fairly alien to the European administration:

> Many of these women, having tasted emancipation, are not satisfied until they have tried as many as ten husbands. It is not the white man who has brought this about. Such has been the practice for long past. It led to murder and war and raids; today it leads to disputes and complaints beyond number, and incidentally at times to a half-crazy commissioner.[190]

During the colonial period, this degree of autonomy was taken by the state to be a threat to the supply of Northern labour. As male outmigration undermined the tenability of the traditional unions based upon mutual assistance, 'wives' were said to have often abandoned their absentee 'husbands'. As Sean Hawkins has explained with reference to court documents discussing marriages in Lawra District, colonial legislation intervened, 'ensuring that women's freedom did not discourage men from "volunteering" for labour recruitment'. Instead, administrators and chiefs redefined marriage and adultery in order to bind women to absent partners.[191] Together with the widespread loss of male labour, growing restrictions on female autonomy had the potential to undermine the nutritional status of dependent children by curtailing previously legitimate forms of food security based on family augmentation and socially reinforced conjugal responsibility. Colonial legislation rescinded these freedoms, leaving women increasingly reliant on spouses who, due to the vagaries of waged employment, were becoming increasingly unreliable.

Although the growth of the migrant economy placed greater demands at the feet of rural women across the North, women were not passive victims of process but provided security for themselves and their children by moving into the space created by colonial reforms. By the 1960s, extra-subsistence trading could be more profitable than, for instance, the local sale of a man's labour. According to Hunter, 'women in possession of a few shillings may buy grain in a distant market, walking many miles in the process, sell it locally, and measure their profit in terms of a calabash (bowl) or so of grain. Wealthier "capitalists" (always women) deal on a bigger scale and make bigger profits.'[192] Women in possession of particular skills or any degree of capital generally lost less weight, or even gained weight, during the lean season.[193] Although courts were ostensibly created by and for male ends, women were increasingly ready to challenge their husbands through these new organs.[194] Others utilised the freedoms and discrepancies left between Christianity and indigenous gender roles, while others still took advantage of the sparse opportunities offered by education.[195]

In general, and as was the case in Asante, colonisation tested the limits of traditional modes of social reproduction and brought about a degree of gender conflict.[196] For instance, following something of an epidemic of 'witchcraft' in Asante, in 1955 the Dagomba experienced an outbreak of 'witch finding' associated with the 'Nana' healing cult.[197] During the Nana witch hunt, younger women levelled accusations against older, wealthier women, referring 'either to the killing of young men or to their being driven away to the coast'.[198] In the past, few Dagomba had left to work in the South, a procession dominated by peoples from further north, 'but now the genealogies record a high percentage ... as "Gone to the Coast"; that is, their locations are not precisely known, in sharp contrast with the contact kept as a rule by Dagomba.'[199] Since the witches were 'women of the households least dependent on the year's crops', the Nana witch hunt may be understood as a generational conflict born from apprehensions over outmigration, the Gold Coast's looming independence, and food security in a changing world:

> The elderly widows are an economic burden on young men who are usually not their own but their brother's sons. Further, elderly wives in large households do not always take much share in the

> heavy work of the household but instead organize the young women who do it ... At a time of year when there is great anxiety about crops and about rain (that is, fear of the future in a subsistence economy), these tensions, it is suggested, found release.[200]

Allegations of witchcraft had long been a gendered form of control. In Gonja, for instance, the characterisation of female witches as evil and male witches as benevolent reflects a pattern of gender relations arranged to deny female freedoms.[201] In Mamprusi, during the early 1990s, a spate of witchcraft allegations have been associated with strained gender relations in a time of increased reliance on cash income. As women increased the range and diversity of their trading, 'the fear of witchcraft has grown as men's dependence on women has increased, and the increasing autonomy of women threatens both men's control of women and the control by senior women of their juniors'.[202] Although the Dagomba witch hunt originated in the anxieties of young women rather than men, it stemmed from similar concerns, from a loss of power or a loss of agency, and from doubts over survival in a changing landscape.

'The real issue,' Megan Vaughan suggests of colonial Africa at large, 'was that with far-reaching changes taking place in economic relations, so enormous strains were placed on both gender and generational relations ... these complex changes were described in terms of degeneration.' Whereas colonial observers saw degeneration in terms of 'uncontrolled sexuality and disease', dependency theorists later recognised migration as 'an element in unequal development, reproducing the same conditions and contributing in this manner to their aggravation'.[203] What took longer to realise, however, was that this peripheral decline was felt most acutely by women and their dependants, left in the midst of a 'reconfigured patriarchy rooted in both indigenous and colonial ideologies'.[204] The colonial period was a time when traditional modes of production and reproduction were refigured by new avenues for capital accumulation and new demands upon the household economy. Colonial legislation and the growth of the market presided over a to-and-fro between the expansion and restriction of female power. Generally, though, demographic shifts under colonial governance burdened women with dual responsibilities over farm and family, undermining both food production and the domestic economy of childrearing. The increasingly difficult lived experiences of young mothers soured the prospect of Northern life for their sisters and daughters, setting the scene for the feminisation of migration and a greater rejection of traditional domesticity throughout Ghana's North (see also Chapters 6 and 8).[205]

With few health workers and sparse reportage, assumptions regarding Northern nutrition were reliant on Purcell's observations that 'gross stigmata of malnutrition in early years … are exceptional, and obvious signs of present illnourishment such as wasting or oedema are rare'.[206] Within a decade, such conclusions were either outdated or built on incomplete understandings of a diverse and diversifying food environment. When a child welfare clinic was finally established in Tamale in the 1950s, it was soon 'overwhelmed' with cases. The sole paediatrician, C.O. Moody, found that 'our ideas on the prevalence of protein deficiencies in children are being revised, we came across many more cases of acute and chronic deficiencies than we had expected to find'.[207] With increasing demands on maternal time and energy, the gendered strains of colonial capitalism were starting to affect nutrition in the savannah, just as in Asante, and probably by much the same mechanism.

Yet in Asante and elsewhere in the South, indigenous capitalism, diversified production, and a politically significant civil society promoted investments in human capital. By nature of its peripheral orientation, the North, on the other hand, was denied political purchase and similar advances in health and education. Even in the Gold Coast's far north-east, where a proneness to Malthusian crises coincided with a uniquely difficult disease environment, the administration recognised that an 'adult and infant mortality rate unchecked by any medical or sanitary improvements has reduced the population below the level at which the farming system based on shifting cultivation can be worked'.[208] At the same time, the social and demographic insurances provided by the relatively insular economic environment of the precolonial nineteenth century were broken down by free market doctrines which promoted new forms of food insecurity, the worst effects of which were, however, partially allayed by colonial relief. Although bounded by the old restraints of a hostile savannah and the new structural impositions of a coercive colonial market, food insecurity was never passively accepted. Granular spatial variations in the volatile nutrition environment have long afforded migration a central place in the mitigation of hunger across the savannah. Denied purchase in other parts of the economy, the colony-wide labour market offered a degree of economic dynamism and afforded an important space in which the Northern poor could exert agency over their own survival. With access to the labour market constrained by age, gender, and ability, the burdens of savannah existence shifted largely onto the women left behind, and insecurity grew among the dependent poor reliant on cross-generational assistance. As was the pattern elsewhere in the Gold Coast, the slow ascendency of cash and capitalism preceded new forms of nutrition insecurity derived as much from the pervasive devaluation of domestic reproduction as from the enduring struggle for food.

Notes

1 Quoted in Paul André Ladouceur, *Chiefs and Politicians: The Politics of Regionalism in Northern Ghana* (London: Longman, 1979), p. 45.
2 Dependency theory analyses of Gold Coast history can be found in Piet Konings, *The State and Rural Class Formation in Ghana: A Comparative Analysis* (London: KPI, 1986); Nii-K. Plange, 'Underdevelopment in Northern Ghana: Natural Causes or Colonial Capitalism?', *Review of African Political Economy*, 15/16 (1979), 4–14; Rhoda E. Howard, *Colonialism and Underdevelopment in Ghana* (London: Croom Helm, 1978).
3 Two classic texts regarding underdevelopment and economic dependency are: André Gunder Frank, *Capitalism and Underdevelopment in Latin America: Historical Studies of Chile and Brazil* (London: Monthly Review, 1967); Amin, *Unequal Development*.
4 Samir Amin, 'Underdevelopment and Dependence in Black Africa – Origins and Contemporary Forms', *The Journal of Modern African Studies*, 10.4 (1972), 503–24 (p. 523).
5 Samir Amin, 'Introduction', in *Modern Migrations in Western Africa*, ed. by Samir Amin (Oxford: Oxford University Press, 1974), pp. 65–151.
6 Jean-François Bayart, *The State in Africa: The Politics of the Belly* (London: Longman, 1993), pp. 2–10.
7 Caldwell, 'Routes'.
8 Caldwell, 'Routes', pp. 173–8. See also John C. Caldwell, 'Education as a Factor in Mortality Decline: An Examination of Nigerian Data', *Population Studies*, 33.3 (1979), 395–413.
9 Caldwell, 'Routes', pp. 182–94.
10 The cultural shortfalls of colonised health and social care have been touched on, with regard to nutrition, in Chapter 1. The best general analysis of these issues is still Vaughan, *Curing Their Ills*.
11 P.A. Twumasi, 'Colonialism and International Health: A Study in Social Change in Ghana', *Social Science & Medicine. Medical Anthropology*, 15B.2 (1981), 147–51 (p. 147).
12 Colbourne et al., 'Medical Survey', p. 289; see also John M. Janzen, *The Quest for Therapy in Lower Zaire* (Berkeley, CA: University of California Press, 1978).
13 K. David Patterson, *Health in Colonial Ghana: Disease, Medicine, and Socio-Economic Change, 1900–1955* (Waltham, MA: Crossroads Press, 1981), p. 77.
14 PRAAD/A/CSO/11/1/355, Deaths following injections, 1934; PRAAD/A/CSO/11/19/12, Anti-trypanosomiasis injections – deaths at Navrongo following 1936–8, PRAAD/A/CSO/11/16/79, Anti-trypanosomiasis injections – deaths following, 1942.
15 Patterson, *Health*, p. 27.
16 B. Bierlich, 'Injections and the Fear of Death: An Essay on the Limits of Biomedicine among the Dagomba of Northern Ghana', *Social Science & Medicine*, 50.5 (2000), 703–13 (p. 707).
17 Caldwell, 'Routes', p. 178.
18 Addae, *Evolution of Modern Medicine*, p. 22.
19 Twumasi, 'Colonialism', p. 147; Addae, *Evolution of Modern Medicine*, p. 29.
20 Twumasi, 'Colonialism', p. 147.
21 Brown, 'Increased Intercommunication', pp. 186–7.
22 Quoted in Addae, *Evolution of Modern Medicine*, p. 72.
23 *MDAR*, 1929/30; based on Moradi, Austin, and Baten, *Heights and Development*, pp. 40–1.
24 This has become an enduring problem in Ghanaian medical education. See John Nott, 'Material History, Historied Materials and the Question of Epistemic Freedom in Ghana's Medical Schools', *Social History of Medicine*, 37.1 (2023), pp. 116–40.
25 Gold Coast Government, *Report of the Commission of Enquiry into the Health Needs of the Gold Coast*, pp. 5, 31.

26 PRAAD/A/CSO/11/6/10, IWC Tamale, 1932, Acting Colonial Secretary, Accra, to Acting Chief Commissioner, Northern Territories, Tamale, 22/11/1932.
27 *MDAR*, 1955, p. 49.
28 *MDAR*, 1954, p. 83.
29 *MDAR*, 1954, p. 143.
30 R. Bagulo Bening, 'The Evolution of the Administrative Boundaries of Northern Ghana, 1898–1965' (unpublished PhD, University of London, 1971), p. 115.
31 Jeff D. Grischow, *Globalisation, Development and Disease in Colonial Northern Ghana, 1906–1960*, WOPAG – Working Paper on Ghana: Historical and Contemporary Studies (Helsinki: Institute of Asian and African Studies, University of Helsinki, 2006), pp. 1–31.
32 David Scott, *Epidemic Disease in Ghana 1901–1960* (London: Oxford University Press, 1965), pp. 103–10.
33 B.B. Waddy, 'Organization and Work of the Gold Coast Medical Field Units', *Transactions of the Royal Society of Tropical Medicine and Hygiene*, 50.4 (1956), 313–43 (pp. 328–31).
34 M.H. Hughes and P.F. Daly, 'Onchocerciasis in the Southern Gold Coast', *Transactions of the Royal Society of Tropical Medicine and Hygiene*, 45.2 (1951), 243–52 (pp. 251–2). On the history of onchocerciasis in Ghana, see K. David Patterson, 'River Blindness in Northern Ghana', in *Disease in African History: An Introductory Survey and Case Studies*, ed. by K. David Patterson and Gerald W. Hartwig (Durham, NC: Duke University Press, 1978), pp. 88–117 (p. 88); David Bannister, 'The Sorcerer's Apprentice: Sleeping Sickness, Onchocerciasis, and Unintended Consequences in Ghana, 1930–60', *The Journal of African History*, 62.1 (2021), pp. 29–57.
35 Patterson, 'River Blindness', pp. 109–10.
36 Patterson, *Health*, p. 101.
37 B.B. Waddy, 'A District Medical Officer in North-West Ghana', in *Health in Tropical Africa During the Colonial Period*, ed. by E.E. Sabben-Clarke, D.J. Bradley, and K. Kirkwood (Oxford: Clarendon Press, 1980), pp. 159–65 (p. 159).
38 PRAAD/A/ADM/11/1/1294, Purcell, 'Report', pp. 12, 112.
39 Gold Coast Government, *1948 Census*.
40 Compare *MDAR*, 1948, p. 16, with Waddy, 'Heights'.
41 Brown, 'Increased Intercommunication'; Komla Tsey and Stephanie D. Short, 'From Headloading to the Iron Horse: The Unequal Health Consequences of Railway Construction and Expansion in the Gold Coast, 1898–1929', *Social Science & Medicine*, 40.5 (1995), 613–21.
42 K. David Patterson, 'The Influenza Epidemic of 1918–19 in the Gold Coast', *Journal of African History*, 24.4 (1983), 485–502 (p. 492).
43 Patterson, 'Influenza', p. 499.
44 Patterson, 'Influenza', p. 502.
45 Sean Hawkins, 'To Pray or Not To Pray: Politics, Medicine, and Conversion among the LoDagaa of Northern Ghana, 1929–1939', *Canadian Journal of African Studies*, 31.1 (1997), 50–85.
46 Waddy, 'North-West', p. 180; Patterson, *Health*, p. 4.
47 Sam Rhodie, 'The Gold Coast Cocoa Hold-Up of 1930–31', *Transactions of the Historical Society of Ghana*, 9 (1968), 105–18; Alence, '1937–1938'.
48 Mahmood Mamdani, *Citizen and Subject: Contemporary Africa and the Legacy of Late Colonialism* (Princeton, NJ: Princeton University Press, 1996), pp. 22, 286–7.
49 Jeff D. Grischow, 'Corruptions of Development in the Countryside of the Northern Territories of the Gold Coast, 1927–57', *The Journal of Peasant Studies*, 26.1 (1998), 139–58 (p. 155).
50 Grischow, 'Corruptions', pp. 150–3. Describing 'Frafras' as one group is a misnomer; the term actually embraces three or four distinct socio-linguistic groups – Gurenshi (including Bosi), Nabdams, and Tallensi – see Fortes, *Dynamics*; Meyer Fortes, *The Web of Kinship among the Tallensi: The Second Part of an Analysis of the Social Structure of a Trans-Volta Tribe* (Oxford: Oxford University Press, 1949).
51 Frederick Gordon Guggisberg, *The Gold Coast: A Review of the Events of 1920–1926 and the Prospects of 1927–1928* (Accra: Government Printer, 1927), pp. 23–4; this is the main argument made by Grischow, most extensively in Jeff D. Grischow, *Shaping Tradition: Civil Society, Community and Development in Colonial Northern Ghana, 1899–1957* (Leiden: Brill, 2006).

52 The history of nationalism and emancipatory politics in the Southern Gold Coast can be found in Allman, *Quills of the Porcupine*; Richard Rathbone, *Nkrumah and the Chiefs: The Politics of Chieftaincy in Ghana, 1951–1960* (Oxford: James Currey, 1999); for the early history of education, see Philip Foster, *Education and Social Change in Ghana* (London: Routledge & Kegan Paul, 1965).
53 Quoted in R. Bagulo Bening, *A History of Education in Northern Ghana, 1907–1976* (Accra: Ghana Universities Press, 1990), pp. 8–9.
54 Bening, 'Evolution', p. 228.
55 Quoted in Bening, *Education*, p. 51.
56 Bening, 'Evolution', pp. 232–3.
57 District Commissioner of Wa, 1922, quoted in Bening, *Education*, p. 49.
58 Bening, 'Evolution', p. 233.
59 Jack Lord, 'Child Labor in the Gold Coast: The Economics of Work, Education, and the Family in Late-Colonial African Childhoods, c. 1940–57', *The Journal of the History of Childhood and Youth*, 4.1 (2011), 88–115 (p. 104).
60 John C. Caldwell, 'Fertility Attitudes in Three Economically Contrasting Rural Regions of Ghana', *Economic Development and Cultural Change*, 15.2 (1967), 217–38 (p. 227).
61 Ghana Government, *1960 Census*.
62 Ghana Government, *1960 Census*.
63 RH/MSS.Afr.S.2003, Fox, 'Memoirs'.
64 PRAAD/Tamale (T)/NRG/8/9/58, Mass Education General, 1964–1975, Report entitled 'Mass Literacy Campaign in Ghana: A Detailed Plan of Action', by Ministry of Social Welfare, 1965. See also Hawkins, *Writing*; Jack Goody, 'Rice–Burning and the Green Revolution in Northern Ghana', *The Journal of Development Studies*, 16.2 (1980), 136–55.
65 Northern Territories Council member J.A. Braimah, 1951. Quoted in Ladouceur, *Chiefs and Politicians*, p. 94.
66 PRAAD/A/ADM/5/3/99, Report of the Select Committee on Federal System of Government and Second Chamber for the Gold Coast, 1955. This is, of course, overly simplistic. See, for instance, Carola Lentz, '"The Time When Politics Came": Ghana's Decolonisation From the Perspective of a Rural Periphery', *Journal of Contemporary African Studies*, 20.2 (2002), 245–74.
67 Moradi, 'Confronting Colonial Legacies', pp. 1113–15; Moradi, Austin, and Baten, *Heights and Development*, p. 23.
68 Gold Coast Government, *Gold Coast Nutrition and Cookery*.
69 Gold Coast Government, *Education Department Annual Report* [*EDAR*], 1934 (Accra: Government Printer, 1935) 1934; *EDAR*, 1954.
70 *MDAR*, 1929; *MDAR*, 1955.
71 C.E. Callwell, *Small Wars: Their Principles and Practice* (London: HMSO, 1896), p. 40.
72 Iliffe, *Famine in Zimbabwe*, pp. 23–4.
73 Keen, *Benefits of Famine*, pp. 28–9; de Waal, *Famine Crimes*, p. 27.
74 Holger Weiss, 'Crop Failures, Food Shortages and Colonial Famine Relief Policies in the Northern Territories of the Gold Coast', *Ghana Studies*, 6 (2003), 5–58 (p. 22).
75 Caroline Elkins, *Britain's Gulag: The Brutal End of Empire in Kenya* (London: Jonathan Cape, 2005), pp. 259–62.
76 Keen, *Benefits of Famine*; de Waal, *Famine Crimes*.
77 For a thorough history of colonial famine relief, see Weiss, 'Crop Failures', pp. 40–8.
78 Weiss, 'Crop Failures', pp. 48–54.
79 TNA/CO/859/115/3, Gold Coast: extracts from informal colonial medical reports, development plans and other papers [pertaining to nutrition], 1944–6. G.H. Gibbs, Chief Commissioner N.T.s, to the Colonial Secretary, 2/2/1944.
80 TNA/CO/859/115/3, Gold Coast: extracts from informal colonial medical reports, development plans and other papers [pertaining to nutrition], 1944–6. S. Culwick, 'Note on discussion with Sir Alan Burns held on 15.5.1944', 16/5/1944. Palm oil was used to combat an apparently widespread deficiency of vitamin A. See *MDAR*, 1931–2, p. 33; *MDAR*, 1940, p. 1.
81 For Ireland, see Cormac Ó Gráda, *Black '47 and Beyond: The Great Irish Famine in History, Economy, and Memory* (Princeton, NJ: Princeton University Press, 1998). For India, see Mike Davis, *Late Victorian Holocausts: El Niño Famines and the Making of the Third World* (London: Verso, 2002), pp. 28–33.

82 PRAAD/A/ADM/11/1/1294, Purcell, 'Report', p. 47.
83 PRAAD/A/ADM/11/1/1294, Purcell, 'Report', p. 47.
84 PRAAD/A/ADM/11/1/1294, Purcell, 'Report', p. 57.
85 H.P. White, 'Internal Exchange of Staple Foods in the Gold Coast', *Economic Geography*, 32.2 (1956), 115–25 (p. 118).
86 Weiss, 'Crop Failures', pp. 10–11.
87 Gold Coast Government, *1931 Census*.
88 Ghana Government, *1960 Census*.
89 Ghana Government, *1960 Census*.
90 NRG/8/2/209, Cattle in Frafra, 1950, Report by Assistant District Commissioner N.O. Dobbs, 'Cattle in Frafra', 11 November 1950, p. 6.
91 PRAAD/A/ADM/11/1/1294, Purcell, 'Report', p. 21.
92 PRAAD/T/NRG/18/8/1, Diet and nutrition (1930–57), Acting Assistant Director of Agriculture, NTs, to Assistant Director of Medical Services, NTs, 'Standards of Nutrition in Farafara [sic.]', 15 April 1952.
93 Keith Hart, 'Migrations and the Opportunity Structure: A Ghanaian Case Study', in *Modern Migrations in Western Africa*, ed. by Samir Amin (Oxford: Oxford University Press, 1974), pp. 321–39 (p. 334).
94 See, for instance, PRAAD/T/NRG/18/1/5, Monthly Food Production Reports, 1952–7.
95 PRAAD/T/NRG/8/11/66, Food Production Drive [Urban Allotments] Including Food Shortages, 1958–62, S. La-Anyane, 'Report on Food Shortage in Northern Ghana', 25/8/1958.
96 Andrew Shepherd, 'Agrarian Change in Northern Ghana: Public Investment, Capitalist Farming and Famine', in *Rural Development in Tropical Africa*, ed. by Judith Heyer, Pepe Roberts, and Gavin Williams (London: Palgrave Macmillan, 1981), pp. 168–92 (p. 185).
97 Sen, *Poverty*, pp. 86–112.
98 Quoted in Bening, 'Evolution', p. 142.
99 Quoted in Bening, 'Evolution', p. 142.
100 Quoted in Bening, 'Evolution', pp. 222–3.
101 Ghana Government, *1960 Census*. See also John C. Caldwell, *African Rural-Urban Migration: The Movement to Ghana's Towns* (Canberra: Australian National University Press, 1969); Enid Schildkrout, *People of the Zongo: The Transformation of Ethnic Identities in Ghana* (Cambridge: Cambridge University Press, 1978).
102 Crisp, *Story of an African Working Class*; Roger G. Thomas, 'Forced Labour in British West Africa: The Case of the Northern Territories of the Gold Coast 1906–1927', *Journal of African History*, 14.1 (1973), 79–103.
103 Hill, *Migrant*.
104 Thomas, 'Forced Labour', pp. 98–9.
105 Minutes of interview between Guggisberg and the Secretary for Mines, 1920, quoted in Thomas, 'Forced Labour', p. 93.
106 Peter R. Gould, *The Development of the Transportation Pattern in Ghana* (Evanston, IL: Department of Geography, Northwestern University, 1960), p. 48.
107 For the history of indirect rule in the Northern Territories, see Grischow, *Shaping Tradition*.
108 Inez Sutton, 'Colonial Agricultural Policy: The Non-Development of the Northern Territories of the Gold Coast', *The International Journal of African Historical Studies*, 22.4 (1989), 637–69 (p. 638).
109 Hawkins, *Writing*, pp. 83–86, 117. It should be noted that a more productive form of local capitalism may not necessarily have been a better outcome for the majority of Northerners. Guggisberg's wagons full of groundnuts, if grown in coordination with a local elite, as in northern Nigeria, may have ultimately contributed to a similarly parasitic form of capitalism which only exacerbated the economic fragility of the savannah economy. See Robert W. Shenton, *The Development of Capitalism in Northern Nigeria* (Toronto: University of Toronto Press, 1986).
110 Waddy, 'Organization', pp. 332–3.
111 Waddy, 'North-West', p. 164.
112 Breschi and Livi Bacci, 'Month of Birth', pp. 161–2.
113 D.R. Brewster and B.M. Greenwood, 'Seasonal Variation of Paediatric Diseases in The Gambia, West Africa', *Annals of Tropical Paediatrics*, 13.2 (1993), 133–46.
114 PRAAD/A/ADM/11/1/1294, Purcell, 'Report', p. 13.

115 John M. Hunter, 'Seasonal Hunger in a Part of the West African Savanna: A Survey of Bodyweights in Nangodi, North-East Ghana', *Transactions of the Institute of British Geographers*, 41 (1967), 167–85.
116 Compare, for instance, PRAAD/T/NRG/8/3/204, Economic Surveys and Reports, 1955–60, D. Masters, 'Structure of the Economy of Tali and Woreboggo in Western Dagomba', c.1955, with PRAAD/T/NRG/8/3/204, Economic Surveys and Reports, 1955–60, D. Masters, 'Janasia (Navrongo) and Zuarensa (Sandema) in the Navrongo District', c.1955.
117 C.O. Moody, 'Malnutrition in Children under Five Years of Age in the Dagomba Villages of Northern Ghana', *The Journal of the Royal Institute of Public Health and Hygiene*, 26 (1963), 224–41 (p. 225).
118 Thomas, 'Forced Labour', pp. 100–2.
119 *MDAR*, 1929–30; 1933–4.
120 'Labour Problems of the Gold Coast Are Being Faced', *West African Review*, December 1942, 18.
121 Thomas, 'Forced Labour', pp. 100–2. See also Raymond Dumett, 'Disease and Mortality among Gold Miners of Ghana: Colonial Government and Mining Company Attitudes and Policies, 1900–1938', *Social Science & Medicine*, 37.2 (1993), 213–32.
122 Iliffe, *African Poor*, p. 7; Richards, *Land, Labour*.
123 Cormac Ó Gráda and Kevin H. O'Rourke, 'Migration as Disaster Relief: Lessons from the Great Irish Famine', *European Review of Economic History*, 1.1 (1997), 3–25.
124 Moore and Vaughan, *Cutting down Trees*.
125 Mary Tiffen, Michael Mortimore, and Francis Gichuki, *More People, Less Erosion: Environmental Recovery in Kenya* (Chichester: Wiley, 1994).
126 Philip D. Curtin, 'Nutrition in African History', in *Hunger and History: The Impact of Changing Food Production and Consumption Patterns on Society*, ed. by Robert I. Rotberg and Theodore K. Rabb (Cambridge: Cambridge University Press, 1985), pp. 173–84.
127 Kponkpogori, Natomah, and Rytz, *Gonja Proverbs*, p. 41.
128 Cardinall, *Northern Territories*, p. 74.
129 Weiss, 'Crop Failures', pp. 15–19.
130 Weiss, 'Crop Failures', pp. 48–54.
131 PRAAD/A/CSO/8/1/12, 'Food supplies in the Northern Territories, 1930–1'.
132 PRAAD/A/ADM/11/1/1294, Purcell, 'Report', p. 27.
133 For a much more thorough analysis of this data, see Jérôme Destombes, 'Nutrition and Chronic Deprivation in the West African Savanna: North-Eastern Ghana, c. 1930–2000' (unpublished PhD, London School of Economics, 2001).
134 Allan, *African Husbandman*, p. 246.
135 Cardinall, *Northern Territories*, p. 1.
136 Cardinall, *Northern Territories*, p. 2.
137 PRAAD/T/NRG/18/8/1, Diet and nutrition (1930–57), Report by C.W. Lynn, Senior Agricultural Superintendent, Department of Agriculture, 'Depopulation of Riverine areas in North Mamprusi: Report on a visit to Sekoti, 8th/9th November, 1942'; Report by C.W. Lynn, Senior Agricultural Superintendent, Department of Agriculture, 'Movements of population in North Mamprusi with particular reference to depopulation along the Red and White Volta Rivers where run north and south', undated, early 1940s.
138 PRAAD/A/CSO/20/6/4, Northern Territories Welfare Committee, 1944–5, 'Agenda for conference of Northern Territories welfare committee meeting', 21/1/1944, pp. 4–5.
139 John M. Hunter, 'River Blindness in Nangodi, Northern Ghana: A Hypothesis of Cyclical Advance and Retreat', *Geographical Review*, 56.3 (1966), 398–416 (pp. 410–16).
140 PRAAD/A/ADM/11/1/1294, Purcell, 'Report', p. 71(f).
141 T.E. Hilton, *Ghana Population Atlas: The Distribution and Density of Population in the Gold Coast and Togoland under United Kingdom Trusteeship* (Edinburgh: Thomas Nelson & Sons for the University of Ghana, 1960), p. 10. Purcell locations related to Table 5.2.
142 Topographic data drawn from United States Geological Survey (USGS) Shuttle Radar Topography Mission (SRTM) <http://www.opendem.info/download_contours.html> [accessed 9 May 2016]. Purcell locations related to Table 5.2.
143 Jérôme Destombes, 'From Long-Term Patterns of Seasonal Hunger to Changing Experiences of Everyday Poverty: Northeastern Ghana, c. 1930–2000', *Journal of African History*, 47.2 (2006), 181–205 (p. 192).

144 PRAAD/A/ADM/11/1/1294, Purcell, 'Report', p. 75.

145 PRAAD/T/NRG/9/19/1, Food shortage in the Upper Region, 1964–9, 'Conditions at Nakon U.R. March 1967', anonymous.

146 PRAAD/T/NRG/18/8/1, Diet and nutrition (1930–57), Report by C.W. Lynn, Senior Agricultural Superintendent, Department of Agriculture, 'Depopulation of Riverine areas in North Mamprusi: Report on a visit to Sekoti, 8th/9th November, 1942'.

147 David A. Cleveland, 'Migration in West Africa: A Savanna Village Perspective', *Africa*, 61.2 (1991), 222–46 (p. 228).

148 PRAAD/A/ADM/11/1/1294, Purcell, 'Report', p. 77.

149 Hunter, 'River Blindness', pp. 405–17.

150 TNA/CO/859/115/3, Gold Coast: extracts from informal colonial medical reports, development plans and other papers [pertaining to nutrition], 1944–6. G.H. Gibbs, Chief Commissioner N.T.s, to the Colonial Secretary, 2/2/1944.

151 Fortes, *Dynamics*, p. 72.

152 Based on PRO/CO/96/751/14, C.W. Lynn, *Agriculture in North Mamprusi* (Accra: Department of Agriculture, 1937), p. 35.

153 Konings, *State*, pp. 249–50.

154 Hart, 'Opportunity', p. 323.

155 Hunter, 'Seasonal Hunger', p. 171.

156 Paul Webber, 'Agrarian Change in Kusasi, North-East Ghana', *Africa*, 66.3 (1996), 437–57 (pp. 442–51).

157 Keith Hart, 'Informal Income Opportunities and Urban Employment in Ghana', *The Journal of Modern African Studies*, 11.1 (1973), 61–89; Hart, 'Opportunity', pp. 328–30.

158 Cleveland, 'Migration', p. 238.

159 Labi and Selormey, *Report*, p. 5.

160 Fortes, *Web of Kinship*, p. 218.

161 TNA/CO/96/751/14, C.W. Lynn, *Agriculture in North Mamprusi* (Accra: Department of Agriculture, 1937), p. 11; Bening, 'Evolution', p. 143.

162 Labi and Selormey, *Report*, p. 5.

163 Jeff D. Grischow, *Tsetse and Trypanosomiasis in the Gold Coast, 1924–1954*, WOPAG – Working Paper on Ghana: Historical and Contemporary Studies (Helsinki: Institute of Asian and African Studies, University of Helsinki, 2005), pp. 1–22 (p. 8); Emmanuel Akyeampong and Samuel Agyei-Mensah, 'Itinerant Gold Mines? Mobility, Sexuality and the Spread of Gonorrhoea and Syphilis in Twentieth Century Ghana', in *Sex and Gender in an Era of AIDS: Ghana at the Turn of the Millennium*, ed. by Christine Oppong, M. Yaa P.A. Oppong, and Irene K. Odotei (Legon, Accra: Sub-Saharan Publishers, 2006), pp. 41–58.

164 Keith Hart, 'The Economic Basis of Tallensi Social History in the Early Twentieth Century', in *Research in Economic Anthropology: An Annual Compilation of Research*, ed. by George Dalton (London: JAI Press, 1978), pp. 185–216.

165 Moradi, 'Confronting Colonial Legacies', pp. 1113–15; Moradi, Austin, and Baten, *Heights and Development*, p. 23; Austin, *Labour*, pp. 424–30.

166 Tiffen, Mortimore, and Gichuki, *More People*; John Murton, 'Population Growth and Poverty in Machakos District, Kenya', *The Geographical Journal*, 165.1 (1999), 37–46.

167 Hawkins, *Writing*, pp. 83–6.

168 Gariba B. Abdul-Korah, '"Ka Biɛ Ba Yor": Labor Migration among the Dagaaba of the Upper West Region of Ghana, 1936–1957', *Nordic Journal of African Studies*, 17.1 (2008), 1–19 (p. 8).

169 Quoted in Hawkins, *Writing*, p. 212.

170 PRAAD/T/NRG/8/17/8, Migrant Labour, 1952–3, 'Annual Report on the Conditions of Labour in the Northern Territories, 1952'.

171 Abdul-Korah, 'Labor Migration'; Gariba B. Abdul-Korah, '"Now If You Have Only Sons You Are Dead": Migration, Gender, and Family Economy in Twentieth Century Northwestern Ghana', *Journal of Asian and African Studies*, 46.4 (2011), 390–403.

172 Gold Coast Government, *1931 Census*; Ghana Government, *1960 Census*.

173 Steven Feierman, 'Struggles for Control: The Social Roots of Health and Healing in Modern Africa', *African Studies Review*, 28.2/3 (1985), 73–147 (pp. 99–105).

174 *MDAR*, 1953, p. 86.

175 PRAAD/A/ADM/11/1/1294, Purcell, 'Report', p. 43.
176 Richards, *Land, Labour*, p. 76.
177 Colbourne et al., 'Medical Survey', p. 282.
178 'Forest country' women averaged 96 per cent of the height and 93 per cent of the weight of men in the sample. In the North, the figures were 94 and 89 per cent respectively. PRAAD/A/ADM/11/1/1294, Purcell, 'Report', pp. 3, 108.
179 Hunter, 'Seasonal Hunger', p. 179.
180 PRAAD/T/NRG/9/19/1, Food shortage in the Upper Region, 1964–9, 'Conditions at Adabeya (Arabie) April, 1967', anonymous.
181 Vaughan, *Story of an African Famine*, pp. 119–47.
182 Fortes and Fortes, 'Food in the Domestic Economy', p. 248.
183 PRAAD/A/ADM/11/1/1294, Purcell, 'Report', p. 58.
184 Rattray, *Hinterland*, p. 138.
185 Meyer Fortes, *Marriage Law among the Tallensi* (Accra: Government Printer, 1937), p. 5.
186 Fortes, *Marriage Law*, p. 9.
187 Fortes, *Marriage Law*, p. 16.
188 PRAAD/A/ADM/11/1/1294, Purcell, 'Report', p. 36.
189 PRAAD/A/ADM/11/1/1294, Purcell, 'Report', p. 58.
190 Cardinall, *Northern Territories*, p. 76. See also Fortes, *Marriage Law*, p. 11.
191 Sean Hawkins, '"The Woman in Question": Marriage and Identity in the Colonial Courts of Northern Ghana, 1907–1954', in *Women in African Colonial Histories*, ed. by Jean Allman, Susan Geiger, and Nakanyike Musisi (Bloomington, IN: Indiana University Press, 2002), pp. 116–43 (p. 123).
192 Hunter, 'Seasonal Hunger', p. 171. This is very similar to the pattern described in the 1930s: Fortes and Fortes, 'Food in the Domestic Economy', p. 246.
193 Hunter, 'Seasonal Hunger', p. 178.
194 Hawkins, 'Marriage'.
195 Andrea Behrends, '"Pogminga": The "Proper Dagara Woman": An Encounter between Christian Thought and Dagara Concepts', *Journal of Religion in Africa*, 32.2 (2002), 231–53.
196 A thorough gender history of a Northern Ghanaian community still needs to be written, although Hawkins has made some headway: Hawkins, *Writing*, pp. 227–76.
197 John Parker, 'Northern Gothic: Witches, Ghosts and Werewolves in the Savanna Hinterland of the Gold Coast, 1900s–1950s', *Africa*, 76.3 (2006), 352–80 (pp. 374–5).
198 David Tait, 'A Sorcery Hunt in Dagomba', *Africa*, 33.2 (1963), 136–47 (pp. 141, 144).
199 Tait, 'Sorcery Hunt', p. 145.
200 Tait, 'Sorcery Hunt', p. 144.
201 Esther Goody, 'Legitimate and Illegitimate Aggression in a West African State', in *Witchcraft Confessions and Accusations*, ed. by Mary Douglas (London: Routledge, 2004), pp. 207–45.
202 Susan Drucker-Brown, 'Mamprusi Witchcraft, Subversion and Changing Gender Relations', *Africa*, 63.4 (1993), 531–49 (p. 548).
203 Vaughan, *Curing Their Ills*, p. 144; Amin, 'Introduction', p. 93.
204 Jean Marie Allman, Susan Geiger, and Nakanyike Musisi, 'Women in African Colonial Histories: An Introduction', in *Women in African Colonial Histories*, ed. by Jean Marie Allman, Susan Geiger, and Nakanyike Musisi (Bloomington, IN: Indiana University Press, 2002), pp. 1–18 (p. 2).
205 Caldwell, *Rural-Urban*; Abdul-Korah, '"Only Sons"'.
206 PRAAD/A/ADM/11/1/1294, Purcell, 'Report', p. 6.
207 PRAAD/T/NRG/8/13/29, Child Welfare Clinic, Tamale, 1954–63, C.O. Moody, Principal Medical Officer, Northern and Upper Regions, to the Secretary to the Regional Commissioner, Tamale, 'Re: Child welfare, ante-natal and post-natal clinics in Tamale', undated, probably mid-1950s.
208 PRAAD/A/CSO/20/6/4, Northern Territories Welfare Committee, 1944–5, 'Agenda for conference of Northern Territories welfare committee meeting', 21/1/1944, p. 4.

6
Feeding Ghanaian independence, c.1957–1983

After spending six weeks in the Gold Coast, Dudley Seers and Dick Ross were confident that they had the measure of the place. Engaged by the outgoing colonial government to assess the viability of self-rule, the two 'typical Keynesian' University of Oxford economists were of the opinion that the Gold Coast economy was 'one of the least complicated in the world' and that the colony's 'main problems should be soon obvious to anyone with professional training'.[1] As they explained in the influential report published in 1952, the year after their short visit, 'if we were forced to sum up the Gold Coast economy in one word, the word we would choose would be "fragile"'. The two primary reasons for this fragility – the two 'special menacing features' of the Gold Coast economy – were the absence of any checks on inflationary spending and the national dependence on cocoa for almost all foreign exchange, the price of which was considered 'one of the most unstable [commodities] in the world's markets'.[2] Fortunately, though, the postwar commodity boom both obscured these shortcomings and presented a means to overcome them. After a decade and a half of low or controlled prices, lasting from the Great Depression to the end of the Second World War, the price of cocoa had gone into sharp ascent. With a little luck and some astute planning, many economists, including Seers and Ross, considered this an opportune moment to capitalise on high market prices and to secure the future of independent Ghana.

However, as another good example of late-colonial hubris, Seers and Ross's bullish conviction of the Gold Coast's economic simplicity was found wanting in practice. Some 30 years after his report was used to plan Ghana's early independent economy, Dudley Seers came to realise that, by 'naively applying a British economic model, without regard to local circumstances', his earlier recommendations, especially the encouragement of liberal state borrowing, had 'disastrous results' for independent Ghana and for the other decolonising states which followed its lead.[3] Writing in the early 1980s, and by then a well-respected and self-reflective figure in the field of development economics, Seers had come to consider his 'own small contribution to the present chaos in Africa'.[4] Economic growth had been steady at first; GDP per capita grew into the early 1970s (except for a brief slump during the late 1960s), and was reflected in improving standards of health and nutrition (see Figure 6.1). However, declining world cocoa prices, political instability, corruption, military governance, and poor economic planning saw Ghana slide into a long malaise. Reflected in declining nutritional status, these years were marked by the return of isolated but acute pockets of famine in the late 1960s and, in the early 1980s, culminated in the near-wholesale collapse of the internal food market and an unprecedented epidemic of nutritional illness.

As one of many planned attempts to right Ghana's macroeconomic shortcomings, the Seers and Ross report represents the beginning of a long period of inconsistent economic planning. Although rarely agreeing on how best to direct the development of Ghanaian independence, the various plans effected between the middle of the 1950s and the early 1980s all recognised the economic fragility which resulted from cocoa

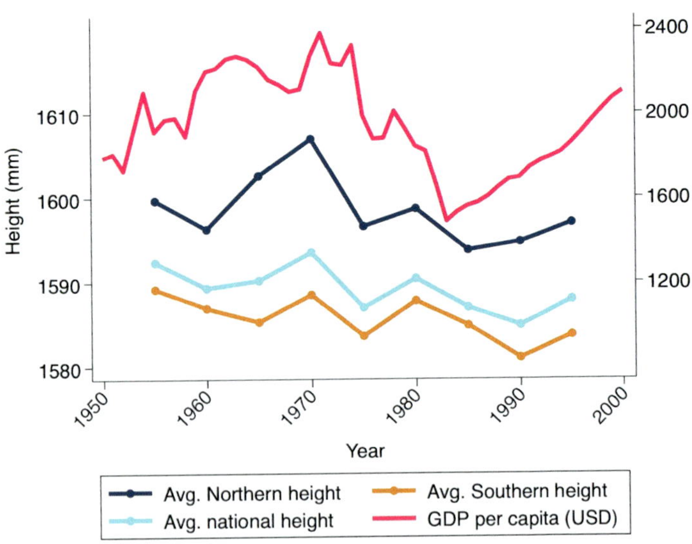

Figure 6.1 Average adult female heights by birth year and GDP/capita, 1953–98.[5]

dependency and the need for economic diversification. Another recurrent feature of independence economics was the tendency to misunderstand, misdirect, or malign the extant systems of food production and distribution necessary for both economic growth and national sovereignty. Beginning this trend, Seers and Ross, for instance, explained that 'no great improvement in productivity can be expected with the present diet'.[6] However, the various economic modernisms pursued in the first decades of decolonisation all struggled to accommodate the relatively unmodern modes of production and distribution which fed the Ghanaian economy throughout the entire period.

There have been several fine histories of Ghana's economic collapse and, although few agree, most lament an opportunity missed. For some, the recent history of newly independent Ghana is 'only a history of shattered dreams' and a case study 'of how not to develop'.[7] Marxist commentators in the 1960s and 1970s, including Nkrumah himself, felt that early attempts to create a truly postcolonial economy were stymied by the conservative military, or by the neo-colonialist workings of international capital.[8] Tony Killick's influential *Development Economics in Action* used Ghana's plight to highlight the weaknesses of 'modernisation theory', then 'centred around an industrialization drive, emphasizing import substitution, structural change and a less open economy … achieved largely through the instrumentalities of the state'.[9] By the 1990s, the likes of Douglas Rimmer and J.H. Frimpong-Ansah began to sideline external economic conditions, instead explaining that Ghana's economic decline was largely the result of the fiscal imprudence and the economic vampirism of successive governments.[10] However, it has also been suggested that such arguments understate the sincerity of these governments, and the political necessity of continued economic growth.[11]

The causes of Ghana's falter and fall are somewhat tangential to the aims of this chapter, which primarily considers the impact of independence economics on the lives of the Ghanaian poor which, in many respects, hardly changed in the decades after independence.[12] However, the erratic trajectory of postcolonial development had various impacts on food economies and domestic arrangements throughout the country. While the macroeconomic environment was clearly reflected in nutritional status, these mechanisms remain unexplored; the precise reasons for nutritional improvement under Nkrumah and nutritional decline in the years afterwards deserve to be untangled.

The roots of famine in the First Republic, c.1957–1966

Food deficits and agricultural decline

Ghana gained its independence slowly. Prior to total emancipation in 1957, the 1951 election earned Nkrumah the position of Leader of Government Business in a cooperative colonial government. Further general elections in 1954 and 1956 established Nkrumah as de facto leader and the strength of the CPP's mandate to rule. Nkrumah's primary policy was the exploitation of high market prices for cocoa in order to implement a relatively hawkish strategy of economic diversification. This sought to transform the country from a subsistence and smallholder-oriented economy to a capitalist one based on wage labour, capable of sustained growth and of providing, in the long term, rising wages. Cocoa farming, as the primary export sector, was squeezed hard in order to fund this modernisation. The Cocoa Marketing Board (CMB) monopolised the purchase of cocoa at set prices, adding vast amounts to government coffers and diverting surpluses towards ambitious state-building projects, alienating much of Asante and contributing to the rise of Asante nationalism in the process.[13] The inherited 1951 First Development Plan – initially designed by colonial governor Sir Charles Arden-Clarke – concentrated almost exclusively on infrastructure and social services and allocated only 5 per cent of its budget to the agricultural sector, restricting the inputs needed to continue colonial-era levels of production.[14] The effects of such policies on food production were clear to W. Arthur Lewis, Nkrumah's special economic advisor and later Nobel laureate. In a 1953 report, Lewis stressed that the 'main obstacle [to diversification] is the fact that agricultural productivity per man is stagnant' and recommended 'vigorous measures to raise food production'.[15]

Following state visits to the USSR, China, and Eastern Europe in 1961, Nkrumah formally adopted socialism, dropped the Second Development Plan written by Lewis, and set his sights on a 'big push' towards rapid industrialisation. However, by the time of the 1963/4 Seven-Year Plan, the planning commission recognised that 'Ghana needs an agricultural revolution as a precondition for the industrial revolution at which policy is aiming eventually'.[16] State involvement in all of the country's major economic activities, including food production, was beginning to turn Ghana into a command economy.[17] Yet investments in agriculture were inefficient and did little to improve marketing networks or to boost production for the mass of peasant cultivators, Ghana's primary food producers. These continued to use traditional, simple tools, and outputs per man failed to improve between 1906 and 1965.[18] This was mainly due to the CPP's concentration on the development of large-scale, state-owned, mechanised farms. Under the 1963/4 plan, state-sector producers – the State Farms Corporation (SFC), the Workers Brigade, and the United Ghana Farmers' Cooperative Council (UGFCC) – were allocated nearly a quarter of the funds set aside for agriculture. However, they farmed less than 1 per cent of agricultural land, contributed as little as 0.5 per cent of the country's food requirements, and underperformed relative to peasant production in both yields per acre and tons per worker.[19] The hastily undertaken mechanisation of these farms was part of this costly failure, with one contemporary agriculturalist noting that 'perhaps nowhere else in the tropics can so many tractors be seen lying in yards or abandoned in the bush'.[20] At the same time, 'the clock stopped on agricultural research', undermining long-term production. Instead, state producers converted research stations into production centres, declaring 'agricultural research a waste of time and money, an irrelevant and unproductive activity associated with men who were only competent to talk and write about food but who could not produce it themselves'.[21]

Agricultural mis-investment had undermined the viability of agricultural expansion in a period of massive population growth. Increasing urbanisation further diminished the productive potential of the countryside. Between 1948 and 1960, Accra's population grew by 181 per cent, Kumasi's by 167 per cent, Sekondi-Takoradi's by 140 per cent, and Tamale's by 83 per cent. The national population only grew by 40 per cent over these same years.[22] With food production lagging behind population growth, food imports became more important throughout the 1960s. However, cocoa, the primary source of foreign exchange, had been falling in price since as early as 1956 and, as the Seven-Year Plan noted, foreign exchange was 'one of the scarcest of the resources needed for Ghana's economic development'.[23] As the country struggled to balance industrial modernisation, an uninterrupted series of budget deficits began in 1960, with money creation used to finance spiralling budgets.[24] These problems were only exacerbated by the decline in local food production. Even in 1957, Ghana was running a significant food deficit but, between 1961 and 1966, the inflation of the cedi and declining agricultural production meant that national spending on food increased from 338 million cedis to 888 million.[25]

At the same time, food marketing and distribution also began to stagnate. In 1967, the economist Rowena Lawson found that:

> Market facilities in the main, large markets of Ghana, in Accra and Kumasi, have not kept pace with the rapid increase in population. Ten years ago a great deal of trade was carried out by itinerant traders who plied their trade on the sidewalks and by 'calling' as they walked around. This is now largely prohibited, yet the main markets in Accra are no larger than they were 20 years ago.[26]

Centralised marketing strategies further reduced competition in the trade in foodstuffs. Through the Ghana National Trading Corporation (GNTC), the state established a virtual monopoly over the marketing and distribution of imported foods and, via various marketing boards, began to exercise influence over the internal marketing of foods as well. However, as with production, state-led marketing efforts struggled to penetrate the relatively isolated food-surplus areas and could not compete with the extant class of self-employed traders that were 'characterised by low labour costs, very little overhead apart from transport costs, and a well-developed entrepreneurship, which operates with a great amount of mobility and flexibility'.[27] Transport efficiency also declined in the early 1960s. Cuts to spending on infrastructure after the 1963/4 plan meant that the construction of feeder roads was curtailed. Due to the shortage of foreign exchange, fewer vehicles were imported and the average age of the national fleet grew as its roadworthiness declined.[28]

As with many other problems in the administration of early independent Ghana, corruption and the widespread misallocation of funds also played a part.[29] Recalling his visit in the early 1960s, Cambridge economist Nicholas Kaldor wrote:

> The ambience of the government was that of a medieval court, flamboyant, extravagant and corrupt. An initially strong financial position, based on Ghana's rapidly expanding cocoa output and the high world price of cocoa, had been dissipated in a grasshopper's summer of waste, extravagance, corruption and prestige projects.[30]

'Hoarders' and 'middlemen' were consistently criticised for driving up the prices of local food, yet state-backed marketers were particularly able to profit given the country's growing dependency on imports. GNTC storekeepers, for instance, were found to 'encourage long queues' and 'privately dispose of some stocks to special customers for a consideration'.[31] Misallocation accompanied a period of dwindling cocoa revenues, when the population was asked to make sacrifices in the name of African socialism. As opposition politician Victor Owosu bravely stated at the time, 'members of the new Ghanaian aristocracy and their hangers-on, who tell them to do this, are fast developing pot bellies and paunches and their wives and sweet-hearts double chins in direct proportion to the rate at which people tighten their belts'.[32]

Cost of living crises and the cost of good nutrition

Swept into power with the 1948 cost of living crisis, Nkrumah lost his position under similar circumstances. Although his ousting, in a bloodless coup in February 1966, was not entirely due to the rapidly rising cost of living, it helps explains why he was not initially missed by many Ghanaians. Agricultural decline had seen food prices increase by around 10 per cent year on year between 1960 and 1966. By the time of the coup, real incomes in Accra were worse than during the 1948 riot, and food supplies had reached their lowest ebb thus far in that century. This fall was only accentuated by memories of earlier affluence. Between 1952 and 1960, the real earnings of African employees had actually risen by 50 per cent, but then, eroded by inflation, they reached a trough in 1966. Government wages followed a similar pattern and the real value of the 1967 minimum wage was only 87 per cent of its 1952 level. However, the period of CPP rule had different effects in the countryside and the town and, between 1952 and 1960, urban real incomes grew by around half while rural real incomes stagnated. Between 1960 and 1967, urban real incomes dropped considerably, whereas rural real incomes rose by 20 per cent (see Figure 6.2).

However, these general patterns did not necessarily present uniformly across either cities or rural areas. For instance, in order to feed Accra in 1965, 'it was decided that as a temporary measure, Regional Commissioners could help by instructing their District Commissioners to arrange foodstuffs buying centres in their Districts and organise the farmers to send their produce to such centres'. Since 'this matter is so urgent' the directors of the SFC, the UGFCC and each District Commissioner were entreated to give it their 'personal attention'.[33] Accra was a touchstone of ferment; it absorbed the greatest amount of formal-sector employment and was the furthest removed from agrarian life. Given the role played by high food prices in the riots which brought Nkrumah to power, a great deal of political capital was expended in keeping Accra fed. Elsewhere, efforts were more reserved. In 1961, for instance, a 'drought the worst of its kind in recent times' was exacerbated by fires and profiteering and led to the 'acute famine which hit Kumasi'.[34] As we will see later, government resources were even less mobile in the famine-prone areas further north.

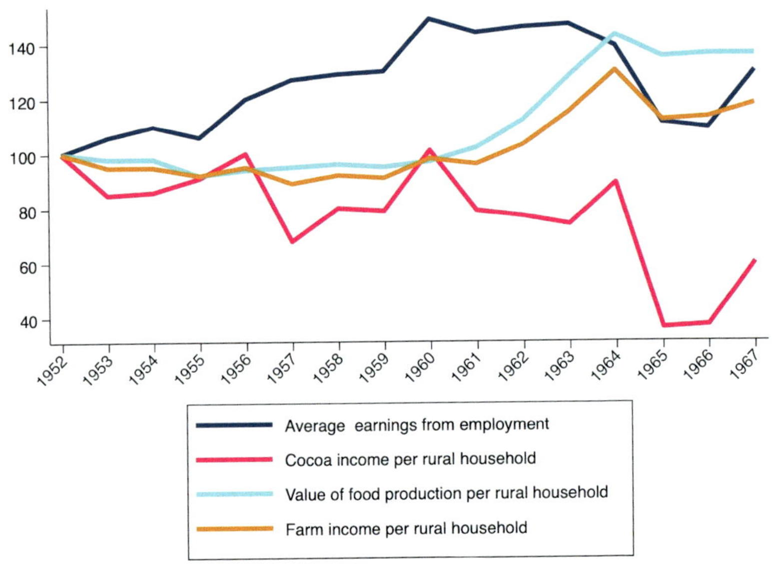

Figure 6.2 Real income trends, 1952–67.[35]

In the countryside, the general pattern may have been that farmers lost out from disinvestment in the early 1960s and benefited from inflation in the later 1960s. Again, though, this was not uniform. The negative impacts of disinvestment were concentrated in the South, where investment had previously been concentrated. By the same token, benefits in later years fell to those involved in the production and transportation of food. Since the sale of food had always been the primary source of income in the North, it may be for this reason that Northern heights increased more quickly during the 1960s, whereas in the South, where nutrition was more dependent upon cash-crops, height increases were more muted (see Figure 6.1). In the North, cost of living increases were a concern in the towns and the perennially hungry upper reaches, but far fewer people were regularly reliant on bought food. Urban communities in the North were also rarely entirely removed from rural life and cannot be thought of in the same respect as Accra. Indeed, the Committee on Price Stabilisation in the Northern Region concluded that food prices grew as a reaction 'to the high cost of controlled consumer goods … [and] to exorbitant rates of interest imposed by the pass-book holders especially on cotton prints, blue drills and khakis', rather than as a result of food-availability decline.[36] Even in the Upper Region, where consistent crop failures meant market prices held greater sway, nutrition indicators appear to have been improving. Although the two surveys are

Table 6.1 Upper Region anthropometric measures, 1939–41 and 1961/2 compared.[37]

	No. examined		Av. height (m)		Av. weight (kg)		Av. BMI	
	Male	Female	Male	Female	Male	Female	Male	Female
1939–41	1,140	829	1.68	1.59	57.1	51.0	20.1	20.2
1961/2	926	994	1.71	1.62	59.3	52.4	20.2	20.0

not entirely comparable, the average heights and weights of men and women increased markedly in the years between the Purcell survey and the National Nutrition Board Survey (see Table 6.1).

Despite this, Northern bureaucrats – usually themselves part of an urban bourgeoisie – regularly complained of 'middlemen' buying at the farm gate, driving up prices and monopolising supply. Some even endorsed blocking and guarding feeder roads to interrupt such trade.[38] The assistant superintendent of police in Wala South, for instance, 'suggested to members [of the district committee] that the most offensive part of the whole show is the women who go on the roads to buy and retail to the consumers'.[39] However, what officials seem to have been really bemoaning was the development of a form of market efficiency which saved producers both time and transport costs, albeit potentially at the expense of market-reliant consumers at the centre. In most respects, food inflation in the 1960s seems to have contributed benefits and brought greater opportunity to an already broadening opportunity structure. These were advantages seized upon most readily by those communities with the least viable export agriculture, especially in the densely populated north-east.[40] 'Comrade Ali Medchu', for instance:

> explained that the first day the [Wala South District] Committee went to the market it saw some guineafowls and other birds but now if you go to the market you will not get anything [at] all because the Zabramas [Zabarimas] and the Frafras have taken the delight to buy and transport them to the South but not to sell to us in the town, at the control price.[41]

However, with food security buoyed by ties to the rural world and growing demands for food further south, by the early 1960s the dynamism of the Northern food economy appears to have been providing a better average standard of living for people in the town in comparison with those in the fields. Across three towns surveyed in the North, wage earners, the self-employed, and petty traders were all seen to be heavier than farmers in their respective communities (see Table 6.2). Infant mortality rates were likewise better in urban areas in the North and South.[42] Conducted around this time, Keith Hart's anthropological work gives substance to this change by explaining that the growth of provincial urbanism provided greater opportunity for those Northern poor impoverished by environmental disadvantage, meaning that, 'as obstacles to migration are removed, it also becomes less necessary'.[43] Absenteeism in Bolgatanga, for instance, was much lower than rural 'Frafra' areas because those from the city were advantaged by their position straddling the urban–rural economy. Hart cites the joke, 'if you find a Bolga man working in the South, he must have been on a trading tip and gone broke'.[44]

Given the continuing predominance of men in both rural–urban migration and cash-crop production, especially in the South, rural women were predisposed to enjoy the improving terms of trade in food during the later 1960s. Almost all of the increase in the agricultural workforce between 1960 and 1970 was down to an increase in female labour. Whereas men's involvement in agriculture increased by 0.4 per cent per year for these years, women's increased by 2.9 per cent.[45] As the traditional arbiters of food production and distribution, rural women and their dependants were poised to benefit from the country's sharpening food deficit. Although the increasing cost of food was largely caused by marketing failures, demographic change, and sectoral disinvestment, the state blamed the greed of 'hoarders' for accentuating and exploiting shortages. In reality, across most of Ghana, food hoarding was conspicuous by its absence, with traders going to considerable lengths

Table 6.2 Weights by occupation, sex, and age group in Northern towns (Damongo, Bolgatanga, and Jirapa).[46]

	Men									
	All		20–9 yrs		30–9 yrs		40–9 yrs		50–9 yrs	
	No.	Weight (kg)	No.	Weight (kg)	No.	Weight (kg)	No.	Weight (kg)	No.	Weight (kg)
Farmers	141	57.6	33	56.7	39	57.2	39	57.6	30	58.1
Wage-earners	61	59.4	30	59.4	18	61.7	9	58.1	4	53.5
Self-employed	263	59.4	98	58.5	110	60.8	44	59.4	11	57.6
Unemployed	44	55.8	23	56.2	10	57.6	7	54.9	4	51.3
	Women									
Housewives	572	52.2	175	52.6	191	51.7	83	51.3	123	51.3
Farmers	45	49.9	16	50.8	15	50.3	11	49.9	3	42.2
Petty traders	160	53.5	45	51.7	60	54.0	30	56.2	25	51.3

to avoid effective ownership of foods which could easily spoil.[47] More often than not, these were specifically gendered attacks, with 'market mammies' and 'queen-mothers' expressly targeted.[48] As the food crisis rumbled into the 1970s, these complaints contained more force. In 1973, the managing director of the state-owned Food Distribution Corporation (FDC) requested that the Upper Region district commissioner 'use [his] good office in stopping the market women from competing with us'.[49] These ideas lent legitimacy to the physical violence women suffered during attacks on markets in Accra, Sekondi, Koforidua, and Kumasi in the wake of Rawlings' 1979 June Revolution.[50]

Unlike food producers, those dependent on cocoa revenue appear to have suffered considerably during this period. 'Extorted' by trading firms and 'the ever present unscrupulous farmers', the average cocoa worker in 1960 Offinso, a rural district north of Kumasi, 'lives the mere bread-line existence ... eats undernourished foods [and] is accommodated in backward environments'.[51] By 1966, cocoa income per rural household was less than 40 per cent of the 1952 level in real terms (see Figure 6.2), with those reliant on waged employment first to suffer from any slowdown in cocoa production. In fact, one early 1960s survey found that cash income in Dagomba villages to the north and east of Tamale 'compares favourably' with the income of labourers on cocoa farms further south.[52] Twenty-five years after the original survey of Akokoaso, the 1970 re-survey found the profitability of cocoa farming in swift decline, especially for small-scale or caretaker farmers. Absentee landowners were said to be 'finding it more and more difficult to get crop share labourers on third share [*abusa*] basis and the system of dividing the crop into two parts is becoming more common'.[53] Others 'complained that they could no longer get good virgin forest', that their cocoa was now too old and uneconomical, or that the expense of inputs had made capsid control an 'almost impossible battle'.[54] Wellbeing was increasingly defined along lines of deepening inequality. In 1933/4, 61 per cent of cocoa farmers produced 21 per cent of the crop and 6 per cent of farmers produced 35 per cent of the total. By 1970, 83 per cent of farmers produced only 12 per cent of the total, while the top 5 per cent of farmers produced 49 per cent.[55]

Similar patterns were found in the cities too, with Gini coefficients (a standard measure of inequality) rising by around 20 per cent between 1956 and 1968.[56] As the cost of food rose, the poorest sections of town society were left less able to enjoy a sufficient diet. This, however, coincided with a shift in the age structure of urban communities, leaving infant nutrition increasingly determined by urban income. In 1967,

40 per cent of the population of Madina, a poor peri-urban area north of Accra, which had not existed even 10 years before, were under 15 years of age. One-fifth were under four.[57] By the time of Caldwell's 1963 demographic survey, long-term migration was the norm, with temporary or seasonal migrants making up only a quarter of the urban migrant community.[58] Families were no longer seen as a check on migration, and whole families began to move together. In Caldwell's survey, only one-sixth of married migrants travelled without their spouses.[59] Urban sex ratios slowly evened out, a greater amount of maternal time was consumed by childcare, and the relative value of domestic service declined (see Chapter 4 for earlier trends). By the late 1960s, the female demographic advantage had clearly waned. Poverty, disease, and malnutrition grew in peri-urban areas swollen with new arrivals. As a 1979 survey of the heights of Accra schoolchildren showed, the advantage enjoyed by the indigenous Ga and the relatively well-provided-for city-dwellers was no longer apparent only 5 miles outside of the city centre.[60] Peri-urban schoolgirls were, on average, 5 cm shorter than their counterparts in the city proper. Living 'within very primitive communities with the barest minimum of social amenities', the short stature of these children was seen to be 'a clear reflection of the effects of unsanitary surroundings, economic poverty, and gross illiteracy'.[61]

Moreover, during the 1960s and more so in the 1970s, many trades previously dominated by female traders were modernised, centralised, or made more capital-intensive, leading to a general decline in previously generous terms of trade.[62] Mirroring broader urban trends, by 1968 the top 10 per cent of traders earned 43 per cent of sectoral income, while the bottom 10 per cent earned only 1.8 per cent.[63] Trading, especially for Southern women, had become a 'natural' way to achieve a maternal ideal which depended more upon financial solubility than time spent caring for children.[64] However, government retrenchment after the 1966 coup increased urban un- and underemployment, with the informal sector taking up much of the slack and leading to increased male competition in previously female-dominated spaces.[65] In 1965, only 6 per cent of school-leavers were without work after 12 months; by 1969, the figure was over 50 per cent.[66] Women were slowly pushed to the margins of urban survival. In late-colonial Accra, Acquah had found that the 'hard core of persons who habitually sleep out ... are mainly Zabarimas (popularly called *kaaya kaaya*, which is a name used for people who carry loads)'.[67] Here the *kaaya kaaya* – later known as the *kayayoo* – were particularly marginal men: 'during police raids in the town centres in September 1953, between forty to fifty people were picked up each night from market stalls, open verandas and the beach. All were men. They were, almost without exception, *kaaya kaaya* men, some of whom were known ex-convicts.'[68] In subsequent years, and continuing into the present, porterage has become ascribed almost exclusively to poor women and girls.[69]

The feminisation of rural–urban migration only became more pronounced in the 1970s, increasing pressures on the informal economy, lowering female economic agency, and increasing the cost of childrearing. The 'crisis fostering' of children whose parents could not afford to care for them became increasingly common, leading some girls into a life of unfree labour.[70] Higher-risk forms of social reproduction led to changes in the epidemiology of malnutrition. By the 1960s, some in the nutrition establishment 'estimate that there is more kwashiorkor among the children of the urban poor than is found even in the forest zone'.[71] In a 1967 paper, Fred Sai, the doyen of Ghanaian epidemiology, claimed that 'it is obvious that children in an urban situation fare nutritionally worse than children in the rural community', with a 'disproportionate percentage of cases of protein-calorie malnutrition occur[ing] in [the] children of immigrants'.[72] Rickets, 'almost unknown in the rural parts of the tropics', was also 'becoming obvious' in cramped, dark shanty towns.[73] Pressured migrant domesticities were exacerbated by a lack of social capital:

> Breast-feeding, which is the rule in rural communities, is losing prestige among most townswomen … [but] immigrant women rapidly assume that to be the right thing to do … Where both the income and educational standards are low, inadequate formula feeds leads to undernutrition in the first year of life.[74]

Concentrated at first among migrant and peri-urban communities, as the urban food situation grew worse in the 1970s, the increasing incidence of marasmus became a more pressing problem throughout Ghanaian towns.[75]

Bottle-feeding was central to this development, facilitating new modes of social reproduction but influenced by educational disparities and fashion as well as by work requirements. A 1967 survey of mothers in an Accra nutrition clinic found that educated mothers were more likely to use bottle feeds earlier in their children's lives. Uneducated mothers continued exclusive breastfeeding until, on average, 6.8 months, 1.4 months longer than educated mothers. Similarly, only 25 per cent of uneducated mothers introduced supplementary food before three months, compared with around 36 per cent of educated mothers.[76] Still, educated mothers were more likely to bring their children to clinics more quickly, were more likely to provide nutritious supplementary food like legumes or eggs, and were more likely to practise the hygienic feeding of supplementary foods. As a result, educated mothers experienced far lower rates of infant mortality.[77] Despite this, education was no panacea against malnutrition, instead granting greater exposure to the conflicting and often opaque nutritional science which swirled around the globalising city, with influences 'ranging from deliberate attempts of nutrition education to commercial food promotion and advertisements'.[78]

In 1970s Uganda, the then global centre of nutrition science, research found that 'between 25 and 30 percent of the variations in nutritional status or recovery of the children attending the outpatient clinics could be attributed to variations in knowledge and the attitudes of the mother'.[79] However, in Ghana as in Uganda, nutrition education was undermined by a conflicted medical apparatus which likely only added to public confusion regarding nutritional health. Commenting on the 'instant success' of a 1965 infant health integration scheme, the paediatrician and public health physician Samuel Ofosu-Amaah noted that 'bottles ran out frequently … this augurs well for the introduction of either plastic or glass containers for which a small fee could be charged'.[80] Such support for bottle-feeding would only serve to antagonise a nutrition community which had begun to form a consensus against the promotion of artificial feeding. Perhaps unsurprisingly, Ofosu-Amaah found that 'from the beginning the demonstrations by the Nutrition Board Team were not welcome to the nursing staff because they thought their own nutrition teaching differed from that of the nutritionists and feared confusing the mothers'.[81] In Northern Ghana, too, the Regional Food and Nutrition Advisory Committee complained of conflicting advice given by Community Health Nurses.[82]

Although artificial feeding was becoming more useful and more popular, it remained unaffordable for the vast majority of mothers. At around this time in Uganda, for instance, the amount of formula needed to entirely replace breastmilk for one child cost around a third of a labourer's salary.[83] The expense of milks and formulas necessitated its dilution, perhaps with unclean water and often until it contained a fraction of the nutritive value of breastmilk, foreshadowing the bouts of gastroenteritis and the epidemic of diarrhoeal marasmus or 'commerciogenic malnutrition', which was most evident in Accra.[84] The situation was probably aggravated in Southern Ghana, where maternal breadwinning and employment outside of the home had long been naturalised as the ideal form of motherhood.[85] And it may have been aggravated again in the late 1960s, when the price of milk substitutes was highly inflated yet maternal employment was both more necessary and less profitable given informal-sector competition. Milk grew into an economically valuable and socially charged commodity. The 1966 Commission of Enquiry into Trade Malpractices specifically highlighted concerns over the cost and dilution of various milk brands.[86] The anthropologist Claire Robertson also paints a scene in the late 1970s, when the urban market had all but collapsed yet a rare quantity of condensed milk was made available, doled out at control prices at one tin per woman. However, 'when it became apparent that there was not enough to go around, the orderly queue dissolved as old rivalries surfaced in loud arguments over who deserved a tin … a fight broke out between two irate traders'.[87]

The ascent of artificial feeding complemented the growth of cash poverty during the First Republic. More children were being born into an increasingly competitive urban economy. The disadvantage suffered by Northern migrants was compounded by a lack of social capital, through linguistic isolation and through localised infrastructural shortfalls. Corruption, on the other hand, concentrated food and nutrition security among those with the greatest social capital. Although the national food deficit may have supported the rural poor in food-surplus areas, it was not enough to remedy rising national hunger. More importantly, thousands in the forest pulled back from cocoa production, stalling the economy further. In something of an indictment of Nkrumah's economic diversification, those furthest removed from food production and the trade in food were precariously placed in the increasingly divergent economy of the 1960s. The 1961/2 nationwide nutrition survey found that male Northerners living in the gold mining town of Tarkwa weighed 61 kg and 'compare[d] very favourably' with their counterparts still living in the North, who averaged around 2 kg less. However, young men left unemployed in Accra weighed only around 55 kg, less even than those unemployed in the North, and more than 7 kg below the Accra average.[88] As formal employment and urban food security fell over the course of the 1960s, life at home may have been the wiser choice, at least for some migrants.[89]

The decline of famine relief

As we have already seen, food security varied vastly across the country. It varied due to ecology, due to the infrastructural deficits born from colonial underdevelopment, and even due to the political value of food solvency in a given population. However, after decades of ignoring and often cheapening Northern hunger, in the 1940s the colonial government established fairly effective mechanisms to underpin food security across the colony. In the Upper Region, where feast and famine could be separated by only a number of miles, the colonial government's greatest direct contribution to famine relief was the extension of its bureaucracy through effective early warning systems and timely famine relief. Although extensive hunger seems to have only returned to Ghana in the years after the 1966 coup, efficient systems of famine prevention were allowed to crumble under Nkrumah, and often at the expense of the country's most vulnerable poor.[90]

During the 1950s, the Agricultural Department was made constantly aware of coming disaster in the North due to detailed monthly reports sent from regional administrators who, in turn, were advised by their districts. These reports noted variations in average rainfall and the price of staple foods at various markets and were used to avert several famines during the late 1950s.[91] However, by the early 1960s these reports appear to have stopped. Instead, famine relief was garnered through informal requests:

> It appears there will be shortage of food and water in the Northern and Upper Regions next year [1962]. *Though no figures are available* [my emphasis] to support this statement, the condition of crops in the fields particularly in parts of the Upper Region points to such a gloomy forecast.[92]

Despite an obvious decline in efficiency, relief was still forthcoming, at least during the first half of the 1960s, and forewarnings were acted upon.[93] However, corruption misdirected limited state supplies. For instance, on requesting food aid for three boarding schools in his district, the education secretary for Western Gonja/Damongo wrote to complain that the regional organiser of the Workers Brigade 'could only give me five bags of konkonte [cassava flour]'. At the same time, 'a Workers Brigade Truck brought eleven bags of grains to one Mallan Issah's house … I cannot imagine why the Regional Organiser has considered one individual more than these three institutions.'[94] It is hard to say how much real suffering was seen during these years; it is likely that the breadth of CPP social services and growing returns from surplus food production outweighed the inefficiencies of state-led relief. However, the infrastructural decline suggested here gives context to the coming hunger of the following decades and, as food became scarcer over the course of the 1960s, acute famines were allowed to fester.

By the late 1960s, as pockets of famine flared up throughout the Upper Region, effective measures to prevent or relieve famine had clearly broken down. In October 1966 it was apparent that, 'owing to the failure of the millet crop, there is a threat of famine in the Region during the dry period between January and the next planting season'.[95] Despite the early recognition of a coming crisis, no proactive measures appear to have been put in place and, by the following March, hunger was quickly spreading. In Nakon, the poorest community surveyed by Purcell, one government investigation asked about the 'present state of the children' and was told 'in no uncertain terms that there are often entire days, or longer, when they have to go without any cooked meals at all'.[96] Conditions in two small hamlets between Nakon and the Sisili River were said to be 'even worse than those prevailing in Nakon'.[97] The 1969 famine in Kulumasa, a village north of Nangodi, provides an example of geospatial poverty exacerbated by the disinvestment and infrastructural decline of the 1960s. According to one report, 'Kulumasa was once a much larger, more important place … where there was once a thriving market, a few pathetic booths persist for local trading on a smaller scale'.[98] Kulumasa's descent into penury was, in part, due to its disease burden, especially the high rate of onchocerciasis. However, in terms of immediate relief and long-term economic solvency, investigators found that the more pressing concern was that Kulumasa's geographic and economic marginalisation had not been addressed in recent years:

> While a Class Three road is marked on the latest road map of Northern Ghana, it does not, in fact, exist … it is doubtful if any vehicle could cross the river during the rains and the people are probably cut off from the main markets, hospital, etc. at this time.[99]

Nkrumah was ousted in early 1966, prior to the famine in Nakon, and had been out of office for three years by 1969. However, the roots of suffering in these areas are clearly historical. Although these problems stretch into the more distant past, the problems of the deeper past were at times either ignored or accentuated by the particularities of CPP governance.

Explaining improvements in nutrition in the First Republic

If food production stagnated, famine relief was less forthcoming, and the cash economy was undermined, how, then, do we explain the apparent improvement in average nutritional status in the 1970s? Perhaps, more than anything, it was due to the earnestness with which the CPP approached social problems in Ghana. As Nkrumah once claimed, 'we shall measure our progress by the improvement in the health of our people ... the welfare of our people is our chief pride, and it is by this that we ask to be judged'.[100]

In keeping with this idea, 36 per cent of the inherited 1951 First Development Plan budget was allocated to social services, another 36 per cent to infrastructure, and only 9 per cent to 'productive activities'.[101] The 1959 Second Development Plan continued along very similar lines, again prioritising 'social overhead capital' such as health, education, and infrastructure in order to stimulate 'directly productive activities' like agriculture and, later, industry.[102] In 1961, hospital fees were abandoned and compulsory primary education was introduced. Healthcare in this period improved considerably, and Accra's Korle Bu Hospital was expanded to welcome student doctors from the long-awaited University of Ghana Medical School in 1962. Focus was also increasingly concentrated on preventive and rural medicine, and considerable effort went towards the expansion of health centres and the training of nurses.[103] With infrastructural improvements, such as the doubling of people served by piped water, an expanded feeder road network, and vastly more doctors and nurses per capita, health outcomes improved significantly.[104] Stillbirths and infant mortality declined steadily into the late 1960s, although with enduring North/South and rural/urban disparities.[105] Following the plan for industrialisation outlined in the 1963/4 Seven-Year Plan, spending on social services and infrastructure declined in favour of productive expenditure. Even so, social services still received 32 per cent of the budget and, since the whole budget was expanded, the dollar amount spent actually increased.[106] Health provisioning continued to improve between 1960 and 1965 but had begun to slow, as had the provision of piped water and the extension of transport infrastructure.[107]

With regard to nutrition specifically, economic advisors had stressed the importance of nutrition as early as the 1950s.[108] Around the same time, the colonial government brought a nutrition officer into the Department of Health while simultaneously setting up a small council on nutrition headed by the Principal Secretary of the Ministry of Agriculture.[109] Nutrition made for populist politics in the Ghanaian context. In 1957, Fred Sai was asked to speak to a radio audience about malnutrition:

> The word 'kwashiorkor' came in very handily because it was known in the capital, and it was used on radio to explain what malnutrition really meant in emotional terms. Before the end of the day, I had been hauled before the Prime Minister to help find out how to go about attacking the problem.[110]

With consultant help from the United Nations (UN), in 1958 the Platt and Mayer nutrition survey was undertaken, with a much more extensive survey carried out in 1961–2, under the direction of an FAO agent, P.L.H. Davey, though this time under the auspices of the government.[111] The resulting National Nutrition Survey is notable for the time at which it was undertaken, as well as for its geographical and theoretical breadth. For instance, more than 3,000 adults were weighed and measured in Northern Ghana alone, extensive dietary surveys were undertaken, and consumption data was compiled, as were the results of thorough medical examinations looking for signs of malnutrition in both adults and children.[112]

Despite political will and able assistance, the nutrition programme was marred by the same culture of corruption and engorged bureaucracy which undermined the broader health programme. The 1970 Konotey-Ahulu Committee investigation into the reimplementation of hospital fees later found that vast amounts of hospital property had gone missing. Accra's Korle Bu Hospital alone had lost 9,380 pieces of linen.[113] In 1959, the National Food and Nutrition Board was formed. However, its first head, a previous minister of agriculture, 'found it necessary to create a food and nutrition empire':

> With little concern for procedures, he recruited well over 100 officers in a few weeks with no job specifications ... Cars were purchased in curious circumstances. Before this show got on the road, the president found out about it and the new recruits were sacked, the cars impounded. The minister was removed.[114]

In 1963 'an effort at resuscitation was made ... but the rot had already set in'.[115] While the initial vigour of the nutrition programme was brought short in the following years, it did steadily expand. By 1959, nutrition and food science was featured in the national primary school syllabus and the main aim of health education programmes, such as the Northern Region Health Education Project, was 'to improve upon the methods of preparation and use of the local foods, the feeding of children by expectant and nursing mothers so as to prevent malnutrition, korshiorkor [sic], anaemia etc.'[116] Even in the farthest reaches, it was said that 'the importance of a balanced diet is commonly understood by the public nowadays'.[117] By 1962, the University of Ghana had opened a Department of Biochemistry, Nutrition and Food Science and, by 1974, there were over 100 domestically trained graduates in nutrition and home science across Ghana.[118]

Under Nkrumah, the social services which had been improving during colonial rule were expanded and reoriented with a tighter focus on the Ghanaian context. The public were better able to recognise and avoid nutritional illness and the medical system was better able to treat it. Though occasionally peddling conflicting information, the medical establishment made significant inroads against nutritional illness caused by taboo, problematic feeding, and short birth spacing. Infant mortality declined as family planning was encouraged and made more readily available. The growing importance of food crops in the rural economy meant that female agency also improved. In these respects, CPP rule promoted many of the social determinants of better health.[119]

Food, famine, and market collapse, c.1966–1983

Explaining the return of famine, c.1966–1972

In February 1966, the National Liberation Council (NLC) took control of Ghana in a bloodless military coup and set out to progressively reverse the economic centralisation of the CPP years. As an African patriot, Nkrumah has been fondly remembered but, as a premier, his rule has been described as leaving behind 'a legacy of economic decline, with a fragile external sector, heavy debts, a delicate fiscal structure, an export sector in which the seeds of destruction had already been sown and state sector industries that were to become a long-term liability'.[120] To deal with its rising national debt, and in lieu of raising taxes, the incoming government drastically reduced recurring public expenditure, introduced school fees, and enforced freezes on public-sector recruitment. The NLC also signed up to IMF advice which included reducing import and export tariffs and devaluing the cedi.[121] The University of Ghana's first African professor, Kofi Busia, and his Progress Party (PP) won the 1969 election to begin the Second Republic, carrying on the NLC's programme of liberalisation. However, Busia's fiscal mismanagement – which aped some aspects of Nkrumah's modernisation programme – reproduced the problems of inflation and rising overseas debt. Again heeding Western advice, Busia implemented another significant currency devaluation. The Second Republic, which was growing increasingly unpopular, was aborted by the military in January 1972, the same month the devaluation became effective.[122]

As was the case in the years after economic liberalisation in the late 1980s (see Chapter 8), economic reforms which were palatable to external investors had troubling social consequences, and only fomented the PP's unpopularity. As explained in a 1973 'post-mortem' of the Second Republic:

> In the villages ... what people noticed about government policy were not the long-term plans – for roads, piped water, electrification and so on – but rather the short-term intensifications of hardship: the rising prices, the imposition of fees for medical treatment at country clinics, the re-imposition of the school fees abolished by Nkrumah.[123]

With regard to nutrition, many of the problems which emerged in the last years of CPP rule continued under the NLC/PP governorship. Cocoa farmers were paid chits instead of cash for produce which had continued to decline in price anyway. The agricultural programme failed to perform, as did the 'emergency task force' established to correct the maldistribution of food, and food prices continued to rise in the cities. As the edifice of the Nkrumah state was peeled away, the civil service was given greater responsibility but with a smaller budget and, after hundreds of civil servants were removed from their posts, far fewer agents.[124] It is probably fair to assume that, under Busia, the spatial and social patterns of malnutrition remained fairly consistent.

Yet the causes of food insecurity which had emerged under Nkrumah were entrenched under NLC/PP government, only now with a fiscal policy which also undermined relief. Famine, in the crude sense of excess mortality due to frank starvation, reappeared as acute if highly localised crises in the last years of the 1960s. Beginning in Nakon, in what was then the Upper Region, in March 1967, epidemic hunger spread significantly into 1969. The after-the-fact approach to famine relief first seen under Nkrumah continued. In late April 1967, Accra was informed that 'the famine and its subsequent implications have extended beyond Nakon and its surrounding villages and further investigations ordered by the Upper Regional Committee of Administration have revealed many large pockets of famine stricken areas due to crop failure'.[125] In March 1967, when state investigations began in Nakon, government weighing programmes indicated moderate to mild underweight throughout the community. The following month, as investigators reached Arabie, average BMIs were even lower, and most of the community was severely underweight according to modern standards (see Table 6.3). Though 'not a famine-stricken area *stricktu sensu* [sic]', the related spike in poverty also played on ethnic divisions and violence flared between the Kusasi and Mamprusi living in Zabugu. Several fatalities resulted and perhaps one hundred people were made homeless due to fires set off following a dispute over a piece of land.[126] It has been suggested that similar ethnic-economic tensions played a role in the 1994/5 'Guinea Fowl War' that accompanied the shift to Structural Adjustment.[127] By June 1967, it was reported that 'the Navrongo War Memorial Hospital is flooded with children suffering from infantile diseases which have emanated from inadequate diets'.[128] In August the administration in Bolgatanga telegrammed Accra to advise that 'food commodities donated by Catholic Relief Service [CRS] not yet received at this end. Famine situation remains unchanged ... please treat urgent'.[129] Despite such requests, as late as December it was said that 'one can hardly get a bag of early millet', even for heavily inflated prices.[130]

In a foreshadowing of later patterns, the vastly underfunded and recently depopulated civil service began to outsource famine relief. Where, under Nkrumah, inefficient state-owned organs of distribution and production were responsible for the movement of food to famine areas, under the NLC/PP governments relief was increasingly drawn from national and international charities. Although famine relief for Nakon arrived fairly quickly, it was largely garnered through donations

Table 6.3 Anthropometric data from Nakon and Arabie, Upper Region, during the 1967 famine.[131]

		Nakon		Arabie	
		No. measured	Average BMI	No. measured	Average BMI
Female	≤16 yrs	14	16.41	9	15.10
	>16 yrs	13	18.30	–	–
	All	27	17.15	9	15.10
Male	≤16 yrs	14	16.55	14	15.65
	>16 yrs	7	17.84	2	17.49
	All	21	16.98	16	15.88
Total		48	17.07	25	15.60

and, even then, 'those who enjoyed this first meal of free food were about 100, half of whom were living skeletons'.[132] The following year, the government entreated the Christian Council of Ghana to provide relief to 'save the souls of the fast-dying people' of Arabie and Nakon.[133] In 1969, the administration again implored the Christian Council to 'kindly use your good office, as a matter of urgency, to supply us with any quantity of food items and used clothings for ... the hunger-stricken and blind people of Kulumasa'.[134] In these years, hunger expanded from isolated flash points to extend across the Upper Region, apparently exceeding the reaches of governmental or even in-country control:

> There are at present, pockets of famine in certain parts of the Upper Region, while other parts face serious threat of famine ... In its effort to meet the situation, the Regional Committee of Administration has issued an appeal to the Government and other Relief Agencies in Ghana viz USAID [United States Agency for International Development], Christian Service Committee.[135]

It is unfair to pin the famines of the late 1960s entirely on NLC/PP governance, the failings of Nkrumah, or colonial underdevelopment; it is a sad irony of African history that the first decades of the postcolonial period coincided with the beginnings of 'a drought of unprecedented severity in recorded history'.[136] Although, rainfall across the Volta basin was more stable in the 1960s than the 1970s and 1980s, environmental conditions were already in decline.[137]

These droughts, however severe, only exacerbated a pattern of political and economic neglect, and the return of hunger to levels which had not been seen since before the 1930s. By June 1969, missionaries teaching in Navrongo wrote to explain that 'the situation is a present hunger, sufficient in one district near here to force people to leave their homes ... A middle school headmaster in a village one of our staff visited last week said that he had never known his people forced to move in forty years.'[138] The teachers had 'little doubt that others who have their eyes open will be trying to reach official sources of help'. Indeed they were: one administrator from Navrongo had written to Bolgatanga to suggest that 'the Ministry of Social Welfare should be made to handle this matter'.[139] Yet government aid remained unforthcoming. One of the teachers noted that 'when I saw Mr. Koomson of Bolgatanaga Social Welfare Office he said the need was great, but the trouble was lack of funds'.[140] It is also not that Mr Koomson had not been trying at all;

if nothing else, he had written to the Christian Council, albeit three months before.

Feeding economic isolationism, c.1972–1983

Under Busia, Ghana's food deficit had only continued to grow. The amount of land under staple crops and the total output of these crops dropped significantly over the course of the 1960s. The years between 1963 and 1971 had seen a 38 per cent increase in food imports, with a 96 per cent increase since 1955.[141] The civil service and the military were among those most affected by steadily rising food prices as well as the loss of supplementary benefits. Spurred partly by this loss of earnings, Colonel Ignatius Acheampong and the National Redemption Council (NRC) overthrew Busia in 1972, instigating a government which would last until 1978. On taking office, Acheampong cited the country's worsening food situation as a justification for the government's suspension of democracy:

> The principle of 'one man, one vote' is meaningless unless it is linked up with the principle of 'one man, one bread'. A government which operates on the basis of ten men, one bread for the broad masses of the people is unjust and unjust rulers do not deserve to be sustained by any theoretical conceptions of democracy.[142]

On these foundations, agricultural reform became the cornerstone of an Nkrumah-inflected, populist, anti-austerity agenda that sought to reverse the economic liberalisation of the NLC/PP governments. The IMF stabilisation programme was abandoned, the cedi was revalued upwards, and import licences and foreign exchange regulations were reinstituted. Dramatically, the NRC repudiated all of the debts incurred by previous governments, effectively shutting itself off from overseas loans and foreign aid. With limited access to credit, imports had to be paid for in advance and reduced to the bare minimum. As a result, the NRC and the Bank of Ghana agreed that state support of industrialisation and economic development could not be considered for several years. Given Ghana's growing reliance on food imports, agricultural reform was both pragmatic and absolutely necessary given this policy trajectory. This started what Frimpong-Ansah describes as perhaps the only period, 'outside the war emergency, when public policy focused on actively promoting the food sector'.[143]

The resulting programme, Operation Feed Yourself (OFY), was imagined as 'a landmark in our struggle for economic emancipation', a green revolution which could reinstall pride in rural work and stem the trend of 'young school leavers who should go into farming ... flocking into the cities to look for white-collar jobs – a legacy of our colonial past'.[144] Alongside propaganda and agricultural outreach, OFY subsidised agricultural inputs (fertiliser and tools), provided tax exemptions for new farms and farms in key markets, and supported government agencies involved in food marketing and distribution. Both OFY and the NRC's broader manifesto were well received throughout the country and, for several years, OFY seemed to be working. Production surged and, according to the historian and politician Albert Adu Boahen,

> by the end of 1974, Ghana had indeed become a more united country than ever before and national pride and confidence has been restored. Agriculture was in full bloom and the Northern and Brong Ahafo regions appeared to have been well set on the road to becoming the granaries of the country.[145]

However, despite early successes, Acheampong's programme to provide 'one man, one bread' was a resounding failure. Beginning in the middle of the 1970s, and continuing into the early 1980s, food prices began to spiral out of control; in 1972, the rate of inflation was already in double digits and increased rapidly to a peak of 116 per cent in 1977.[146] The FAO production index suggests that general agricultural production increased by 16 per cent between 1969 and 1980 but had ultimately declined by 15 per cent on a per capita basis.[147] The World Bank's influential Berg Report found that the total production of both food and non-food agriculture fell between 1969 and 1979.[148] Hunger returned more forcefully to larger parts of the North and malnutrition reached epidemic proportions in the South as the health system collapsed. In Ghana today, Acheampong is judged to be the worst of the country's despots. As Boahen concludes, 'his was the worst reign – one of disaster, deprivation, degeneration and stagnation, if not retrogression – that this country has ever known'.[149] How, though, did an administration dedicated to the reinvigoration of the agricultural sector lead instead to its total collapse?

In many respects, OFY followed in Nkrumah's agricultural missteps, only the NRC went further. For instance, in the first years of the programme a considerable amount of government capital was invested into large-scale operations which proved as inefficient under Acheampong as they had been under Nkrumah. In 1967, the NLC had reduced state involvement in agriculture, cutting the number of SFC farms from 123 to 62, dissolving the UGFCC, and moving its agricultural machinery to the Ministry of Agriculture's extension division. However, under OFY, state-owned farms were reinvested in.[150] The Food Production Corporation (FPC) – which had grown out of the Agricultural Wing of the Workers Brigade – received around half of OFY's corporation loans in 1972, and around a quarter again the following year.[151] Yet poor repayment performances and a practice of misapplying funds earmarked for agricultural inputs prompted the Agricultural Development Bank (ADB) to discontinue the granting of loans to these corporations. Almost immediately, the ADB complained that 'it was a common practice of these corporations to divert such funds to the payment of old debts, personal allowances, salaries, and the acquisition of other capital items not having any immediate bearing on production'.[152] As under the CPP, questionable management had an impact on yields, which were generally below the countrywide average.[153] Targeted acreages declined by as much as half over the course of the programme, implying that 'either the government has reduced its goals in line with reality, or is embarrassed at its apparent inability to meet a realistic goal which it set for itself'.[154] Although research into agriculture was greater under OFY than it was under the CPP, it emphasised commercial and forest crops. Despite producing most of the country's staple foods, the savannah zone received only 20 per cent of the food-crop research projects. By contrast, the forest zone received 53 per cent of food-crop research projects.[155]

At the same time as state production was underperforming, the government was expanding its monopoly on distribution, which was still considerably less efficient than non-state distributors. Even in the early 1970s, when OFY was seeing some progress, organisations obliged to buy from the FDC, like schools and colleges, complained that the FDC provides a 'disappointingly meagre quantity of foodstuffs at cut throat prices'.[156] The headmaster of Bawku Secondary School found FDC prices 'much higher than prices initially charged by former food suppliers' and worried of coming food deficits if prices were to increase in the lean season.[157] Though the government recognised a 'crisis of confidence' in government distribution, C.D. Benni, the Commissioner for Information, thought that 'our countrymen are not suited to the idea of "suffering a little" or "bearing temporary inconveniences"' and that 'it would not be right to tell Ghanaians and the world at large about these shortages which have become a perennial problem'.[158]

Where capital was made available for private agriculture, it was generally concentrated among a new form of 'progressive' farmer. According to Colonel F.G. Bernasko, the NRC's Commissioner for Agriculture,

> [the] Operation Feed Yourself programme (through incentives such as credit facilities, technical advisory services, land clearing as well as harvesting services) has opened the way for many Ghanaians in the top stratum of society to go into farming. Did anyone ever imagine that eminent lawyers, doctors, senior army and police officers, university lecturers, top civil servants and company managers would ever engage in crop and livestock farming? Again, chiefs in the country are making farming lands available to prospective farmers in amounts (that is, acreages) never before thought possible. Such lands are now being given more and more to people of other ethnic groups, people who but a short while ago were referred to as 'foreigners'.[159]

By putting agricultural extension in the hands of an already relatively affluent bourgeoisie, OFY's financing of private agriculture did nothing to expand food security or production capacity for peasant farmers. Instead, OFY's funding structure refined previous patterns of inequality and food insecurity, especially considering that most large-scale food farms were producing for export.[160]

The promotion of 'foreigner' or 'stranger' farmers also had troubling effects, especially in the North. As Jack Goody has explained with specific reference to rice farming around Tamale, those able to invest in mechanised, commercial food-cropping which used high-yielding grain represented a particular and privileged minority.[161] What resulted were increasingly inequitable opportunities to cultivate the limited amount of land in shallow river valleys which was appropriate for rice cropping. The large-scale, shifting cultivation of perhaps several hundreds of acres rendered land quickly worthless in the medium term, moving cultivation further from the marketplace. Since government loans could only be granted if land ownership was properly documented, the literate Northern elite were able to exploit the educational backwardness of the North, utilising literacy to secure land rights in a bureaucratic system which 'clearly places the unschooled at a very definite disadvantage and turns them from non-literates into illiterates'.[162] Initially, 'progressive' farmers were mainly Dagomba, residents of urban areas such as Tamale or Yendi. Most were artisans affiliated with the colonial government or members of the UGFCC, and most retained jobs in trade or government. However, since 1973, more Southerners, mainly army officers and civil servants, joined as absentee farmers under the patronage of the NRC.[163] The uneven and occasionally ill-gotten advantages enjoyed by these elites were quite evident to the local poor, the response of whom was the spontaneous burning of rice fields which, according to Goody, represented 'a reaction against the development of inequality, the kind of inequality that derives from the green revolution'.[164] What was left behind was a 'dual agrarian system' which concentrated the bulk of investment on a small cadre of farmers, spreading investment capital thinly over a much greater number of peasant growers.[165]

The multi-decadal drought which began in the late 1960s also only grew in severity throughout the 1970s.[166] However, government policy did little to ameliorate climatic conditions, especially in land-poor areas. The sporadic bouts of famine which had re-emerged in the late 1960s only became more severe under Acheampong, with the first named postcolonial famines occurring in Kusasi in 1974 and 1977.[167] Although rice farming concentrated capital away from peasants, it did bring new cash-earning possibilities for the Northern Region, where land was still relatively abundant. However, agricultural investment was almost entirely absent from the Upper Region, where only two small valleys were found suitable for rice farming and two irrigation schemes were installed, with limited regional impact.[168] The reorientation of the Northern economy under the NRC represented 'an unmitigated disaster' for Upper Region peasants, with 'uneven development' a neglectful conspiracy which allowed famine to once again 'proletarianise a substantial number of north-easterners'.[169] During the 1970s, labour and any surplus food flowed out of land-short areas in order to feed the hungry at home and the growing markets in Bolgatanga and the Northern Region. In June 1977, for instance, in the midst of acute famine, about a thousand bags of produce were transported from Bawku to Bolgatanga each day. The ban on exports put in place by the Bawku District chief executive was overruled by the regional commissioner, who conceded only a nominal one cedi tax per bag. By August there was plenty of food available in Bolgatanga, if at inflated prices, but little in Bawku.[170] Government relief was also not forthcoming; instead, the presence of hunger was officially denied and relief restricted. In Kusasi, between 55 and 80 per cent of children were reported as underweight by July 1977, compared with 35 per cent in July 1973.[171] Poor rains and poor governance brought hunger to a great many during these years. Crop failures were more widespread than usual and modern relief less forthcoming. Traditional insurances had been undermined by steadily mounting population pressures, and the countrywide decline in cash employment will have been keenly felt.

Prior to this, the global increase in cocoa prices had, for a time, shielded the country from the inevitable crisis of foreign exchange.

The relatively short-lived boom, which peaked in 1974–5, allowed the government to print cedis in order to increase state spending, much of which went on patronage building and placating powerful actors in the military and police. As cocoa prices again dropped, they left an expenditure structure which could not be followed in later years, setting Ghana on its path towards national bankruptcy.[172] The agricultural sector was already short of inputs – even in 1974 the country's entire supply of fertiliser would only have covered 52 per cent of the area under rice alone – however, these shortages only increased in the following years.[173] The agricultural sector slowed and then stalled, and acreages and production declined.[174]

Such shortages also contributed to the collapse of healthcare. In the 1975 Ashanti Health Services report, A.K. Ghosh, then Regional Medical Officer of Health, describes the extent to which public health and the infrastructural underpinnings of good health had been undermined. For instance, in Kumasi, 'conservancy and cesspool emptiers are so few that they cannot possibly cope with the volume of work. As a result septic tank latrines are sometimes so full that the floors are covered with partially digested excreta.'[175] Curative medicine was also gravely damaged 'by permanently recurrent shortages':

> Nurses and doctors readily improvised whenever necessary in order to cope with shortages of various items, but a limit is set to this initiative. The results of the chronic recurrent shortage are slowness of various surgical and clinical procedures, frustration of the nursing and medical staff, general decline in efficiency, and in some cases, loss of interest.[176]

These were problems which also affected the nutrition programme. In the 1950s, the popularity of new nutrition clinics had 'overwhelmed' them with patients.[177] Into the 1960s, malnutrition clinics still sought to provide supplementation and relief for mothers burdened by multiparous births or financial handicaps.[178] However, later in the decade, 'the interest of the villagers in reporting to [the] clinic was waning due to the unavailability of powdered milk, oil and second hand clothing'.[179] By 1975, 'mothers appear to be reluctant in bringing their malnourished children to this special [nutrition] clinic'. However, increased attendance at particular welfare clinics coincided with nutrients supplied by the CRS.[180] As Allman found in colonial Asante, Ghanaian mothers 'participated in mothercraft exercises largely on their own terms'.[181] However, if the costs of attendance at these clinics dropped relative to their benefits, the use of such services naturally waned. Following public-service cuts in the later 1960s and input shortages during the 1970s, the state could no longer provide the curative medicine mothers wanted; simultaneously, the medical community also lost the stage from which they had disseminated advice.

In the same 1975 report, Ghosh lamented that 'the Public Health Nursing Service was faced with an up-hill task', as 'the two Kombi V.W. busses sent to the region some years ago are now unserviceable and off the road with no attempt being made to replace them'.[182] In contrast with the increasingly austere Health Service, Acheampong's government had been dubbed *'Fa woto begye Golf'* ('Bring your backside for a Golf') for the liberality with which government officials were said to give away Volkswagens to their lovers.[183] Under Acheampong, corruption reached lofty heights and opulence in the centre came to define his rule as much as shortage at the fringe. Import licences and foreign-exchange allocations became symbols of government largesse and fed an already parasitic state at the expense of the country's poor.[184] The visibility of corrupt accumulation by officials discouraged public involvement in legitimate trade and promoted a beat-them-all culture of survival known as *kalabule*, removing any incentive to participate in the formal economy.[185] The black market swelled and, following the revaluation of the cedi and government 'management' of exchange rates, huge amounts of produce were smuggled out of the country. With real prices four times higher in Côte d'Ivoire and Togo and no incentives to encourage the legitimate sale of cocoa, as much as 17 per cent of Ghana's annual cocoa harvest was smuggled out of the country in 1977/8 alone.[186] In Asante, farmers too far from the borders to profit from smuggling reduced their investment in cocoa and grew more food crops, some of which were also smuggled abroad to side-step price fixes. Intraregional trade broke down, with grain shortages in the South largely the result of smuggling in the North.[187] Even government-sponsored rice farmers banded together to create a private rice market.[188]

Combined with the collapse of the health system, the collapse of the food economy preceded a dramatic epidemic of clinical malnutrition in the 1980s. In 1964, 6.3 per cent of the nearly twenty thousand children seen over a six-month period at Kumasi's Maternal and Child Health Centre presented with protein-energy malnutrition, with 2.9 per cent 'mainly kwashiorkor' cases.[189] Between 1970 and 1975, nearly 17 per cent of inpatients in Agogo Hospital's paediatric department were seen with either kwashiorkor or marasmus (see Table 6.4). Though these figures are not necessarily comparable, the singular dataset collected by Jeltje van der Mei, a Dutch paediatrician who had worked for 26 years in Ashanti-Akim, confirms the dramatic increase in malnutrition over the course of the 1970s (see Tables 6.4 and 6.5).[190] Between 1970 and 1975, kwashiorkor was fairly common but not particularly severe, with an inpatient death rate of 6.4 per cent. Marasmus also followed a similar pattern. However, between 1977 and 1982, kwashiorkor brought more patients and caused more deaths in Agogo Hospital than any other disease. Between these two periods, there was a 110 per cent increase in kwashiorkor patients, with the far higher 1977–82 death rate of 19.8 contributing to a 522 per cent increase in kwashiorkor deaths between these two periods. Marasmus deaths increased too, although only by 74.3 per cent. Still, the death rate for marasmic children increased from 8.4 to 15.4. Interestingly, where marasmus was a growing concern in the cities, marasmus patients dropped by 5.5 per cent in Agogo, suggesting a return to precolonial patterns of malnutrition less related to early and improper weaning.[191] Perhaps, as was the case in preindustrial Europe, market decline freed up maternal time, restricted access to supplementary foods, encouraged lower fertility, and facilitated longer periods of breastfeeding.[192]

Though nutritional status declined across the country (see Figure 6.1), in the late 1970s and early 1980s the primary concern in rural Asante was clearly kwashiorkor. This can perhaps be partly ascribed to the dietary substitutions seen during this period. Listing concerns over feeder roads and distribution failures, the Commissioner for Agriculture, Colonel Bernasko, implored the public to produce more foods which could be preserved for longer, especially *gari* (roasted cassava) and *konkonte* (cassava flour).[193] It is likely that, during these years, cassava replaced yam and plantain in *fufu*, while maize paps, like *kenkey,* disappeared entirely. *Konkonte* is seen to be particularly dangerous – especially as a weaning food – because it can be easily stretched into a thin gruel which fills stomachs but cannot feed growth. In the North, too, the acceptance of *gari* has been said to derive from these years, when traders in the north sold what little grain they had produced and instead bought cassava.[194] At the same time as forest staples were being substituted out of Akan cooking, those living in Asante also lacked the purchasing power to command the high-protein grains and pulses which were now being smuggled out of the North, leading to a flurry of accusatory letters between regional administrations and to the militarisation of regional borders.[195] However, epidemic kwashiorkor in Ashanti-Akim did not result simply from food decline and dietary substitution in the late 1970s – it was also influenced

Table 6.4 Rank order of paediatric admissions for primary diseases in Ashanti-Akim – three study periods between 1970 and 1988.[196]

Rank	Period 1 1970–5			Period 2 1977–82			Period 3 1983–8			Percentage change			
		n	%		n	%		n	%		Period 1–2	Period 2–3	Period 1–3
1	RTI	562	12.3	Kwash	825	15.0	RTI	1,519	17.3	An	31.2	48.6	140.8
2	Mar	418	9.1	RTI	622	11.3	Msls	1,215	13.8	DD	10.1	−32.6	−11.3
3	DD	417	9.1	Msls	549	10.0	Kwash	1,133	12.9	Kwash	109.9	186.8	188.3
4	Msls	411	9.0	DD	459	8.3	Mal	704	8.0	Mal	4.1	150.5	160.7
5	Kwash	393	8.6	Mar	395	7.2	An	378	4.3	Mar	−5.5	−8.9	−13.9
6	Mal	270	5.9	Mal	281	5.1	DD	370	4.2	Men	−27.7	150.5	7.4
7	Men	242	5.3	An	206	3.7	Mar	360	4.1	Msls	33.6	121.3	195.6
8	An	157	3.4	Men	175	3.2	Men	260	3.0	RTI	10.7	144.2	170.3
–	Others	1,706	37.3	Others	1,991	36.2	Others	2,841	32.4	Others	16.7	42.7	66.5
–	Total	4,576	100	Total	5,503	100	Total	8,780	100	Total	20.3	59.5	91.9

Table 6.5 Rank order of paediatric deaths and case fatality rates for primary diseases in Ashanti-Akim – three study periods between 1970 and 1988.[197]

	Rank order deaths																
	Period 1 1970–5			Period 2 1977–82			Period 3 1983–8			Percentage change				Case fatality rate			
Rank		n	%		n	%		n	%		Per. 1–2	Per. 2–3	Per. 1–3		1970–5	1977–82	1983–8
1	Msls	59	10.8	Kwash	163	23.0	Kwash	203	22.8	An	45.5	31.3	90.9	An	14.0	15.5	11.1
2	Men	54	9.9	Msls	71	10.0	RTI	100	11.2	DD	–12.2	–19.4	–29.3	DD	9.8	7.8	7.8
3	RTI	54	9.9	RTI	63	8.9	Msls	98	11.0	Kwash	552.0	24.5	712.0	Kwash	6.4	19.8	17.9
4	DD	41	7.5	Mar	61	8.6	Men	57	6.4	Mal	42.3	18.9	69.2	Mal	9.6	15.4	6.3
5	Mar	35	6.4	Mal	37	5.2	Mar	64	7.2	Mar	74.3	4.9	82.9	Mar	8.4	15.4	17.8
6	Mal	26	4.8	DD	36	5.1	Mal	44	4.9	Men	–50.0	111.1	5.6	Men	22.3	15.4	21.9
7	Kwash	25	4.6	An	32	4.5	An	42	4.7	Msls	20.3	38.0	66.1	Msls	14.4	12.9	8.1
8	An	22	4.0	Men	27	3.8	DD	29	3.3	RTI	16.7	58.7	85.2	RTI	9.6	10.1	6.6
–	Others	229	42.0	Others	220	31.0	Others	253	28.4	Others	-3.9	15.0	10.5	Others	13.4	11.0	8.9
–	Total	545	100	Total	710	100	Total	890	100	Total	30.3	25.4	63.3	Total	11.9	12.9	10.1

by the ecology of forest agriculture and the particularities of Asante food culture and Asante childrearing.

Both the food shortage of the 1970s and the recent course of Asante history combined to compound Asante's cultural and ecological predisposition to protein deficiency. Over the course of the twentieth century, population growth and cocoa's incursions into the forest had also led to a marked decline in biodiversity and the food and nutrition security which had accompanied the forest ecosystem. In terms of bushmeat, for instance, in 1956 it was said that 'bushmeat forms an important protein source at least for families in the rural areas of Ghana'. However, the price of bushmeat increased by 25 per cent between 1956 and 1963, leading to more intensive hunting during which 'smaller species besides big game are also ... intensively hunted and have gained prominence in the bush trade'.[198] By 1966, 36 per cent of all meat consumed in the country was bushmeat.[199] However, overhunting ultimately led to a decline in bushmeat availability. Fruit agriculture also declined with the expansion and maturation of tall cocoa orchards, as did self-seeded fruit trees and, with this, the viability of foraging for food. Fruits and animals could still be found deeper in the bush, but they cost more in terms of time and energy, and rewards were uncertain. By the late 1970s it is probably safe to assume that the food and nutrition security previously offered by the richness of the forest had declined significantly and was no longer amenable to many.

It is also likely that the densely populated, cocoa-dependent area around Agogo was particularly unfortunate in this respect. Elsewhere, as in the Brong-Ahafo village of Hani, lower population densities and a lower dependency upon cash-cropping facilitated a swifter return to subsistence. Here, cottage industries, such as potters and blacksmiths, re-emerged to make and fix the tools which would have been imported but were now too expensive to buy, the number of homes increased from 67 to 100, and school attendances jumped by 100 per cent. Remarkably, the people of Hani judged themselves and their neighbours better off in 1980 than they had been in 1970.[200] Even at the height of economic crisis, most rural families and villages remained food-secure. Hunger in the countryside was greatest in highly specialised areas which were least able to revert to food production.[201] It was those areas most skewed towards capitalist agriculture which were the most at risk. For some at least, and perhaps for some around Agogo, the 'broad forest rent' which had previously ensured food security and economic advantage had been latterly undermined by the degree to which it had facilitated capitalist development.[202]

As was the case in Asante during the 1960s cost of living crisis, those dependent upon bought food were particularly at risk of forfeiting their nutrition in view of market decline. For instance, as early as 1973, there was said to be an 'acute' food shortage in the large mining town of Obuasi.[203] By May 1977, and following the government's attempts at regulating the prices paid for maize, it was reported that 'all spots in Kumasi noted for the sale of *kenkey* have become virtually deserted … [this] situation causing grave concern among general public'.[204] In a survey undertaken in Asante during OFY, 93 per cent of non-farmers – ranging from architects to clerks to housewives – said that they could not easily feed their families and claimed that between 80 and 90 per cent of personal income went on food.[205] Asante farmers were also asked, 'Do you feel that today you can easily feed yourself and your family?' Seventy-six per cent of the farmers responded negatively, leading the surveyors to the rhetorical question, 'If a large majority of farmers cannot feed themselves and their families, how then can they satisfy the appetites of an entire population?'[206] By the late 1970s they simply could not, and those dependent upon the market were left stranded as the market shrank from view. In 1972, Robertson explained that 'a person entering Salaga Market [in Accra] is usually overcome, first by the smell of fish, and second by the incredible press of people'. By 1978 she saw it 'somnolent with half of the stalls empty, low stocks of goods, and very few customers' – the end of a 'long process of unbenign neglect'.[207]

1983, and how Ghana got there

In a prescient 1974 speech, A.A. Kwapong, the vice chancellor of the University of Ghana, explained that 'hunger is not yet a serious problem in Ghana, but with our rising population, the world-wide inflation and the greatly increased cost of imported food commodities, a spell of unfavourable climatic conditions in addition can plunge us into disaster'.[208] Ghana was already in the midst of its worst drought for decades but, in 1983, rainfall across the Volta basin reached its lowest figure for a generation; a million Ghanaians living in Nigeria (then around 10 per cent of the population) were repatriated into a food economy which had scant ability to feed them; to cap off the crisis, wildfires destroyed an already-deficient harvest across Southern Ghana.[209]

The years leading up to 1983 saw patterns of hunger and malnutrition further strained by political fragility. Before brewing social tensions could escalate into violence, in July 1978 Acheampong was overthrown by members of his own military leadership, the Supreme Military Council (SMC). Yet, as Frimpong-Ansah has explained, 'the pressures within the economy that led to Acheampong's removal could not be assumed to have evaporated with his departure. Governments were reinstalled and removed depending upon what they could deliver from whatever resources that remained.'[210] Though attempting some limp reform, the SMC was too closely allied to the previous government to supress urban discontent and, in June 1979, Jerry John Rawlings and a band of junior military officers, the Armed Forces Revolutionary Council (AFRC), took power for the first time. Their brief but brutal rule had little long-term economic impact and neither did Hilla Limann's incoming democratically elected government, largely because Rawlings seized power again in 1981. Rawlings' now overtly Marxist government, the Provisional National Defence Council (PNDC), focused on redistribution and market control rather than addressing flaws in production. 'Economic criminals' were broadly defined; traders were beaten, fined, or imprisoned; bank accounts exceeding an arbitrary allowance were redistributed; and large denomination banknotes were abruptly taken out of circulation.[211] But Ghana's long-fermented economic decay was brought to a head by the insurmountable problems of 1983. Rebuffed by the increasingly isolationist Soviet Union, the ideological allies of the PNDC, Rawlings had little choice but to submit to the IMF's Structural Adjustment Programme (SAP) and rapid market liberalisation. Initially seen by some in the PNDC as analogous with Lenin's retreat from War Communism, Structural Adjustment has, however, set the course of national development ever since.[212]

Although the extreme events of 1983 may be seen to have forced Rawlings' hand, severe food shortages were almost inevitable given the extent of the market failure. The food market had all but collapsed in the immediate wake of Rawlings' first revolution. The confiscation of foodstuffs en route to market, the sale of food by police and soldiers at arbitrarily low prices, and savage attacks on food sellers had an 'immediate' and 'catastrophic' effect on urban food supplies. Perishable vegetables disappeared within days, while grains, beans, and pulses only lasted until traders had exhausted their current stocks.[213] Direct assaults on merchants simply accelerated a trajectory which was already in place. Those reliant on the market suffered, while those able to withdraw from it took their opportunity to do so. During this period it was farmers, not traders, that determined food supply. Food which would rot quickly came to market, whereas that which could be left on the plant or in the ground stayed there until it could be safely sold or, as was increasingly the case, bartered.[214] PNDC attempts to strong-arm a command economy in support of an insubstantial proletariat ignored the will and mass of the rural peasantry, as well as the degree of antipathy towards the revolutionary aims which had only made the rural poor poorer in the short term.

Marking the peak of postcolonial malaise and the then lowest point in terms of nationwide nutritional status (see Figure 6.1), 1983 and the spiralling food crises of preceding years were markedly different from previous periods of want. Epidemic malnutrition during these years represented a new form of dearth which resulted from market contraction and was concentrated among the market-dependent proletariat. In terms of the rather clinical 'intensity scales' defined by Howe and Devereux, these might be considered famine years. Given comparable anthropometric figures for the later 1980s and early 1990s (see Chapter 7), it seems plausible that the incidence of clinical wasting (weight-for-height <-2SDs from the international standard) may have exceeded the 20 per cent threshold forwarded by Howe and Devereux, at least in certain areas and among certain groups. Excess mortality also surely increased, perhaps also to the 1 per 10,000 per day apparently suggestive of famine conditions. Where it did increase, it will have been concentrated among children, and resulted primarily from the dramatic rise of severe oedematous malnutrition, another indicator of famine (see Tables 6.4 and 6.5).[215] However, in the cruder but more emotive 'classic' sense, characterised by the presence of death from frank starvation, famine was absent during these years.[216] It is grimly ironic that the breadth and depth of nutrition insecurity – born from an ever-increasing dependence upon bought food – probably contributed to significantly more excess mortality than the isolated food insecurity and periodic starvation seen in the North during previous years.

More properly, 1983 represents the drawn-out zenith of a food crisis particular to the political economy of the preceding years. Whereas, in pursuit of better-organised relief, migration usually flows from the country to the city during periods of food shortage, by the late 1970s the food situation was rather worse in Southern cities than in the surrounding countryside.[217] The repatriation of migrants from Nigeria also suggests that the source of long-distance migration during this period of contraction was previously affluent, market-dependent communities in the cocoa belt. UN data show that 32 per cent of returning Ghanaians were moving to the Ashanti Region and 18 per cent to the Eastern Region. The Central, Western, and Greater Accra Regions together accounted for another 32 per cent, with the Volta and Brong-Ahafo Regions taking 7 per cent each. The Northern and Upper Regions only received 2 per cent of returnees each.[218] In the North, longitudinal analyses of migration and rainfall suggest that the period of worst environmental stress, the late 1970s and early 1980s, was actually a time of reduced outmigration, as political and economic factors outweighed environmental ones.[219] Although, in the north-west, these years have entered collective memory as a period of particular hardship and hunger, there does not seem to be evidence of either widespread or localised starvation. Instead, those suffering poor harvests reverted to traditional coping measures, including localised migration in pursuit of cash employment or food aid.[220]

In some respects, the reasons for Ghana's economic decline, the return of famine in the 1960s and 1970s, and the dramatic decline of nutritional status are deeply rooted in its history. A legacy of colonialism and outward-facing development made it difficult for independent Ghana to address its internal concerns without upsetting its long-standing orientation within an insidious global system. While these are important considerations, colonial crimes cannot entirely negate those of successive independent administrations. Poor economic planning in the immediate postcolonial period undermined agricultural development in a time of economic promise and climatic good fortune. Instead, successive development agendas consistently overlooked peasant production as a driver of development and the foundation of the Ghanaian economy. Not only did this do little to buoy national food security, but the promotion of progressive farmers also established a petite bourgeoisie and exaggerated the polarisation of Ghanaian society at the expense of a disenfranchised rural poor. Moreover, agrarian collapse did nothing to arrest the population pressures and population movements which further upset rural productivity. Although it is not necessarily wrong to view hunger and nutritional stress during these years as Malthusian crises, Malthusian explanations remain wrongheaded. Ghana's depleted agrarian population resulted from governmental neglect rather than untenable population growth. If drinking water, electricity, and healthcare are absent in rural areas, and if roads are poor or often impassable, it is unlikely that an agrarian lifestyle will attract or retain populations vigorous enough to stimulate efficient capitalist production. More direct assaults on the economic agency of peasant producers under the PNDC only served to further alienate these key elements of national food security. But life in the towns was not necessarily any better either. Although the political expediency of urban populations and the greater provision of infrastructure allowed for a degree of social security, food security became increasingly strained and nutritional status declined in conjunction with the national food economy and urban public health.

Drought accentuated this decline but did not cause it. It was, instead, caused by a continuation of colonial politics, a politics of neglect which emphasised extraction at the expense of social reproduction. Perhaps it is best to see the faulting history of Ghana's post-independence growth as a crisis of capitalism, where the undervalued traditional-agrarian system propped up an inefficient capitalist one. This was a system which left those farthest removed from the precapitalist economy, and at the margins of capitalist production, the most likely to suffer as internal contradictions came to a head. At the same time, those operating at the points of friction, where the two systems intersected, were the most likely to take the blame. Middlemen and, more commonly, women were targeted because of their visibility, because they plied the gap between these two economies, and because their trade was seen to exploit the inconsistencies of the postcolonial state. However, the fact that successive governments were wont to hold them up as the cause of Ghana's troubles only attests to the culpability of the state itself. In this respect, the destruction of Makola market in August 1979 is a more telling culmination of postcolonial malaise than the apex of the economic crisis four years later. As market women in Accra were publicly beaten and a Kumasi cloth trader was shot for 'profiteering' – her baby first removed from her back – *The Ghanaian Times*, then a mouthpiece of the PNDC, endorsed a 'happy tragedy' for the 'worker, the common man', the physical destruction of a food market which had long since collapsed.[221] What the PNDC failed to concede, however, was the marginal importance of 'the worker' for the maintenance of the divergent postcolonial economy.

Notes

1 Dudley Seers and Claud Richard Ross, *Report on Financial and Physical Problems of Development in the Gold Coast* (Accra: Office of the Government Statistician, 1952), p. 170. Thirty years after the fact, 'typical Keynesian' is how Seers came to describe his own advice to Nkrumah. See Dudley Seers, *The Political Economy of Nationalism* (Oxford: Oxford University Press, 1983), p. 187. This and the following paragraphs are heavily informed by Margaret Mary Lipscomb, 'Changing Meanings of Development: Dudley Seers – An Intellectual Biography' (unpublished PhD, University of Southampton, 1993), pp. 49–64. Lipscomb's PhD represents the most detailed consideration of Seers's contribution to economic thought in general and Ghanaian development in particular.

2 Seers and Ross, *Report on Financial and Physical Problems*, pp. 1–3.

3 Seers, *Political Economy*, p. 187.

4 Seers, *Political Economy*, p. 187.
5 GDHS, 1988–2014; GDP/c from Jutta Bolt and Jan Luiten van Zanden, 'The First Update of the Maddison Project: Re-Estimating growth before 1820', 2013 <https://www.clio-infra.eu/datasets/select/indictorr/288/> [accessed 16 November 2014]. Heights taken as five-year averages of women aged between 16 and 60 years at the time of the survey. Inspired by Moradi and Baten, 'Inequality'.
6 Seers and Ross, *Report on Financial and Physical Problems*, p. 99.
7 Michael Roemer, 'Ghana 1950–80: Missed Opportunities', in *World Economic Growth: Case Studies of Developed and Developing Nations*, ed. by Arnold C. Harberger (San Francisco, CA: ICS Press, 1984), pp. 201–26 (p. 202).
8 Robert Beck Fitch and Mary Oppenheimer, *Ghana: End of an Illusion* (London: Monthly Review Press, 1968); Kwame Nkrumah, *Neo-Colonialism: The Last Stage of Imperialism* (London: Panaf, 1965).
9 Tony Killick, *Development Economics in Action: A Study of Economic Policies in Ghana* (London: Heinemann, 1978), p. 2.
10 Douglas Rimmer, *Staying Poor: Ghana's Political Economy, 1950–1990* (Oxford: Pergamon Press, 1992); J.H. Frimpong-Ansah, *The Vampire State in Africa: The Political Economy of Decline in Ghana* (London: James Currey, 1991).
11 Gareth Austin, 'National Poverty and the "Vampire State" in Ghana: A Review Article', *Journal of International Development*, 8.4 (1996), 553–73.
12 Rimmer, *Staying Poor*, p. 6.
13 Frimpong-Ansah, *Vampire State*, pp. 73–92. On Asante nationalism and the need for so many elections, see Allman, *Quills of the Porcupine*.
14 Gold Coast Government, *The Development Plan, 1951: Being a Plan for the Economic and Social Development of the Gold Coast as Approved by the Legislative Assembly, September 1951* (Accra: Government Printer, 1951).
15 W. Arthur Lewis, *Report on Industrialisation and the Gold Coast* (Accra: Government Printer, 1953), p. 4.
16 Ghana Government, *Seven-Year Plan for National Reconstruction and Development: Financial Years 1963/64–1969/70* (Accra: Office of the Planning Commission, 1964), p. 56.
17 Killick, *Development Economics*, p. 48.
18 Ferdinand Stoces, 'Agricultural Production in Ghana, 1955–65', *The Economic Bulletin of Ghana*, 10.3 (1966), 3–32 (p. 10).
19 Gerardo Serra, 'From Scattered Data to Ideological Education: Economics, Statistics and the State in Ghana, 1948–1966' (unpublished PhD, London School of Economics, 2015), pp. 208–12; Killick, *Development Economics*, pp. 193–4.
20 J. Gordon, quoted in Serra, 'Scattered Data', p. 212.
21 S. La-Anyane, 'Research in Agriculture in Relation to National Economic Development', in *Scientific Research in Ghana: Proceedings of the Workshop on Research Priorities and Problems in the Execution of Research in Ghana* (Washington, D.C.: National Academy of Sciences, 1971).
22 Gold Coast Government, *1948 Census*; Ghana Government, *1960 Census*.
23 Ghana Government, *Seven-Year Plan*, pp. 61, 56.
24 Naseem Ahmad, *Deficit Financing, Inflation and Capital Formation: The Ghanaian Experience 1960–65* (Munich: Weltforum Verlag, 1970), p. 24.
25 Ghana Government, *Economic Survey, 1968* (Accra: Government Printer, 1969).
26 Rowena M. Lawson, 'The Distributive System in Ghana: A Review Article', *The Journal of Development Studies*, 3.2 (1967), 195–205 (p. 201).
27 Lawson, 'Distributive', p. 199. For the organisation of marketing in Kumasi, see Clark, *Onions*, pp. 42–7.
28 Killick, *Development Economics*, p. 189.
29 For an account of corruption under Nkrumah, see Herbert H. Werlin, 'The Consequences of Corruption: The Ghanaian Experience', *Political Science Quarterly*, 88.1 (1973), 71–85.
30 Quoted in Serra, 'Scattered Data', p. 215.
31 Ghana Government, *Report of the Commission of Enquiry into Trade Malpractices in Ghana* (Ghana: Ministry of Information, 1965), p. 29.
32 Quoted in T. Peter Omari, *Kwame Nkrumah: The Anatomy of an African Dictatorship* (London: C. Hurst & Co., 1970), p. 90.

33 PRAAD/T/NRG/8/37/5, Food Storage in Northern Region, 1962–6, Circular letter from F.A. Jantuah, Minister of Agriculture, 21/7/1965.
34 PRAAD/K/ARG/2/1/61, Cost of living enquiry, 1960–1, J. Owusu, Chairman of the Kumasi Municipal Council, to O. Owusu–Afriyie, Ashanti Regional Commissioner, 22/6/1961.
35 Adapted from J.B. Knight, 'Rural-Urban Income Comparisons and Migration in Ghana', *Bulletin of the Oxford University Institute of Economics & Statistics*, 34.2 (1972), 199–228 (p. 213).
36 PRAAD/T/NRG/8/37/5, Food Storage in Northern Region, 1962–6, 'Findings of the Committee on Prize [sic] Stabilization in the Northern Region', 15/9/1965.
37 PRAAD/A/ADM/11/1/1294, Purcell, 'Report'; Ghana Government, *The Nutrition of Adults in Northern Ghana: A Report of the National Nutrition Survey of the National Food and Nutrition Board* (Accra: Mimeo., 1962).
38 PRAAD/T/NRG/8/37/5, Food Storage in Northern Region, 1962–6, 'Minutes of the Bimbilla District Store-keepers, bakers and foodstuffs traders with the District Commissioner', 14/1/1966.
39 PRAAD/T/NRG/9/19/1, Food shortage in the Upper Region, 1964–9, 'Distribution of foodstuffs, Wala South District Committee minutes', 29/7/1965.
40 Hart, 'Opportunity'.
41 PRAAD/T/NRG/9/19/1, Food shortage in the Upper Region, 1964–9, 'Distribution of foodstuffs, Wala South District Committee minutes', 29/7/1965.
42 S.K. Gaisie, 'Levels and Patterns of Infant and Child Mortality in Ghana', *Demography*, 12.1 (1975), 21–34 (p. 29).
43 Hart, 'Informal', p. 332.
44 Hart, 'Tallensi', p. 334.
45 Killick, *Development Economics*, pp. 77, 195.
46 Ghana Government, *The Nutrition of Adults in Northern Ghana.*
47 Gracia Clark, 'Food Traders and Food Security in Ghana', in *The Political Economy of African Famine*, ed. by Richard Erskine Downs, Donna O. Kerner, and Stephen P. Reyna (London: Gordon and Breach, 1991), pp. 227–56 (pp. 234–5).
48 Ghana Government, *Trade Malpractices*, pp. 10–13.
49 PRAAD/T/NRG/9/4/68, Ghana Food Distribution Corporation, 1972–3, Col. E.M Osei-Wusu, Managing Director, Ghana Food Distribution Corporation, Accra, to Regional Commissioner, Upper Region, Bolgatanga, 28/3/1973, 'Purchase of tomatoes and rice in the upper region'.
50 Claire Robertson, 'The Death of Makola and Other Tragedies', *Canadian Journal of African Studies*, 17.3 (1983), 469–95.
51 PRAAD/K/ARG/2/1/61, Cost of living enquiry, 1960–1, Ashanti District Commissioner, 14/10/1960, 'Viewpoint from Offinso District, Ashanti'.
52 Allan, *African Husbandman*, p. 240.
53 C. Okali and R.A. Kotey, *Akokoaso: A Resurvey* (Legon, Accra: University of Ghana, 1971), p. 43.
54 Okali and Kotey, *Akokoaso*, pp. 11, 17, 28.
55 Okali and Kotey, *Akokoaso*, pp. 18–19.
56 Kodwo Ewusi, *The Distribution of Monetary Incomes in Ghana* (Legon, Accra: University of Ghana, 1971), p. 95.
57 Nelson Otu Addo, Margaret Peil, and A.K. Quarcoo, *Madina Survey: A Study of the Structure and Development of a Contemporary Sub-Urban Settlement* (Legon, Accra: University of Ghana, 1967), p. 39.
58 Caldwell, *Rural-Urban*, p. 41.
59 Caldwell, *Rural-Urban*, pp. 85, 127.
60 Fiawoo, 'Physical Growth'.
61 Fiawoo, 'Physical Growth', pp. 311, 303.
62 Robertson, *Sharing*, pp. 75–122; V.K. Nyanteng and G.J. Van Apeldoorn, *The Farmer and the Marketing of Foodstuffs* (Legon, Accra: University of Ghana, 1971), p. 48; J. North, *Women in National Development in Ghana* (Washington, D.C.: USAID, 1975), p. 43.
63 Kodwo Ewusi, *Economic Inequality in Ghana* (Legon, Accra: University of Ghana, 1977), p. 73.
64 Gracia Clark, 'Mothering, Work, and Gender in Urban Asante Ideology and Practice', *American Anthropologist*, 101.4 (1999), 717–29.

65 As Hart explains, an increase in informal employment was not necessarily bad for individuals, or for the broader urban economy. However, it seems unlikely that it benefited women or their children. See Hart, 'Informal'. For a similar pattern in the years following SAP, see Ragnhild Overå, 'When Men Do Women's Work: Structural Adjustment, Unemployment and Changing Gender Relations in the Informal Economy of Accra, Ghana', *The Journal of Modern African Studies*, 45.4 (2007), 539–63.
66 Keith Bezanson, cited in Killick, *Development Economics*, p. 98.
67 Acquah, *Accra Survey*, p. 53.
68 Acquah, *Accra Survey*, p. 54.
69 Seema Agarwal, *Bearing the Weight: The Kayayoo, Ghana's Working Girl Child* (Legon, Accra: University of Ghana, 1997).
70 Roger Sanjek, 'Maid Servants and Market Women's Apprentices in Adabraka', in *At Work in Homes: Household Workers in World Perspective*, ed. by Roger Sanjek and Shellee Cohen (Washington, D.C.: American Anthropological Association, 1990), pp. 35–62.
71 S.A. Boone, *Survey of Contemporary Ghana: Nutrition in Ghana* (Accra: Nutrition Research Unit, undated c.1965), p. 7.
72 Fred T. Sai, 'The Impact of Urban Life on the Diets of Rural Immigrants and Its Repercussions on the Nutritional Status of the Community', *Ghana Medical Journal*, 6.4 (1967), pp. 134–9 (p. 137).
73 Sai, 'Urban Life', p. 137.
74 Sai, 'Urban Life', p. 137.
75 Fred T. Sai, 'Nutrition in Ghana', in *Nutrition and National Policy*, ed. by Beverly Winikoff (Cambridge, MA: MIT Press, 1978), pp. 81–107 (p. 97).
76 Florence E. Dovlo, *A Study of Infant Feeding Practices in Accra*, FRI Research Bulletin (Accra: Food Research Institute, 1968), p. 5.
77 Dovlo, *Infant Feeding Practices*, pp. 9–10.
78 Dovlo, *Infant Feeding Practices*, p. 3.
79 Jan Hoorweg and Ian McDowell, *Evaluation of Nutrition Education in Africa: Community Research in Uganda, 1971–1972* (The Hague: Mouton, 1979), p. 94.
80 S. Ofosu-Amaah, 'The Maternal and Child Health Services in Ghana', *Ghana Medical Journal*, 6.2 (1967), 51–9 (p. 57).
81 Ofosu-Amaah, 'Maternal and Child Health Services', p. 57.
82 PRAAD/T/NRG/8/6/57, Ghana Food and Nutrition Board, 1964–8, 'Minutes of First Meeting of Regional Food and Nutrition Advisory Committee', 4/2/1966, Regional Office, Tamale.
83 F.J. Bennett and J.P. Stanfield, 'The Clinical Conditions and Aetiology of Malnutrition in Uganda', in *Nutrition and Food in an African Economy*, ed. by V.F. Amann, D.G.R. Belshaw, and J.P. Stanfield (Kampala: Department of Rural Economy, Makerere Library, 1972), pp. 1–9 (p. 4).
84 D.B. Jelliffe, 'Commerciogenic Malnutrition?'; Williams, *Milk*; Welbourn, 'Bottle Feeding'.
85 Clark, 'Mothering'.
86 Ghana Government, *Trade Malpractices*, p. 29.
87 Robertson, 'Makola', p. 471.
88 Cited in Sai, 'Urban Life', p. 138.
89 This follows a similar pattern as that seen in Uganda. See Nott, 'Malnutrition in a Modernising Economy'.
90 This argument expands on the conclusions forwarded by Weiss and Grischow. See Weiss, 'Crop Failures'; Jeff D. Grischow and Holger Weiss, 'Colonial Famine Relief and Development Policies: Towards an Environmental History of Northern Ghana', *Global Environment*, 7/8 (2012), 50–97.
91 Weiss, 'Crop Failures', pp. 48–54.
92 PRAAD/T/NRG/8/37/4: Food Shortage and Storage in the Northern Region 1959–62, Chief Agricultural Officer to Ministry of Agriculture, 'Food and water situation in the Northern and Upper Regions', 16/11/1961.
93 Detailed in PRAAD/T/NRG/8/37/4, Food Shortage and Storage in the Northern Region 1959–62; PRAAD/T/NRG/8/37/5, Food Storage in Northern Region, 1962–6.
94 PRAAD/T/NRG/8/37/5, Food Storage in Northern Region, 1962–6, Education Secretary for Western Gonja/Damongo to the Secretary to the Regional Commissioner, Tamale, 'Sales of foodstuffs, Workers Brigade, Damongo', 9/6/1962.

95 PRAAD/T/NRG/9/19/1, Food shortage in the Upper Region, 1964–9, Circular letter from D.K. Ntosuoh, Regional Administrative Officer, 'Food shortage in the Upper Region', 15/10/1966.
96 PRAAD/T/NRG/9/19/1, Food shortage in the Upper Region, 1964–9, 'Conditions at Nakon U.R. March 1967', anonymous.
97 PRAAD/T/NRG/9/19/1, 'Conditions at Nakon'.
98 PRAAD/T/NRG/9/19/1, Food shortage in the Upper Region, 1964–9, T.M. McRae, R.A. Abbatey and Rev. G. Anoa, 'Report on Kulumasa', undated, c. March 1969.
99 PRAAD/T/NRG/9/19/1, 'Report on Kulumasa'.
100 Kwame Nkrumah, *Axioms of Kwame Nkrumah* (London: Panaf, 1969), p. 51.
101 Rimmer, *Staying Poor*, p. 62.
102 Killick, *Development Economics*, pp. 44–5.
103 See, for instance, Mary Opare and Judy E. Mill, 'The Evolution of Nursing Education in a Postindependence Context: Ghana from 1957 to 1970', *Western Journal of Nursing Research*, 22.8 (2000), 936–44.
104 Ghana Government, *Seven-Year Plan*, p. 26.
105 PRAAD/K/ARG/2/8/69, Ministry of Health, 1964–75, J.L.Q. van der Puije, Regional Senior Medical Officer, *Annual Report for Ashanti*, 1964, pp. 10–11; Gaisie, 'Levels and Patterns'; G.M.K. Kpedekpo, *Studies on Vital Registration Data from the Compulsory Registration Areas of Ghana, 1962–1967* (Legon, Accra: University of Ghana, 1970).
106 Killick, *Development Economics*, pp. 53–4; Rimmer, *Staying Poor*, pp. 85–6.
107 Killick, *Development Economics*, pp. 74–5.
108 Seers and Ross, *Report on Financial and Physical Problems*; Lewis, *Report*.
109 Sai, 'Nutrition in Ghana', p. 97.
110 Sai, 'Nutrition in Ghana', p. 99.
111 B.S. Platt and Jean Mayer, *Report of a Joint FAO/WHO Mission to Ghana* (Rome: WHO/FAO, 1959); F.T. Sai, P.L.H. Davey, and P. Whitby, 'A National Food and Nutrition Survey Project', *Postgraduate Medical Journal*, 38.436 (1962), 112–20.
112 Sadly, much of the detailed reportage which evidently resulted from this survey appears to have been lost. The government never published the data and only one of the detailed mimeographed reports remains.
113 F.I.D. Konotey-Ahulu, *Report of the Committee Appointed to Investigate Hospital Fees, 1970* (Accra: Government Printer, 1973).
114 Sai, 'Nutrition in Ghana', p. 101.
115 Sai, 'Nutrition in Ghana', p. 101.
116 PRAAD/T/NRG/8/13/29, Child Welfare Clinic, Tamale, 1954–63, 'Primary School Hygiene Syllabus'; PRAAD/T/NRG/8/13/40, Health Education, 1959–65, 'Northern Region Health Education Project Report', 22 March 1960.
117 PRAAD/T/NRG/8/13/29, Child Welfare Clinic, Tamale, 1954–63, C.S. Hoffman, Medical Officer, Wa, to Principal Medical Officer, Ministry of Health, Tamale, 20/7/1959, 'Recommendations to improve supplies of fresh fruit to the population of Northern Ghana without financial help from the government.'
118 W.B. Morgan, 'Food Imports of West Africa', *Economic Geography*, 39.4 (1963), 351–62 (p. 358); Sai, 'Nutrition in Ghana', p. 98.
119 Caldwell, 'Routes'.
120 Frimpong-Ansah, *Vampire State*, p. 97.
121 For an interesting collection of sources detailing IMF involvement in 1966–9, see Eboe Hutchful, *The IMF and Ghana: The Confidential Record* (London: ZED Books, 1987).
122 Frimpong-Ansah, *Vampire State*, pp. 99–108.
123 David Goldsworthy, 'Ghana's Second Republic: A Post-Mortem', *African Affairs*, 72.286 (1973), 8–25 (p. 14).
124 Victor T. Le Vine, 'Autopsy on a Régime: Ghana's Civilian Interregnum 1969–72', *The Journal of Modern African Studies*, 25.1 (1987), 169–78.
125 PRAAD/T/NRG/9/19/1, Food shortage in the Upper Region, 1964–9, K.G. Asimenu, Acting Regional Administrative Officer to Principal Secretary, Ministry of Labour and Social Welfare, Accra, 'Famine and Ill-health at Nakong and its surrounding villages', 26/4/1967.
126 PRAAD/T/NRG/9/19/1, Food shortage in the Upper Region, 1964–9, V.A. Yetumy, Assistant Community Development Officer, to the Principal Community Development Officer,

Bolgatanga, 'A Report of the Social Survey of Zabugu Conflagration and its Victims Relief Programme', 12/5/1967.

127 Jay Oelbaum, *Spatial Poverty Traps and Ethnic Conflict Traps: Lessons from Northern Ghana's 'Blood Yams'* (London: Overseas Development Institute, 2010).

128 PRAAD/T/NRG/9/19/2, Food shortage in the Upper Region, 1969–70, A.B. Salih, District Administrative Officer, Navrongo, to the Regional Chief Executive, Upper Region, 14/7/1969.

129 PRAAD/T/NRG/9/19/2, Food shortage in the Upper Region, 1969–70, Upterritory Bolgatanga to Principal Secretary, Ministry of Economic Affairs, Accra, 22/8/1969.

130 PRAAD/T/NRG/9/19/2, Food shortage in the Upper Region, 1969–70, Adam Zangbeo, Bawku-Naba, to the Chairman, Regional Administration, Upper Region, 'Shortage of Grains in the District', 2/12/1969.

131 PRAAD/T/NRG/9/19/1, Food shortage in the Upper Region, 1964–9, 'Conditions at Nakon U.R. March 1967', anonymous; 'Conditions at Adabeya (Arabie) April, 1967', anonymous.

132 PRAAD/T/NRG/9/19/1, Food shortage in the Upper Region, 1964–9, M.A. Larkai, Principal Community Development Officer, 'Progress report – famine village of Nakong', 13/3/1967.

133 PRAAD/T/NRG/9/19/1, Food shortage in the Upper Region, 1964–9, W.H. Koomson, Principal Community Development Officer and Regional Head of Department to the Christian Council Representative, Tamale, 'Famine at Arabi and Nankon', 20/6/1968.

134 PRAAD/T/NRG/9/19/1, Food shortage in the Upper Region, 1964–9, W.H. Koomson, Principal Community Development Officer and Regional Head of Department, to the Regional Representative, Christian Service Centre, Tamale, 'Famine at Kulumasa', 8/3/1969.

135 PRAAD/T/NRG/9/19/2, Food shortage in the Upper Region, 1969–70, Circular from I.B. Ashun, Regional Chief Executive, Upper Region, 'Threat of Famine – Upper Region', 16/7/1969.

136 Ning Zeng, 'Drought in the Sahel', *Science*, 302.5647 (2003), 999–1000 (p. 999).

137 I. Masih et al., 'A Review of Droughts on the African Continent: A Geospatial and Long-Term Perspective', *Hydrol. Earth Syst. Sci.*, 18.9 (2014), 3635–49; Raymond Kasei, Bernd Diekkrüger, and Constanze Leemhuis, 'Drought Frequency in the Volta Basin of West Africa', *Sustainability Science*, 5.1 (2009), 89–97.

138 PRAAD/T/NRG/9/19/2, Food shortage in the Upper Region, 1969–70, Judith and Chris [surname unknown, Navrongo School headteachers] to Carol [surname unknown], 23/6/1969.

139 PRAAD/T/NRG/9/19/2, Food shortage in the Upper Region, 1969–70, A.B. Salih, District Administrative Officer, Navrongo, to the Regional Chief Executive, Upper Region, 14/7/1969.

140 PRAAD/T/NRG/9/19/2, Food shortage in the Upper Region, 1969–70, Letter from Navrongo School headteachers.

141 R. Orraca-Tetteh, 'Effects of Rapid Population Growth in Ghana on Nutritional Needs', in *Symposium on Implications of Population Trends for Policy Measures in West Africa*, ed. by N.O. Addo et al., Ghana Population Studies No. 3 (Legon, Accra: University of Ghana, 1971), pp. 57–68.

142 I.K. Acheampong, *Two Years in Office of Colonel Ignatius Kutu Acheampong, 13th January 1972–12th January 1974* (Accra: Office of the Press Secretary to the National Redemption Council, 1974), pp. 9–10.

143 Frimpong-Ansah, *Vampire State*, p. 109.

144 F.G. Bernasko, 'Opening Address: Ghana's Operation Feed Yourself Programme', in *Food and Population: Ghana's Operation Feed Yourself Programme – A Case Study, Report of the 26th Annual New Year School of the Institute of Adult Education, 30 December 1974–8 January 1975*, ed. by Kwa O. Hagan, University of Ghana (Legon, Accra: University of Ghana, 1975), p. 20.

145 Albert Adu Boahen, *The Ghanaian Sphinx: Reflections on the Contemporary History of Ghana 1972–1987* (Accra: Ghana Academy of Arts and Sciences, 1989), pp. 8–9.

146 Jon Kraus, 'The Political Economy of Agrarian Regression in Ghana', in *Africa's Agrarian Crisis: The Roots of Famine*, ed. by Stephen K. Commins, Michael F. Lofchie, and Rhys Payne (Boulder, CO: Lynne Rienner, 1986), p. 105.

147 FAO, *FAO Production Yearbook* (Rome: FAO, 1980), pp. 75–80.

148 Elliot Berg, *Accelerated Development in Sub-Saharan Africa: An Agenda for Action* (Washington, D.C.: World Bank, 1981), pp. 1–217 (p. 50).

149 Boahen, *Ghanaian Sphinx*, p. 19.

150 Felix I. Nweke, 'Direct Governmental Production in Agriculture in Ghana: Consequences for Food Production and Consumption, 1960–1966 and 1967–1975', *Food Policy*, 3.3 (1978), 202–8 (p. 205).
151 Janet Girdner et al., 'Ghana's Agricultural Food Policy: Operation Feed Yourself', *Food Policy*, 5.1 (1980), 14–25 (p. 18).
152 Quoted in Girdner et al., 'Ghana's Agricultural Food Policy', p. 18.
153 Nweke, 'Governmental Production', p. 205.
154 Girdner et al., 'Ghana's Agricultural Food Policy', p. 18.
155 Felix I. Nweke, 'The Organisation of Agricultural Research in Ghana: Priorities, Problems, Implications for Domestic Food Production and Policy Issues', *Agricultural Administration*, 6.1 (1979), 19–29.
156 PRAAD/T/NRG/9/4/68, Ghana Food Distribution Corporation, 1972–3, S.A. Mumuni, Principal, Kanton Training College, Tumu, Upper Region, to the Regional Administrative Officer, Bolgatanga, Upper Region, 15/12/1972, 'Operations of the Food Development Corporation in the Region'.
157 PRAAD/T/NRG/9/4/68, Ghana Food Distribution Corporation, R.A. Ajene, Headmaster, Bawku Secondary School, Bawku, Upper Region, to the Regional Administrative Officer, Bolgatanga, Upper Region, 15/12/1972, 'Operations of the Food Development Corporation in the Region'.
158 PRAAD/K/ARG/2/8/111, Ministry of Agriculture, 1973–4, C.D. Benni, Commissioner for Information, to F.G. Bernasko, Commissioner for Agriculture, 10/5/1973, 'Complaints about rising food prices'; PRAAD/K/ARG/2/12/17, Operation Feed Yourself, First Phase (Vol. 1), 1972–3, D.K. Addo, Commissioner for Agriculture, to all Regional Commissioners, 19/10/1972, 'Movement of foodstuffs around the regions'.
159 Bernasko, 'Opening Address', p. 23.
160 Girdner et al., 'Ghana's Agricultural Food Policy', p. 20.
161 Goody, 'Rice-Burning'. Rice farming is discussed extensively in Konings, *State*, pp. 140–236.
162 Girdner et al., 'Ghana's Agricultural Food Policy', pp. 19–20; Goody, 'Rice-Burning', p. 146. See also Hawkins, *Writing*.
163 Shepherd, 'Agrarian Change', p. 173.
164 Goody, 'Rice-Burning', p. 149.
165 Shepherd, 'Agrarian Change', p. 174.
166 E. Ofori-Sarpong, *Impact of Drought in Ghana and Upper Volta, 1970–1977* (Legon, Accra: University of Ghana, 1980). For the climate history of Ghana and West Africa, see T.M. Shanahan et al., 'Atlantic Forcing of Persistent Drought in West Africa', *Science*, 324.5925 (2009), 377–80; Kasei, Diekkrüger, and Leemhuis, 'Drought Frequency'.
167 These were bad years for record-keeping. The almost universal absence of archival sources from the 1970s and early 1980s makes it difficult to verify these claims or assess the extent of this hunger. However, as he wrote in the late 1970s, there is no reason to doubt Shepherd's narrative for these years. See Shepherd, 'Agrarian Change', p. 182.
168 Even these Konings denounces as 'a veritable colonial cheap labour policy in a post-colonial guise': Konings, *State*, p. 327.
169 Shepherd, 'Agrarian Change', p. 181.
170 Shepherd, 'Agrarian Change', pp. 184–5.
171 Shepherd, 'Agrarian Change', p. 183.
172 The reasons behind this decline are complex and the period lacks in-depth research. Good starting points are Frimpong-Ansah, *Vampire State*, pp. 109–10; Dan-Bright S. Dzorgbo, *Ghana in Search of Development: The Challenge of Governance, Economic Management and Institution Building* (Aldershot: Ashgate, 2001), pp. 236–37.
173 Nweke, 'Agricultural Research', p. 20.
174 See, for instance, PRAAD/K/ARG/2/12/27, Operation Feed Yourself, Third Phase (Vol. 4), 1973–7, Speech by Brigadier N.A. Odartey-Wellington, Commissioner for Agriculture, 11/2/1977.
175 PRAAD/K/ARG/2/8/69, Ministry of Health, 1964–75, A.K. Ghosh, Regional Medical Officer of Health, *Ashanti Region Health Services Annual Report*, 1975, p. 21.
176 PRAAD/K/ARG/2/8/69, Ghosh, p. 49.
177 PRAAD/T/NRG/8/13/29, Child Welfare Clinic, Tamale, 1954–63, Moody to Secretary to the Regional Commissioner.

178 PRAAD/K/ARG/2/8/69, van der Puije, p. 20.

179 PRAAD/T/NRG/8/6/57, Ghana Food and Nutrition Board, 1964–8, 'Minutes of First Meeting of Regional Food and Nutrition Advisory Committee', 4/2/1966, Regional Office, Tamale.

180 PRAAD/K/ARG/2/8/69, Ghosh, p. 24.

181 Allman, 'Making Mothers', p. 40.

182 PRAAD/K/ARG/2/8/69, Ghosh, p. 24.

183 Akyeampong, 'Urbanization', p. 230.

184 Naomi Chazan, *An Anatomy of Ghanaian Politics: Managing Political Recession 1969–1982* (Boulder, CO: Westview Press, 1983), p. 181; Rimmer, *Staying Poor*, pp. 134–5.

185 It is thought that *kalabule* comes from the Hausa 'kara bude', meaning 'hide it'. See Chazan, *Anatomy*, pp. 194–7.

186 Paul Nugent, 'Educating Rawlings: The Evolution of Government Strategy Towards Smuggling', in *Ghana: The Political Economy of Recovery*, ed. by Donald S. Rothchild (Boulder, CO: Lynne Rienner, 1991), pp. 69–84 (p. 72).

187 PRAAD/K/ARG/2/8/118, Food Distribution Corporation, 1974–7, R.K. Zumah Regional Commissioner, Northern Region, to the Secretary of the SMC, Accra, 14/10/1976, 'Flow of foodstuffs from the region'.

188 Shepherd, 'Agrarian Change', p. 179.

189 PRAAD/K/ARG/2/8/69, van der Puije, pp. 10–11.

190 Jeltje van der Mei, '26 Years of Paediatric Practice in Rural Ghana: Child Health in Ashanti-Akim District, Working towards a Comprehensive Approach' (unpublished PhD, University of Groningen, 2005).

191 Sai, 'Nutrition in Ghana', p. 97.

192 Breschi and Livi Bacci, 'Month of Birth', pp. 161–2.

193 PRAAD/K/ARG/2/8/111, Ministry of Agriculture, 1973–4, F.G. Bernasko, Commissioner for Agriculture to C.D. Benni, Commissioner for Information, 2/5/1973, 'Complaints about rising food prices'.

194 Clark, 'Food Traders', p. 249.

195 PRAAD/K/ARG/2/8/118, Food Distribution Corporation, 1974–7, R.K. Zumah Regional Commissioner, Northern Region, to the Secretary of the SMC, Accra, 14/10/1976, 'Flow of foodstuffs from the region'; PRAAD/K/ARG/2/8/118, Food Distribution Corporation, 1974–7, Y. Boachie, Regional Commissioner, FDC to Regional Commissioner, Ashanti, 10/11/1976, 'Seizure of maize at the regional border checkpoints'; PRAAD/K/ARG/2/8/118, L.K. Kodkiku, Regional Commissioner, Ashanti, to Deputy Commissioner of Police, Ashanti, 18/11/1976, 'Haulage of maize to and from Kumasi'.

196 Data drawn from van der Mei, '26 Years', pp. 85–6. RTI = respiratory tract infection; DD = diarrhoeal diseases; Kwash = kwashiorkor, including marasmic kwashiorkor; Mar = marasmus; Mal = malaria; Msls = measles; Men = meningitis; An = anaemia, including sickle cell disease.

197 Data drawn from van der Mei, '26 Years', pp. 86–7. Acronyms the same as in n. 196 above.

198 E.O.A. Asibey, 'Utilisation of Wildlife in Ghana', *The Ghana Farmer*, 9.3 (1965), 91–3 (p. 91).

199 B. Volta, 'The Future of Ghana's Wildlife', *The Ghana Farmer*, 15.1 (1971), 30–5 (p. 30).

200 Merrick Posnansky, 'How Ghana's Crisis Affects a Village', *West Africa*, 1 December 1980, pp. 2418–40.

201 Clark, 'Food Traders', pp. 244–5.

202 Austin, *Labour*, pp. 10–12.

203 PRAAD/K/ARG/2/12/25, Operation Feed Yourself, Second Phase (Vol. 1), 1973, B.E. Laing, District Administration Officer, Obuasi, to the Regional Officer, FDC, Ashanti, 7/6/1973, 'Food Shortage at Obuasi'.

204 PRAAD/K/ARG/2/8/118, Food Distribution Corporation, 1974–7, G.S. Aggor, SECPOL Ashanti to SECPOL Headquarters, 3/5/1977, 'SITREP'.

205 Girdner et al., 'Ghana's Agricultural Food Policy', p. 22.

206 Girdner et al., 'Ghana's Agricultural Food Policy', p. 21.

207 Robertson, 'Makola', pp. 470–1.

208 A.A. Kwapong, 'Vice-Chancellor's Welcome Address', in *Food and Population: Ghana's Operation Feed Yourself Programme – A Case Study. Report of the 26th Annual New Year School*

of the Institute of Adult Education, 30 December 1974–8 January 1975, ed. by Kwa O. Hagan (Legon, Accra: University of Ghana, 1975), pp. 15–19 (p. 18).

209 E. Ofori-Sarpong, 'The 1981–1983 Drought in Ghana', *Singapore Journal of Tropical Geography*, 7.2 (1986), 108–27.

210 Frimpong-Ansah, *Vampire State*, p. 111.

211 Dzorgbo, *Ghana in Search of Development*, pp. 256–78.

212 Don Robotham, 'The Ghana Problem', *Labour, Capital and Society*, 21.1 (1988), 12–35.

213 Clark, 'Food Traders', p. 243.

214 Clark, 'Food Traders', pp. 244–5.

215 Howe and Devereux, 'Famine Intensity'.

216 Ó Gráda, *Famine*, pp. 6–7.

217 Ó Gráda, *Famine*, p. 84; PRAAD/K/ARG/2/8/118, Food Distribution Corporation, 1974–7, G.S. Aggor, SECPOL Ashanti to SECPOL Headquarters, 3/5/1977, 'SITREP'.

218 With only one coastal land border officially open, Brydon's straw poll of returnees in Volta suggests that as many as 18 per cent of returnees arrived along bush paths. It can probably be assumed that this number was considerably higher further north and lower in regions further from land borders. See Lynne Brydon, 'Ghanaian Responses to the Nigerian Expulsions of 1983', *African Affairs*, 84.337 (1985), 561–85 (pp. 570–1, 578).

219 Kees van der Geest, 'North-South Migration in Ghana: What Role for the Environment?', *International Migration*, 49.S1 (2011), 69–94.

220 Kees van der Geest, *We're Managing!: Climate Change and Livelihood Vulnerability in Northwest Ghana* (Leiden: African Studies Centre, 2004).

221 Quoted in Robertson, 'Makola', p. 469.

7
Towards a political economy of postcolonial nutrition

One of the remarkable things about the history of nutritional science following the end of empire is how long it took for anything to change. The science of nutrition stagnated during the first decades of decolonisation and was so heavily influenced by the politics and personnel of colonial rule that it could not easily break from them. The internationalist approach to medicine which stepped into the space left by retreating colonial regimes continued to look backwards and Westwards, appropriating many of the ideas which had informed, or misinformed, previous generations of physicians. In this environment, the reductive concentration protein which had characterised colonial-era nutrition endured. Well into the 1970s, and as in earlier decades, this protein myopia distracted from the social and economic determinants of diet and deficiency. Later derided as the 'great protein fiasco', the tragedy caused by the continued promotion of breastmilk substitutes was compounded during these years by an often farcical new array of heavily engineered high-protein foods.

While nutritionists were building on reductive, technical ideas regarding deficiency, social and political scientists were developing similarly technical approaches to African hunger. Informed by intellectual developments within nutritional science, as well as evolving anxieties around demographic change and 'overpopulation', ostensibly new approaches to nutrition were broadly rooted in the same classical liberal economics which had underlined colonial development. As concerns around a global lack of dietary protein started to fade, a renewed interest in Malthusian explanations of hunger instead encouraged population-level analyses and demographic interventions against malnutrition. The economic depression which spread across the continent in the 1970s and 1980s combined with the waning of Soviet influence, the return of Malthus, and a renewed faith in free market solutions to poverty and hunger. It was in this very particular environment that treatments for malnutrition were eventually reappraised and ultimately revolutionised, with the biology of deficiency more keenly understood and mortality rates dramatically reduced.

Stepping back from the specific history of nutrition in Ghana, this chapter details the international currents of scientific discourse which have shaped the medicine of malnutrition since the 1960s. While this provides some context to the story which has been laid out in earlier chapters, it is the period following the 1983 crisis and the onset of Structural Adjustment – a time of growing internationalist involvement in Ghanaian health and nutrition programming – that was most obviously shaped by the debates which are detailed here. In much the same way that colonial nutrition research reflected the political preoccupations of colonial government, the recent revolution in nutritional medicine reflects the political economy of neoliberal Africa. Echoing the modernist, technical, and reductive approaches which had long ignored the structural causes of malnutrition, nutritional science in the postcolony has remained largely subordinate to the political economy in which it evolved.[1]

Looking past protein, eventually: the durability of colonial medicine in postcolonial Africa

As early as the 1950s, the first cracks in the colonial formulation of kwashiorkor were starting to show. The concentration on kwashiorkor as Africa's greatest nutritional deficiency, and as a simple problem of protein, had been heavily informed by the culture and politics of empire while simultaneously oblivious to the social and medical implications of colonisation (see Chapter 2). Given that this relatively apolitical conceptualisation of kwashiorkor provided colonial governments with a degree of absolution, it is little surprise that the protein-deficiency hypothesis garnered its earliest criticisms from the postcolonial world. Speaking against the WHO's conclusions, Nevin Scrimshaw explained to a FAO/WHO-sponsored nutrition conference in 1953 that 'in INCAP [the Institute of Nutrition for Central America and Panama] we are far from convinced that the biochemical changes encountered [in kwashiorkor patients] are specific to protein malnutrition; rather they seem to be non-specific'.[2]

This contrasted with the more prevalent opinion that kwashiorkor was simply the most extreme form of a widespread protein deficit. Concerns regarding the 'impending protein crisis' were such that the UN's Protein Advisory Group (PAG) was created in 1955 in order to 'fight to close the protein gap'.[3] By 1962, Marcel Autret, then director of the FAO's nutrition division, explained that, in the organisation's view, 'the number one problem … for national agricultural departments is the production of protein foods of good quality'.[4] Although the winds of change were beginning to sweep away colonial governments, they did little to change the direction of medical thinking in Africa, and former colonial officers continued to dictate the direction of nutrition research long into independence. As the Ghanaian public health pioneer Fred Sai explained in the 1970s, reflecting on his work with Ghana's early nutrition programme, 'you can overthrow a government very much more readily that you can change members of the civil service'.[5]

In this environment, and in the shadow of the 'impending protein crisis', international agencies and Western governments concentrated on the high-tech production of protein foods. In what Tom Scott-Smith describes as the 'high-modernist' approach to nutrition, researchers around the world continued the trend previously displayed in works like *Gold Coast Nutrition and Cookery* and strove to construct culturally alien high-protein 'foodstuffs' which played into the continuing dislocation of nutrition from food. British Petroleum, for instance, created Single-Cell Proteins grown on oil, while others created Leaf-Protein Concentrates, green jelly-like substances which were produced by putting inedible leaves through a centrifuge. Fish-Protein Concentrate, offal left over from filleting or the whole of a 'junk fish' proved fairly popular. Chlorella was less so, comprising a single-cell form of algae which was grown on sewage. Nonetheless, as food grown entirely on waste, it did represent the crowning achievement of modernist nutrition and is still available, marketed as a health food.[6] The modernist obsession seeped into burgeoning African academies too, with Fred Sai and other members of Ghana's nutrition community showing considerable interest in technical approaches to protein deficiency, and with a mind to population growth.[7]

Slowly, though, the relative position of protein and calories in global nutrition was reconsidered. Dietary histories of kwashiorkor patients were reassessed and found to generally be deficient in calories as well as protein and, following a series of publications questioning the degree of protein needed to prevent and treat kwashiorkor in infants, the UN system slashed its recommended protein allowances.[8] The estimated requirements of protein for a one-year-old were, for instance, dropped to 1.1 g/kg a day in 1965, down markedly from the 2.0 g/kg a day recommended by the 1957 report.[9] Despite this, even in 1970 it was reported that 'the FAO as part of its Indicative World Plan for Agricultural Development (IWP), continue to be pessimistic [about the supply of protein] for most parts of the developing world'.[10]

It was only following a number of pointed publications written by Donald McLaren in the later 1960s that the growing incidence of marasmus was highlighted as a more pressing nutritional problem than any worldwide protein deficit. In 1966, McLaren explained that:

> The future is fraught with danger and at present we are ill-prepared to meet it. Marasmus is already underestimated, and all the indications are that it is rapidly on the increase as an epiphenomenon of the half-assimilated modernising process engulfing the developing regions of the world. On the other hand, kwashiorkor, under the same influences, is dying out.[11]

In 1974, McLaren famously suggested that the overt concentration on kwashiorkor should be considered a 'great protein fiasco' which had undervalued non-Western diets while simultaneously ignoring localised patterns of endemic marasmus.[12] McLaren's criticism of this trajectory was, at the 1966 International Congress of Nutrition, immediately met with 'public rejoinders from "the establishment" defending the party line'. However, 'in private I was told by many delegates that they agreed but were afraid to say so aloud for fear of having their support cut off'.[13]

Epidemic marasmus continued to spread into the postcolonial world as breastmilk substitutes, promoted overtly at first by retreating imperial governments, were given the tacit approval of those internationalist organisations which had grown to occupy their space in the postcolonial world.[14] Poorly regulated markets combined with poorly equipped medical systems to open the door to European manufacturers of baby foods. Nestlé employees dressed as nurses plied maternity wards in order to push breastmilk substitutes onto new and expectant mothers, while the budding mass media similarly advised them to 'choose Cow and Gate milk food for your baby and watch him thrive from the very first bottle'.[15] Despite their internationalist mandates, UNICEF, the FAO, and the WHO were loath to speak out against predatory marketing strategies. Vigorous criticism from such organisations could be recognised as economic interventionism and an attack on those free market doctrines pursued by their primary state sponsors. Instead, and as late as 1973, the UN PAG advised that 'in any country lacking breastmilk substitutes, it is urgent that infant formulas be developed and introduced'.[16]

In the mid-1970s, following the increasingly barbed arguments of McLaren and others, the protein bubble eventually burst. The UN, previously principal scaremonger for 'a world protein problem', made no mention of any global protein deficit during its 1974 World Food Conference.[17] The next year, in a word-for-word reversal of the conclusions made in *Nutrition in the Colonial Empire*, two prominent British nutritionists (both of whom had cut their teeth under imperial administrations), explained in an article in *Nature* that 'the problem is mainly one of quantity rather than quality of food', clarifying that 'the protein gap is a myth, and that what really exists, even for vulnerable groups, is a food gap and an energy gap'.[18] The epidemiology of marasmus was soon re-evaluated and the pathology of kwashiorkor soon reconsidered, with one 1980 study concluding 'that energy was generally a limiting nutrient before protein'.[19] By the mid-1980s, the pursuit of expensive, technical solutions to protein deficiency in resource-poor settings was receiving unreserved criticism in the medical press. One project pursuing the development of the 'winged bean' was denounced by LSHTM faculty members as constituting part of 'a continuing process of justifying scientific enthusiasms by the drawing of facile and tenuous links between research which is intellectually exciting to the investigator and problems which are of sufficient public concern to make it politically attractive to devote funds to them'.[20]

The biology of kwashiorkor remained scientifically interesting, though, primarily because of the complicated pathology of the oedema seen in kwashiorkor. Studies into the presentation of adult 'famine oedema' had long discounted the exclusive influence of protein, since swelling also appeared in patients with no history of low-protein diets.[21] Drawing from these studies, Michael Golden – one of the nutritionists most intimately involved with the development of modern therapeutic foods – concluded in a 1982 *Lancet* article that 'no independent effect of protein intake on either loss or accumulation of oedema could be demonstrated'.[22] The explanation that kwashiorkor results simply from inadequate protein intake was apparently oversimplistic, and a considerable amount of contradictory evidence led Golden, among others, to conclude that 'oedematous malnutrition in the child or adult is not caused by protein deficiency; such a concept can lead to fatal therapeutic error in oedematous malnutrition treatment'. This article goes on to suggest that a shortage of antioxidants was the cause of oedematous malnutrition, something disputed by a 2005 study which concluded that the administration of antioxidants failed to prevent the onset of kwashiorkor in over 2,000 Malawian preschool children.[23] Other researchers doubting the position of simple protein deficiency in the aetiology of kwashiorkor have forwarded 'dysadaption', mycotoxins, or other free radical damage as the ultimate cause.[24] In any case, the place of protein in the aetiology of kwashiorkor is far from simple, and far from settled. Sadly, relatively little of this later kwashiorkor research was considered in the context of public health. Though the protein bubble may have burst, the othering of African illness and some of the earlier fetishisation of kwashiorkor remained. In a short reply to this new debate, the eminent Ghanaian physician Felix Konotey-Ahulu reminded the international community to look beyond the reductive concentration on diet and to consider the social aetiology of malnutrition, explaining, in a 1994 letter to *The Lancet*, that 'those of us who grew up in the kwashiorkor belt and who have also had the benefit of an excellent medical education cannot help but caution our ministries of health and of social welfare about the danger of missing the social pathology wood for the trees of free radicals and leukotrienes.'[25]

With a broad base in imperial medicine, the trajectory of nutrition research even into the 1970s can be seen as a continuation of the same paternalistic biopolitics which had distorted the 'discovery' of malnutrition in the colonial world. The perceptions of African dietary deficiencies established under colonial rule and in the context of colonial power extended well beyond the period of direct imperial intervention as part of a scientific tradition informed by the imperialist invention of a specific form of malnutrition. The preoccupation with protein in Africa was a politically reactive scientific construction and, by continuing to codify malnutrition as a problem of ecology or understanding well into independence, this formulation understated the role of social and economic change and undermined the development of preventive measures.

The reductive concentration on protein in postcolonial Africa should, therefore, be seen as part of a linear intellectual history beginning with the 1939 publication of *Nutrition in the Colonial Empire*. The 'protein fiasco' can be considered a continuation of the same thought process which allowed the Colonial Office to ignore the possibility that malnutrition was a structural, social problem resulting from the partial integration of Africa into the globalised economy and instead reframe it as an ecological, technical problem which could only be tackled by globalised science.[26] Nutritional science in the twentieth century is, then, inseparable from the earlier politics of colonialism. It is a long-standing convention within the philosophy of science that scientific discovery and understanding is often muddied by the establishment of its own worth. The further science progresses away from each initial discovery, the harder it is to understand the science of that discovery and the processes which had led to it. Even in the postcolonial period, nutritional intervention was built on under-criticised conclusions about nutrition which were largely formed in the skewed scientific environment of tropical medicine and colonial rule.[27] Driven by competition and informed by the socio-political environment, scientific fact does not simply exist in the natural world but is instead created by consensus and maintained by a network of social, cultural, and political alliances. The consensus regarding protein malnutrition was formed in the particular cultural context of imperial Africa and was strengthened by the networks of Western researchers which continue to underpin perseverant ideas regarding African exceptionalism and justify European authority over Africa.

Malthus and malnutrition

During the colonial period, kwashiorkor research was pursued because it was scientifically interesting and promoted as politically passive – an inevitable consequence of a generalised African food environment. However, Western approaches to nutrition in Africa changed quickly in the postcolonial climate, where responsibility for African hunger could be less readily ascribed to the actions of European polities. As with the construction of endemic protein deficiency in earlier years, understandings of African malnutrition developed in conjunction with the post-colonial political discourse. The refiguring of African deficiency into a problem of calories cannot be divorced from these external political conditions. In the same way that protein was a biopolitical object manipulated both consciously and subconsciously by colonial administrators, calories, food aid and famine relief were utilised as biopolitical objects and agents for the control and coercion of postcolonial governments. The political ascendency of neo-Malthusian thinking in the later twentieth century coincided with postcolonial conflict, economic decline, and the African food crisis in order to colour the science of nutrition. It is, perhaps more than anything else, the politics of African populations that has determined the modern history of nutrition in Africa.

Demography has long been an essential part of the scientific and social-scientific discourse around poverty and hunger in Africa. Although inconsistent, demographic anxieties and population politics shaped colonial planning across the continent.[28] During the early years of colonial rule it was generally assumed that African populations were declining, in terms of both size and vigour, and that only through imperial intervention might improvements be seen. In extremely invasive regimes, as in the Belgian Congo, colonial governments and expatriate companies explicitly promoted high birth rates and short birth spacing through financial incentives.[29] However, as Africa's population exploded under the relative stability of colonial government, demographers began to construct a view of Africa's population growth as unsustainable and overreaching the ecological restraints of a poorly endowed continent. Encouraged by the increasing incidence of drought and famine, in the 1970s something of a consensus was formed along these lines.[30] 'Overpopulation' has since become a recurring motif in modern discourses regarding Africa, while 'population pressure' is still often used to explain high continental burdens of poverty, famine, and disease.[31] Narrowly framed as a ratio of food production to population, given Africa's limited industrialisation the neo-Malthusian conceptualisation of African hunger could be addressed either through the expansion of food production or through population control. In practice, this meant either a 'green revolution' which could expand agricultural capacity through the introduction of new crop varieties, or the widespread adoption of contraception. In both cases, and as was the case with the colonised epidemiology of 'endemic' kwashiorkor, postcolonial hunger could only be solved through technical fixes generally peddled by Western governments and promoted by Western initiative.[32]

In the 1940s and 1950s some agencies, including John Boyd Orr's FAO, favoured addressing problems of food production and distribution and assumed that the deployment of Western science could establish a world of plenty, where equitable food supply and mortality reduction would regulate standards of living and precede a natural fertility decline.[33] Others, such as the increasingly powerful Rockefeller-funded Population Council, sought to curb population growth through fertility control.[34] Using the 'transition model', demographers at first assumed that fertility decline would follow the preindustrial European pattern, resulting from improved socioeconomic conditions and falling mortality rates. However, the social precursors to mortality and fertility declines in the nation states of preindustrial Europe – exemplified by conflict and famine prevention and improvements in health and agriculture – were often absent in the tumultuous political environment of postcolonial Africa. As many African countries began to record economic growth with little indication of fertility decline, demographers instead began to assume that population growth might actually undo the benefits of development and that fertility had to first be reduced in order to make room for development.[35] This rather negated a modernist or welfarist approach to food reform. What instead emerged was a view of African poverty and hunger which problematised female fertility rather than social and economic inequality or the inequitable distribution of food. This narrative suited Western agendas, emphasising the extension of Western medicine and the positive effects of mortality reduction while simultaneously ignoring recent changes to food production and food security.

Given the growing consensus regarding the solution to Africa's 'population problem', it did not take long for Western agencies to intervene in African population policy. However, the new conceptualisation of African hunger was born from troubling scientific principles.[36] Eugenicist and often explicitly racialised approaches to contraception had formed the foundations of early family planning initiatives. For instance, the foremost voices in American contraception colluded to explicitly target black fertility. Margaret Sanger, founder of the American Birth Control League, and Clarence Gamble, founder of the Pathfinder Fund and heir to the Procter and Gamble soap company fortune, created the 'Negro Project' which claimed that 'the mass of Negroes, particularly in the South, still breed carelessly and disastrously'.[37] In South Africa, where African women generally had higher fertility rates than European women, African fertility was a particular worry for the future of Apartheid.[38]

Following the Second World War, eugenics largely fell out of vogue. However, ecology and environmentalism picked up neo-Malthusian critiques of high-fertility populations and have run with them ever since. Hugely popular works such as Stanford University ecologist Paul Ehrlich's *The Population Bomb* startled audiences, highlighting the ecological impact of overpopulation and making sombre predictions regarding upcoming global catastrophe. Written in 1968, *The Population Bomb* had sold over three million copies by 1978.[39] University of California biologist Garrett Hardin's influential 1968 *Science* paper, 'The Tragedy of the Commons', gave a philosophical framework to these new concerns. Hardin suggested that welfarism and access to commonly held property or land was at the root of the population problem, going on to ask 'how shall we deal with the family, the religion, the race, or the class ... that adopts overbreeding as a policy to secure its own aggrandizement?'[40]

'The Tragedy of the Commons' stigmatised the ambitions of the poor – it was eugenic, anti-democratic, and anti-socialist, and gave rousing justification for the moral authority of class stratification, private property, and capital accumulation. It fitted perfectly into Cold War political and economic theory and later neoliberal demographic thinking, which, as early as the 1950s, had prompted the World Bank to expressly warn loan-seeking countries about the economic impacts of unfettered population growth.[41]

The spreading neo-Malthusianism typified by Hardin was already enshrined in the Cold War containment policies pursued by Western governments and their internationalist agents, who saw overpopulation as the source of the conditions which attracted peasants to communism.[42] Population control measures became an increasingly important and consistent feature of European and North American foreign policy and national security planning.[43] In the 1950s, and with the tacit approval of Western governments, private groups such as the International Planned Parenthood Federation (IPPF) and the Pathfinder Fund began to establish birth control clinics across Africa. By the 1960s, the United States Agency for International Development (USAID) and the British Ministry of Overseas Development began to directly fund birth control programmes, often explicitly tying the provision of food aid to the implementation of population control programmes.[44] Here, Western financing of fertility manipulation plays into the debate concerning 'soft power', non-governmental organisation (NGO) involvement in Africa, and the erosion of state sovereignty by wealthy non-state actors.[45] More generally, the coercive implementation of family planning programmes can be seen as a continuation of the domestic engineering first attempted by colonial governments.[46]

Host countries, however, were not entirely convinced that fertility management was necessary. Although Ghana's official attempt at population control began in 1969, Sai explained that, at the 1974 Bucharest World Population Conference, 'African countries attended in some strength; but they attended in some strength to present the view that population did not fit into African aspirations or African development'.[47] Despite this, by the 1980s virtually every nation in sub-Saharan Africa had implemented family planning programmes, largely at the behest of Western donors.[48] In more recent years, climate change has further promoted Western pressure on African nations to impose population controls, despite the fact that Africa is a net victim of climate crisis.

The enduring absence of fertility decline was initially understood as an inconsistency between the preference for a smaller family and the knowledge needed to limit family size. Largely unquestioned until the late 1980s, the 'KAP-gap' (KAP being 'knowledge, attitude, and practice') emphasised an unmet need for family planning services even though 'the overwhelming majority of women who want no more children or who want to postpone fertility ... are behaving in a manner consistent with that goal'.[49] Overpopulation, and, by extension, malnutrition, was, therefore, conceptualised as the result of educational shortcomings, social backwardness, political intransigence, and an often uniquely African failure to adapt or modernise. In reality, as anthropological research on African populations has since shown, fertility generally responds to the culturally specific internal logics of childbearing as pertains to value, health, timing, or honour.[50] Rational calculations regarding family size were a muted part of the Western demographic transition too, but it is only recent scholarship which has illuminated this.[51]

Changes in demographic thought both reflected and informed contemporary changes in nutritional science. Beginning in the 1950s, the feminisation and Africanisation of African medical services had contributed to a discourse which gave greater consideration to the social and economic causes of nutritional illness, many of which were understood to be tied to the trials of motherhood in modern Africa.[52] Doctors across the continent began to consider the interaction between malnutrition and poverty and the ways that urbanisation and economic modernisation were interrupting the social and demographic mechanisms which had previously prevented malnutrition.[53] Influenced by increasingly socialised and gender-conscious perspectives, contraception was understood by many in Africa as a vital tool to combat malnutrition in a modernising economy. Following on from his nutrition work, Fred Sai, for instance, became a vocal crusader for the use of contraception in Africa, eventually becoming president of the IPPF.[54] The extension of family planning to poor communities can undoubtedly grant women valuable agency over their own childbearing. However, as a policy measure against malnutrition, the extension of family planning services was another technical fix for a symptom of colonial underdevelopment and postcolonial malaise. It did little to address the root causes of malnutrition and instead actively helped to obscure structural shortcomings by giving credence to neo-Malthusian narratives of African hunger.

Malthusian thinking also combined with a continental food crisis which was as much political as it was ecological. The food deficit seen in Ghana was matched across the continent, with per capita food output dropping by around 1 per cent per year between the 1960s and the mid-1980s, when the decline started to slow.[55] This justified the neo-Malthusian model of African hunger and the need for family planning, while also apparently necessitating overseas involvement in African food security. Elsewhere, in Asia or South America, hotter spots in the Cold War, agricultural modernisation was the primary method promoted by Western governments in order to stem population pressure and leftist insurgency.[56] In Africa, however, the green revolution never really took off. Stymied by hostile environments and unsuitable variants of high-yielding crops, output from experimental farms was usually quite poor.[57] Nor did green revolution techniques suit the craft of African peasant production, which deftly utilises a wide range of crops adapted to small variations in soil and climate.[58] More generally, though, the political will which brought the green revolution (as well as its social and economic problems) to Asia and South America was largely absent from Africa. Instead, African food security was propped up with foreign food. In 1954 the US Agricultural Trade Development and Assistance Act, commonly known as PL480 or 'Food for Peace', came into being, soon becoming integral to US foreign policy as well as an important outlet for surplus agricultural produce.[59] PL480 initially aimed to dispose of surplus commodities either in the form of humanitarian assistance or as subsidised food for friendly countries. However, as NGOs began running autonomous food distribution programmes during the 1960s, PL480 also found a ready market for fortified and blended foods made from soy or skimmed milk and built on modernist, technical approaches to malnutrition.[60]

Through fertility manipulation and the extension of food aid, Western agencies formulated technocratic attacks on African hunger without the explicit authority of the host states. The politics of population gave the intellectual impetus for these developments. Over the course of the twentieth century, demography problematised 'overpopulation' as an issue of women's fertility for which Western contraceptive innovation was the best solution. Nutritional science followed suit, in turn targeting a reformulated conceptualisation of African malnutrition as a symptom of overpopulation. In the same way that kwashiorkor was a racialised and othered form of deficiency in an ostensibly universalist science, 'overpopulation' and, by extension, hunger were understood as problems of African otherness, results of incomplete modernisation and a particularly African inability to adapt. This conceptualisation of African deficiency allowed for the continuation of the expatriate-led, technical approaches to malnutrition which had defined colonial developments in nutritional science. Perhaps more importantly, the return of Malthusian explanations for political and economic shortcomings set the stage for the neoliberal economic reforms of the 1980s, and for the very particular approach to nutrition care which grew up under the free market framework.

The international development of neoliberal nutrition

Neo-Malthusianism is an important intellectual touchstone for neoliberal economics. For neo-Malthusians and for free market fundamentalists, famine is a natural check on populations exceeding their means. Given a chance – and adequate access to fertility limitation – the invisible hand could balance these populations. However, statist interventions in the market, usually in terms of unwarranted redistributive transfers, were understood to have allowed populations to swell beyond their natural bounds, resulting in poverty, malnutrition, and environmental degradation. Although natural and perhaps necessary to some observers, starvation was still just as repugnant in the globalised political economy as it was under British governance. However, unlike under empire, where the narrative of African exceptionalism clouded the political realities of African hunger, internationalist approaches to postcolonial poverty normalised a view that independent African states could not provide for their subjects but immersion into the globalised economy could. In the postcolony, hunger ultimately justified the neoliberal project, the outsourcing of famine relief, and the circumvention of state authority over the broad biopolitics of food and nutrition.

In the 1980s, the conditionalities tied to IMF and World Bank loans brought African economies more fully into the global marketplace. States undertaking SAPs have been encouraged to support market-led development by reducing taxation, leaving less tax revenue available for the subsidisation of public services and healthcare programmes. This process increased the presence of NGO and charity bodies in African healthcare and nutrition management. As we will see in the next chapter, the first generation of adjustment policies did little to shore up nutrition security for marginalised groups, leading eventually to the UNICEF proposal of 'adjustment with a human face' and the World Bank's 'food security approach' in the late 1980s.[61] However, as Alex de Waal explains in his now classic account of modern hunger, this approach 'focuses on the social and economic dimensions and excludes the political. Structural adjustment involved a tremendous reconfiguring of political power and responsibility.' Perhaps more importantly, 'it has reinforced the trends towards treating famine as a technical economic issue rather than a political one'.[62] Malnutrition was treated in much the same way, echoing the colonial construction of malnutrition.[63]

However, that is not to say that internationalist technical approaches to nutrition were unsuccessful. At the start of the 1990s inpatient mortality rates were between 20 and 30 per cent – the same rates as the 1950s – despite known protocols which could drop mortality to as little as 1 to 5 per cent.[64] By 1993 the widespread failure to translate clinical knowledge into practice was being condemned as 'nutrition malpractice'.[65] Regarding the state of kwashiorkor research in 1994, McLaren wrote:

> Two things greatly impressed me – how little original work has been done in the past two decades and how little progress has been made towards controlling kwashiorkor. The two could be linked, but an "off with the old and on with the new" attitude will not help.[66]

Seeing as the primary thrust of nutrition research had been fatally undermined, nutrition research was languishing in the years after the 'protein fiasco'. However, the dramatic reduction of state-based nutrition programmes and the sharp rise of malnutrition which generally accompanied the neoliberal political economy gave nutritionists renewed purpose and new space in which to operate. Partly as a result of this, the greatest technical successes in nutrition intervention and the cure of severe protein energy malnutrition only began to emerge in the late 1990s and early 2000s.

There can be no doubt that these were among the most laudable medical advances against the human tragedy of malnutrition. Realising that calorie deficits had to be addressed in conjunction with protein deficiencies, by the early 1990s high-energy milk-based formulas were seen to provide effective treatment. F-75 and F-100 provided a relatively low amount of protein but proved their worth in the initial treatment of severe malnutrition (F-75) and in catch-up growth (F-100), eventually forming a central part of WHO treatment guidelines.[67] By the mid-2000s, 'community-based' solutions to malnutrition became more viable due to the formulation of home-based treatments, generally consisting of single-serve sachets of Ready-to-use therapeutic food (RUTF).[68] Oil-based RUTFs – the most successful and well-known of which is Plumpy'nut – were more appropriate for at-home use than those which used water and could easily harbour bacteria, although F-75 is still generally used among inpatients.[69] Community-based management of acute malnutrition (CMAM) is now pursued by many health ministries as an efficient and cost-effective treatment for malnutrition. It utilises the triage of malnourished children, using mid-upper arm circumference (MUAC) bands and the diagnosis of potential complications, so that most patients can now be deemed 'uncomplicated' and treated as outpatients, saving hospitals bed space and staff time. This system has also proved popular with parents, who no longer have to give their child up to a far-away clinic for weeks at a time, saving time and contributing to a lower loss of earnings.[70]

The home-based palliative approach, using RUTFs, has slashed malnutrition mortality and has been rightly heralded as a revolution in nutritional science. However, there are enduring concerns relating to the social, political, and historical contexts in which new nutrition treatments are utilised.[71] In the West, the high-modernist approach to the imagined protein shortage quickly dissipated. Heavily constructed foods soon became grotesque and eventually a thing of popular dystopian fiction: the amphetamine-laced milk 'Moloko Plus' in Anthony Burgess's 1962 novel *A Clockwork Orange* or 'Soylent Green', the high-protein ration made from human remains in the classic 1973 sci-fi film of the same name.[72] This thinking presaged the more recent 'eco-dietetics' or 'food quality' paradigm shift which has moved understandings of nutrition away from the science of nutrients in favour of a more holistic approach to diet rooted in environmentalism or evolutionary anthropology.[73] In many postcolonial countries, however, modernist and technical approaches to deficiency were much more resilient and simply shifted with the science of the day. Protein foods were initially manufactured from surplus food residues by big European companies, exploiting hunger and malnutrition in the space created by the narrative of the protein gap. In conjunction with the Peruvian government and the FAO, Nestlé made Peruvita. Unigate worked with UNICEF in Northern Nigeria to produce Arlac. Coca-Cola made Saci, a high-protein drink in Brazil. Glaxo produced the peanut-based Amama in Nigeria.[74] Manufactured under licence in France 1994, Plumpy'nut is nothing new but its innovative oil base and its restrictive licensing earned its enduring status as well as questions regarding the ethics of intellectual property in the realm of humanitarian relief.[75] Plumpy'nut is simply a successful outlier in the long history of commercialised aid, propagated by Western industrial concerns and skewed by scientific preoccupations.[76] For instance, when PL480 was passed in 1954 it was envisaged as a precursor to the development of a profitable market for agricultural surpluses.[77] Constructed from those same surpluses, 'nutraceutical' foods now also contribute to these ends. Initially marketed to the third sector, they are now sold directly to the world's poor as a food-free solution to the symptoms of their own poverty.[78]

However, Plumpy'nut has also endured because it perfectly complements the political economy of Africa's adjustment era. Like MUAC bands and CMAM protocols, the efficacy of Plumpy'nut – which aims to bring a child to their target weight in 6 to 10 weeks – has caused its deification among humanitarian organisations at the same time as it undermines the state by suggesting that technology and the free market can better fill its space.[79] Hospital treatments for malnutrition had been lacking in any case but, established in response to the diminished capacity of the state to provide even these services, CMAM and Plumpy'nut have begun to make state-run nutrition programmes an irrelevancy. RUTFs are an effective palliative to hunger but they also normalise the idea that neither national health services nor their attendant food economies can provide adequate nutrition security, thus justifying the position of internationalist organs which can.[80]

Again, we can return to Foucault to consider these changes. Tom Scott-Smith suggests that discussing nutrition supplements with reference to 'biopower' lacks relevance in refugee or crisis contexts 'because many humanitarian activities operate not through a dispersed, productive power, but in the opposite manner: in a way that is top-down, controlling, and paternalistic'.[81] However, in non-crisis contexts, where nutrition care forms an important aspect of everyday maternal and child health programmes, biopower becomes more relevant. As part of an ordinary pursuit of health, RUTFs and internationalist organisations move into the space and appropriate the power which might have been wielded by a functioning healthcare system. It should therefore be no surprise that RUTFs and CMAM grew in prominence under neoliberal governments. They facilitated an increasingly inequitable economy with minimal state involvement in an increasingly individualistic social environment. The irony of 'community-based' approaches to malnutrition, served in individual, sealed sachets and donated by foreign governments or aid agencies, is particularly tragic when we consider kwashiorkor in its original context, as a disease of social disintegration. In the same way as bottled milk some 50 years earlier, RUTFs have become a crutch to help bear the growing weight of childrearing in modern Africa. Malnutrition is a symptom of a complex of social, political, and economic failures, and nutritional science can only ever address malnutrition as a symptom of structural shortcomings. Sadly, by doing so, it also abets its continuing causation.

Born from tropical medicine, arranged through colonial networks, and based upon the imperialistic othering of African diet, postcolonial nutrition shares a great deal with colonial nutrition at the international level. As Sasson and Vernon have explained with reference to the organisation of postcolonial famine relief agencies, 'these experts did not always serve the purpose of the British government and were thus not necessarily neo-colonial'. However, they continued to operate 'on a system of knowledge which was cost-effective and aimed at creating self-governing subjects'.[82] In much the same way, postcolonial developments in food security and nutrition care were born from colonial knowledge and postcolonial anxieties and were largely designed to circumvent state involvement. Given the tumultuous political environment which characterised much of postcolonial Africa, this is not necessarily surprising. The MRC's primary overseas nutrition unit was, for instance, uprooted from Kampala as a result of the Amin regime, eventually relocating to The Gambia in 1973.[83] Clearly, African political agency also had the potential to disrupt the biopolitics previously regulated by tropical medicine and the health provisioning offered by various colonial states. This does not necessarily mean that postcolonial science was neo-colonial but, in much the same way as under colonial government, scientific approaches to hunger and malnutrition had to operate in the space they were granted by contemporary political economies. The enduring dominance of Western academies, with respect to medicine, demography, economics, and biology, skewed any debate by forwarding technical fixes and Western involvement as solutions to structural problems born from social disruption. All too often, internationalist approaches addressed hunger and malnutrition in ahistorical and apolitical terms which failed to look beyond narrow economic understandings of food and nutrition insecurity. Flourishing first under colonial rule, the technical approach to famine, food security, and malnutrition peaked with the spread of neoliberal governance. This, as de Waal again explains, is part of a trend which 'obscures the contradiction between the neoliberal enterprise and the historical fact that effective action against famine has always been achieved by interventionist social and economic programmes'.[84]

Notes

1 This chapter is a revised version of John Nott, '"How Little Progress"? A Political Economy of Postcolonial Nutrition', *Population and Development Review*, 44.4 (2018), 771–91.

2 *Protein Malnutrition: Proceedings of a Conference in Jamaica, 1953*, ed. by J.C. Waterlow (Cambridge: Cambridge University Press for the FAO, WHO and Josiah Macy Jr. Foundation, 1955), p. 4.

3 FAO/WHO/UNICEF Protein Advisory Group, *Lives in Peril: Protein and the Child.* (Rome: FAO, World Food Problems, no. 12, 1970), p. 51; Carpenter, *Protein and Energy*, p. 162. Similar

concerns were also expressed by the colonial medical administration in late 1930s and early 1940s Uganda but cannot be divorced from the colonial context. Scrimshaw is presenting the view of nutritionists.

4 M. Autret, 'Protein Malnutrition and the FAO Viewpoint', in *Progress in Meeting Protein Needs of Infants and Pre-School Children: Proceedings of an International Conference Held in Washington, D.C., August 21–24, 1960. Under the Auspices of the Committee on Protein Malnutrition, Food and Nutrition Board, and the Nutrition Study Section, National Institutes of Health*, ed. by National Academy of Sciences (Washington, D.C.: National Academy of Sciences, 1961), pp. 537–43 (p. 537).

5 Sai, 'Nutrition in Ghana', p. 100.

6 Tom Scott-Smith, 'Defining Hunger, Redefining Food: Humanitarianism in the Twentieth Century' (unpublished DPhil, University of Oxford, 2014), pp. 165–91.

7 Fred T. Sai, 'Introducing New Foods Against Protein Deficiency', *Nutrition Reviews*, 18.12 (1960), 353–5; D.R. MacGregor, *Non-Traditional Food Sources for Feeding Increasing Populations: An Inaugural Lecture Delivered on Thursday, 26th October 1972, at the University of Ghana, Legon* (Accra: University of Ghana, 1972).

8 Carpenter, *Protein and Energy*, pp. 180–203.

9 FAO Committee on Protein Requirements, *Protein Requirements* (Rome: FAO Nutritional Studies, no. 16, 1957); FAO/WHO Expert Group, *Protein Requirements* (Geneva: WHO Technical Report, no. 301, 1965).

10 FAO/WHO/UNICEF Protein Advisory Group, *Lives in Peril*, p. 41.

11 D.S. McLaren, 'A Fresh Look at Protein-Calorie Malnutrition', *The Lancet*, 288.7461 (1966), 485–88 (p. 488).

12 D.S. McLaren, 'The Great Protein Fiasco', *The Lancet*, 304.7872 (1974), 93–6.

13 McLaren, 'Fiasco', p. 94.

14 Gabrielle Palmer, *The Politics of Breastfeeding: When Breasts Are Bad for Business* (London: Pinter & Martin, 2009), pp. 238–59.

15 Mike Muller, *The Baby Killer: A War on Want Investigation into the Promotion and Sale of Powdered Milks in the Third World* (London: War on Want, 1974), p. 10.

16 'Promotion of special foods (infant formula and processed protein foods) for vulnerable groups', PAG statement no. 23, 18 July 1972, revised 28 November 1973. Quoted in Andrew Chetley, *The Politics of Baby Foods* (London: F. Pinter, 1986), p. 41.

17 United Nations, *Report of the World Food Conference, Rome, 5–16th November 1974* (New York: United Nations Press, 1975); Kenneth J. Carpenter, 'A Short History of Nutritional Science: Part 4 (1945–1985)', *The Journal of Nutrition*, 133.11 (2003), 3331–42 (p. 3337).

18 J.C. Waterlow and P.R. Payne, 'The Protein Gap', *Nature*, 258.5531 (1975), 113–17.

19 J. Landman and A.A. Jackson, 'The Role of Protein Deficiency in the Aetiology of Kwashiorkor', *The West Indian Medical Journal*, 29.4 (1980), 229–38.

20 C.J.K. Henry, P.A. Donachie, and J.P.W. Rivers, 'The Winged Bean: Will the Wonder Crop Be Another Flop?', *Ecology of Food and Nutrition*, 16.4 (1985), 331–8; Carpenter, 'Part 4', p. 3337.

21 McCance, 'History'; Keys et al., *Biology of Human Starvation*, pp. 74, 921–65.

22 M.H. Golden, 'Protein Deficiency, Energy Deficiency, and the Oedema of Malnutrition', *The Lancet*, 1.8284 (1982), 1261–5 (p. 1264).

23 M.H. Golden, 'Oedematous Malnutrition', *British Medical Bulletin*, 54.2 (1998), 433–4 (p. 433); Heather Ciliberto et al., 'Antioxidant Supplementation for the Prevention of Kwashiorkor in Malawian Children: Randomised, Double Blind, Placebo Controlled Trial', *BMJ*, 330.7500 (2005), 1109–11.

24 Truswell, 'Protein-Energy Malnutrition', p. 304.

25 F.I.D. Konotey-Ahulu, 'Issues in Kwashiorkor', *The Lancet*, 343.8896 (1994), 548.

26 Worboys, 'Discovery', p. 221.

27 Bruno Latour, *Science in Action: How to Follow Scientists and Engineers through Society* (Milton Keynes: Open University Press, 1987), pp. 2–3.

28 For the inconsistent history of demography and population politics in imperial settings, see Karl Ittmann, *A Problem of Great Importance: Population, Race, and Power in the British Empire, 1918–1973* (Berkeley, CA: University of California Press, 2014); Samuël Coghe, *Population Politics in the Tropics: Demography, Health and Transimperialism in Colonial Angola* (Cambridge: Cambridge University Press, 2022). For more general histories of demography,

see Alison Bashford, *Global Population: History, Geopolitics, and Life on Earth* (New York: Columbia University Press, 2014); Emily Klancher Merchant, 'Prediction and Control: Global Population, Population Science, and Population Politics in the Twentieth Century' (unpublished PhD, University of Michigan, 2015).

29 Hunt, '"Le Bebe En Brousse"'.

30 See, for instance, Robert W. Steel, 'Problems of Population Pressure in Tropical Africa', *Transactions of the Institute of British Geographers*, 49 (1970), 1–14.

31 For example, Iliffe, *African Poor*, pp. 253–4.

32 Karl Ittmann, '"Where Nature Dominates Man": Demographic Ideas and Policy in British Colonial Africa, 1890–1970', in *The Demographics of Empire*, ed. by Karl Ittmann, Dennis D. Cordell, and Gregory H. Maddox (Athens, OH: Ohio University Press, 2010), pp. 59–88 (p. 76).

33 Bashford, *Global Population*, p. 303.

34 Merchant, 'Prediction and Control', p. 319.

35 Simon Szreter, 'The Idea of Demographic Transition and the Study of Fertility Change: A Critical Intellectual History', *Population and Development Review*, 19.4 (1993), 659–701.

36 Ittmann, *Problem*, pp. 147–76.

37 'Negro project' proposal, quoted in Linda Perlman Gordon, *Woman's Body, Woman's Right: Birth Control in America* (New York: Penguin, 1990), p. 328.

38 See, for instance, Susanne Klausen, 'The Race Welfare Society: Eugenics and Birth Control in Johannesburg, 1930–40', in *Science and Society in Southern Africa*, ed. by Saul Dubow (Manchester: Manchester University Press, 2000), pp. 164–87.

39 Merchant, 'Prediction and Control', p. 442.

40 Garrett Hardin, 'The Tragedy of the Commons', *Science*, 162.3859 (1968), 1243–8 (p. 1246). This view was also commonly held in late-colonial Africa, with freehold land tenure considered the necessary response to population growth environmental decline. See, for instance, Hugh Dow, *East Africa Royal Commission 1953–1955 Report* (London: HMSO, 1955).

41 Merchant, 'Prediction and Control', pp. 324–7.

42 Ittmann, *Problem*, p. 171.

43 On the earlier, varied history of population politics, see Ittmann, *Problem*; Coghe, *Population Politics in the Tropics*.

44 Ittmann, '"Where Nature"', p. 75.

45 Firoze Manji and Carl O'Coill, 'The Missionary Position: NGOs and Development in Africa', *International Affairs*, 78.3 (2002), 567–83.

46 Agnes Czerwinski Riedmann, *Science That Colonizes: A Critique of Fertility Studies in Africa* (Philadelphia, PA: Temple University Press, 1993).

47 Fred T. Sai, 'Changing Perspectives of Population in Africa and International Responses', *African Affairs*, 87.347 (1988), 267–76 (p. 270).

48 Sai, 'Changing Perspectives'.

49 Charles F. Westoff, 'Is the KAP-Gap Real?', *Population and Development Review*, 14.2 (1988), 225–32 (p. 232). See also John Bongaarts, 'The KAP-Gap and the Unmet Need for Contraception', *Population and Development Review*, 17.2 (1991), 293–313.

50 Caroline Bledsoe, *Contingent Lives: Fertility, Time, and Aging in West Africa* (Chicago, IL: University of Chicago Press, 2002); Jennifer Johnson-Hanks, *Uncertain Honor: Modern Motherhood in an African Crisis* (Chicago, IL: University of Chicago Press, 2006).

51 Kate Fisher, *Birth Control, Sex, and Marriage in Britain 1918–1960* (Oxford: Oxford University Press, 2006).

52 Iliffe, *East African Doctors*, p. 141.

53 See, for instance, Sai, 'Urban Life'; Welbourn, 'Bottle Feeding'.

54 Fred T. Sai, *Dr Fred Sai Speaks Out* (London: International Planned Parenthood Federation, 1994).

55 Jean-Philippe Platteau, 'The Food Crisis in Africa: A Comparative Structural Analysis', in *The Political Economy of Hunger: Volume 2, Famine Prevention*, ed. by Jean Drèze and Amartya Sen (Oxford: Oxford University Press, 1991), pp. 279–388.

56 John H. Perkins, *Geopolitics and the Green Revolution: Wheat, Genes, and the Cold War* (Oxford: Oxford University Press, 1997).

57 R.E. Evenson and D. Gollin, 'Assessing the Impact of the Green Revolution, 1960 to 2000', *Science*, 300.5620 (2003), 758–62.

58 John Iliffe, *Africans: The History of a Continent* (Cambridge: Cambridge University Press, 1995), p. 266.
59 See Vernon W. Ruttan, 'The Politics of U.S. Food Aid Policy: A Historical Review', in *Why Food Aid?*, ed. by Vernon W. Ruttan (Baltimore, MD: Johns Hopkins University Press, 1993), pp. 2–38; Jennifer Clapp, *Hunger in the Balance: The New Politics of International Food Aid* (Ithaca, NY: Cornell University Press, 2012).
60 Tom Scott-Smith, 'Beyond the "Raw" and the "Cooked": A History of Fortified Blended Foods', *Disasters*, 39.2 (2015), 244–60 (pp. 254–6).
61 World Bank, *Poverty and Hunger: Issues and Options for Food Security in Developing Countries.* (Washington, D.C.: World Bank, 1986); *Adjustment with a Human Face*, ed. by Giovanni Andrea Cornia, Richard Jolly, and Frances Stewart, 2 vols (Oxford: Clarendon Press, 1987).
62 de Waal, *Famine Crimes*, p. 54.
63 Worboys, 'Discovery', p. 221.
64 C. Schofield and A. Ashworth, 'Why Have Mortality Rates for Severe Malnutrition Remained so High?', *Bulletin of the World Health Organization*, 74.2 (1996), 223–29.
65 A. Berg, 'Sliding toward Nutrition Malpractice: Time to Reconsider and Redeploy', *The American Journal of Clinical Nutrition*, 57.1 (1993), 3–7.
66 D.S. McLaren, 'Issues in Kwashiorkor', *The Lancet*, 343 (1994), 548–9 (p. 549).
67 Golden, 'Development of Concepts', p. 2121S; WHO, *Management of Severe Malnutrition: A Manual for Physicians and Other Senior Health Workers* (Geneva: World Health Organization, 1999).
68 Ann Ashworth, 'Efficacy and Effectiveness of Community-Based Treatment of Severe Malnutrition', *Food and Nutrition Bulletin*, 27.3 (2006), S24–48.
69 André Briend et al., 'Ready-to-Use Therapeutic Food for Treatment of Marasmus', *The Lancet*, 353.9166 (1999), 1767–8.
70 For an excellent survey article regarding recent changes in malnutrition care, see Collins et al., 'Management'.
71 See especially, Tom Scott-Smith, 'The Fetishism of Humanitarian Objects and the Management of Malnutrition in Emergencies', *Third World Quarterly*, 34.5 (2013), 913–28; Tom Scott-Smith, 'Control and Biopower in Contemporary Humanitarian Aid: The Case of Supplementary Feeding', *Journal of Refugee Studies*, 28.1 (2014), 1–17. For the contextualisation of Plumpy'nut, see also Peter Redfield, 'Bioexpectations: Life Technologies as Humanitarian Goods', *Public Culture*, 24.1 66 (2012), 157–84 (pp. 166–70).
72 Scott-Smith, 'Defining Hunger', p. 181.
73 In later years, these ideas have been exported to Africa – again largely through technical projects pursued by NGOs – as part of the food sovereignty and anti-GMO movements. Although there is no room here, these are developments which deserve historical consideration. See Scrinis, *Nutritionism*; Rebrovick, 'Politics of Diet: "Eco-Dietetics"'.
74 Carpenter, *Protein and Energy*, pp. 172–5; Scott-Smith, 'Defining Hunger', p. 213.
75 For instance, Jim Motavalli, 'Let Them Eat Plumpy'Nut', *Foreign Policy*, 8 October 2009 <https://foreignpolicy.com/2009/10/08/let-them-eat-plumpynut/> [accessed 15 June 2016].
76 Scott-Smith, 'Defining Hunger', p. 333.
77 Ruttan, 'Politics'.
78 Street, 'Food as Pharma'.
79 Scott-Smith, 'Fetishism', p. 926; Tom Scott-Smith, 'Humanitarian Neophilia: The "Innovation Turn" and Its Implications', *Third World Quarterly*, 37.12 (2016), 2229–51 (p. 2237).
80 Redfield, 'Bioexpectations', p. 170.
81 Scott-Smith, 'Biopower', p. 25.
82 Tehila Sasson and James Vernon, 'Practising the British Way of Famine: Technologies of Relief, 1770–1985', *European Review of History: Revue Européenne d'histoire*, 22.6 (2015), 860–72 (p. 868).
83 This history is detailed in Tappan, 'Mwanamugimu'.
84 de Waal, *Famine Crimes*, p. 54.

8
Neoliberal nutrition, c.1983–2000

In 1908, the physician and eugenicist Caleb Saleeby's criticism of municipal milk depots in Britain concluded that 'there is no State womb, there are no State breasts, there is no real substitute for the beauty of individual motherhood'.[1] In the context of 'biopolitics' and mounting concerns around 'national efficiency', these ideas were not particularly popular at the time.[2] In fact, by 1943, then Prime Minister Winston Churchill announced that 'there is no finer investment for a community than putting milk into babies'.[3] However, with the emergence of neoliberalism and the promotion of private-sector solutions to problems of public health, during the 1970s and 1980s ideas similar to Saleeby's started to gain traction. In fact, it was the 1971 abandonment of Britain's free school milk programme which earned Margaret Thatcher – then Education Secretary and later one of the greatest proponents of small-state, free market development – her 'milk snatcher' sobriquet.[4]

Neoliberalism might be defined as the retreat of the state from the provision of milk, or healthcare, education, social security, or any other aspect of domestic reproduction. Under the neoliberal model these 'commodities', and human wellbeing in general, is best provided by the advancement of entrepreneurial freedom, personal rights over private property, an unencumbered market, and the free movement of capital. Following the global economic downturn of the 1970s, and the ensuing global debt crisis, economic elites and prominent governments moved away from Keynesian interventionism and towards a neoliberal doctrine which suggested that the benefits of an unbridled market would eventually 'trickle down' to the poor. In a hugely influential 1981 World Bank paper, Elliot Berg explained that Africa's economic crisis derived from excess government involvement in the economy, from protectionism and price subsidisation.[5] Named for the home of the IMF, the World Bank and the US Department of the Treasury, the Washington Consensus formed around these ideas, ultimately dictating the terms by which the IMF would finance reconstruction in poor countries recovering from the economic crises of previous decades. What emerged were the SAPs, which, by 1991, had been implemented in 30 African states.[6]

In Ghana, Structural Adjustment began in April 1983. In the middle of an acute and accelerating economic crisis, and in order to qualify for World Bank loans, the PNDC implemented the IMF's plans for sweeping economic reform. These included immediate 'stabilisation' policies to quickly fix macroeconomic imbalances and longer-term 'adjustment' policies to encourage investment, improve economic efficiency, and promote sustainable growth. The Economic Recovery Programme (ERP), as Ghana's programme of Structural Adjustment became known, included massive social service cuts and staff retrenchment, exchange rate adjustment through the discrete devaluation of the cedi, the abandonment of domestic price controls, privatisation of state-owned enterprise, a huge export drive, rehabilitation of economic infrastructure, and the broadening of the tax base. Macroeconomic growth under adjustment began strongly, and the budget deficits which had haunted previous governments were replaced with a small surplus by the late 1980s. Rapid and consistent GDP/capita growth in the 20 years following adjustment was matched by similarly significant reductions in inflation, repairs to structural imbalances, growth in the provision of goods and services, generation of donor confidence, and the attraction of foreign investment.[7] In terms of how the ERP reformed the macroeconomy, Ghana has been regarded as the World Bank's 'star pupil' and has been referred to as the model for African adjustment.[8]

Despite providing macroeconomic growth and political stability, adjustment policies in Ghana had troubling social consequences.[9] Among them was the enduring prevalence of childhood malnutrition. The Growth Surveillance System of the Catholic Relief Service (CRS) – the only nutrition monitoring system in place during the early 1980s – saw a decline in the nutritional status of Ghanaian children attending child welfare clinics over a short period immediately after adjustment. In 1980, 36 per cent of children aged 7 to 42 months were below 80 per cent of the US National Centre for Health Statistics (NCHS) weight-for-age (underweight) standard. By 1983, at the height of economic crisis, this figure exceeded 50 per cent.[10] Although CRS measurements of clinic attendees suggests that, by 1986, nutritional status had returned to the 1980 level, a national nutrition survey undertaken by the Ghana Government in conjunction with UNICEF found that 58 per cent of children under five years were below 80 per cent of the NCHS weight-for-age standards. This was roughly double the figure found in the 1961–2 National Nutrition Survey. More troubling still was the 8 per cent of children across the country suffering from clinical manifestations of malnutrition – marasmus or kwashiorkor – an incidence around twice as high as was seen in other low-income countries at the time. The epidemiology of malnutrition during these years continued along the north–south nutrition divide, with 64 per cent of children underweight in the savannah and 48 per cent in the coastal zone. By 1989, the World Bank's conclusion regarding malnutrition in Ghana was that 'the problem is serious and getting worse'.[11]

In many respects, Structural Adjustment's impact on the aetiology and epidemiology of malnutrition echoes the effects of colonisation as seen during the first decades of the twentieth century, and as detailed in the first chapters of this book. The abandonment of statist social insurances and the promotion of the productive economy demanded cash-earning and increased market involvement. The highly individualised pursuit of capital influenced the value of social reproduction, domestic labour, and subsistence industry, and created space for familial and gender conflict, new forms of poverty, and social and spatial inequality. Cultural responses to this economic transformation included changes to food cultures and cultures of eating and of caring.[12] Patterns of deficiency reflected these broad social, economic, and cultural shifts. A notable point of departure from the trends observed during the 1930s and 1940s is the sheer quantity of data produced to describe, understand, and improve nutrition in Ghana and throughout the 'Global South'. Since the late 1980s, and increasingly since the Millennium Development Goals were set in 2000, it has become impossible to parse the history of nutrition from the 'audit cultures' which have characterised a new and increasingly global governmentality.[13] As a distinct characteristic of neoliberal nutrition, the pursuit of and deference to statistics has provided a remarkable resource for both historical epidemiology and economic history. However, this phenomenon also demands some explanation as to why statistics have assumed such prominence, and some consideration as to the epidemiological and epistemic limits of metrics for the study of health in general and nutritional health in particular.

Metrics and malnutrition

With significant limitations on governmental expenditure and a diminished national capacity to check the pattern of worsening nutrition, overseas governments and internationalist organisations began to survey the problem instead. Conducted at regular intervals, the large-scale, cross-sectional surveillance programmes conducted in Ghana since the onset of Structural Adjustment have included: the Ghana Living Standards Surveys (GLSS), a World Bank Living Standards Measurement Study (LSMS); the Ghana Demographic and Health Surveys (GDHSs), part of the worldwide USAID-funded DHS series; and the Multiple Indicator Cluster Surveys (MICS), a similar survey run by UNICEF. Much as in the 1930s, when Purcell and other colonial surveyors sought to analyse the deterioration of nutritional health in the wake of colonisation, the massive expansion of nutrition surveillance in the period following Structural Adjustment was part of the broader framing of malnutrition as a technical problem to be solved by technical solutions, rather than a more fundamental political-economic concern (see Chapters 2 and 7).

Both the surveys of the 1930s and those beginning in the 1980s pursued the quantification of nutrition through the collection of anthropometric data, taking the heights and weights of both children and adults in order to suggest spatial, social, and demographic variations in the incidence of malnutrition. However, unlike colonial-era surveillance, much of which had been conducted in a piecemeal manner and was not readily comparable, these new surveys strove to collect standard anthropometric indices in order to allow comparison across time and space. Of particular relevance are BMI, a relatively simple derivation of weight and height measurements which is taken to suggest under- or overweightness, and the more complex and problematic calculation of child growth standards. Unlike BMI, a static measurement, albeit one which has its own troubling history, child growth suggests whether a given child at a given age is above or below a specific growth curve derived from a specific reference population.[14] Surveys like the DHS – probably the most influential extant health surveillance programme – have contributed these biological data to a growing ecosystem of quantified social surveillance. As 'technologies of counting that form global knowledge', this new pursuit of metrics is, according to Vincanne Adams, 'imagined to offer uniform and standardized conversations about how best to intervene, how best to conceptualize health and disease, how best to both count and be accountable, and how best to pay for it all'.[15]

The standardisation of nutrition indicators has allowed for the correlation of anthropometry with numberless other standardised economic, demographic, and biological metrics, offering ostensibly consistent and focused insight into the demographic and microeconomic determinants of nutritional stress.[16] In providing new data for geographical comparison, as well as new means to chart temporal trends in nutrition, this glut of anthropometric data has dominated nutrition epidemiology since the 1980s. Unlike the more fragmentary research of the 1930s, these figures and the methods employed in their construction have become central actors in the recent history of nutrition. While conscious that data are never neutral – always deriving from and contributing to some political purpose – the ubiquity and durability of anthropometrics in contemporary epidemiology mean that these data must be engaged with on their own terms.[17] Indeed, it is only by doing so that we might 'show how the act of data collection becomes always and invariably political'.[18]

The terms of particular significance in contemporary nutrition surveillance are as follows: 'acute' malnutrition, or 'wasting', is classified as low weight-for-height; 'chronic' malnutrition, or 'stunting', is defined as a low height-for-age; 'clinical' malnutrition is usually taken to begin at two standard deviations (SDs) below the WHO's 2006 Multicentre Growth Reference Study (MGRS) reference median. A now-standard curve for plotting childhood growth, the MGRS came into being in order to reorient anthropometric standards away from predominantly White north-Atlantic populations. Children presenting with measurements between two and three SDs below these WHO standards may be considered 'moderately' malnourished, with 'severe' malnutrition beginning at three SDs below. The population's average nutritional status can be taken as the mean deviation from the WHO standard.

Using the four DHS surveys undertaken in Ghana between 1988 and 2003 – the data which is most widely used in contemporary nutrition epidemiology – there are some clear and consistent nationwide patterns. Both acute and chronic malnutrition were more common in the North than the South, in the countryside than the city, and among poor rather than wealthy families. Stunting was considerably more common than wasting, and average height-for-age figures deviate further from WHO standards than weight-for-height, suggesting that sustained undernutrition, rather than periodic severe shortfalls, was the dominant pattern.

More specific results for our areas of particular interest – Greater Accra, the Ashanti Region, and the savannah regions – are less apparent, and it should also be borne in mind that the amalgamated Northern data hides significant variation across individual regions (see Figures 8.1 to 8.4). However, there are some clear if superficial trends. Aside from in the North – which saw a sharp decline in the average weight-for-height and increasing levels of moderate but not severe wasting between 1988 and 1993 – average weight-for-height figures generally improved during these years, with regional disparities narrowing into the 2000s. Yet these average figures hide the incidence of clinical wasting, which rose steadily in Accra in particular, with consistent increases of severe wasting too. Despite a steady fall in the aggregated incidence of clinical wasting, the number of severely wasted children in Ashanti also increased between 1988 and 2003. Perhaps surprisingly, only Northern Ghana saw a net decline in severe wasting over these years. Although nutrition indicators for the average child in Greater Accra and the Ashanti Region improved, the parallel increase in extreme wasting may well speak to a trend of growing inequality. As an indicator of long-term malnutrition, average height-for-age figures are more reflective of the incidence of clinical stunting. Average height-for-age measures for all three areas improved between 1988 and 1998, before falling slightly between 1998 and 2003. Clinical chronic malnutrition also follows this general pattern, aside from in the Ashanti Region, where, in 2003, clinical stunting and average deviation from the WHO height-for-age standard actually worsened against the 1988 figure.

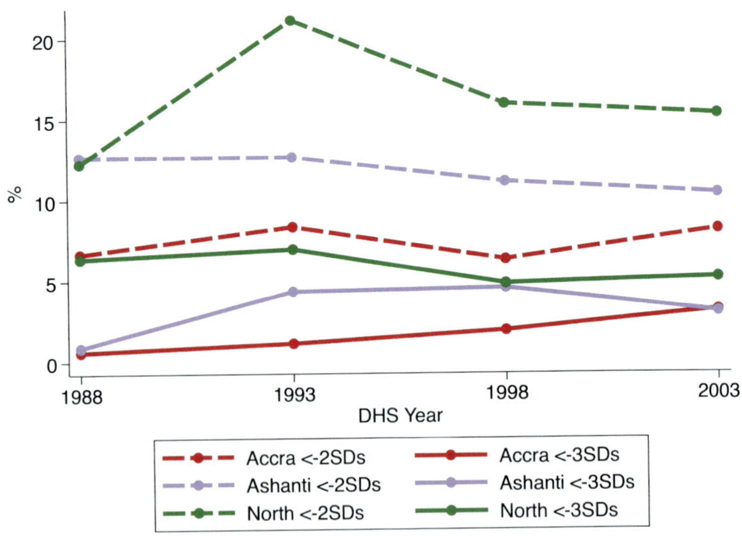

Figure 8.1 Incidence of wasting (weight-for-height) for children <36 months in the North, Ashanti, and Accra as SDs from WHO median, 1988–2003.[19]

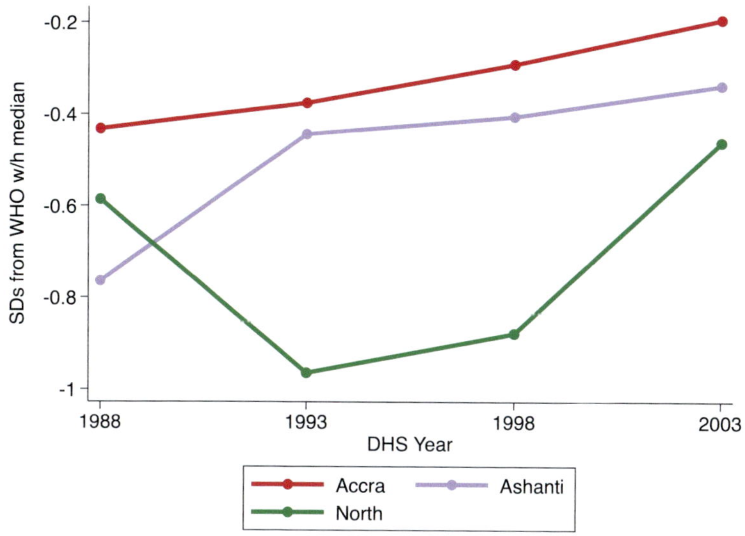

Figure 8.2 Average weight-for-height figures for children <36 months as mean SDs from WHO median, 1988–2003.[20]

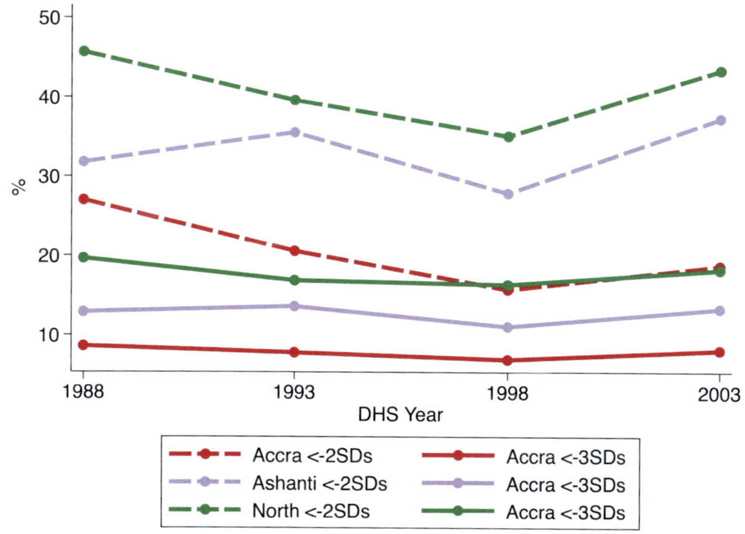

Figure 8.3 Incidence of stunting (weight-for-height) for children <36 months in the North, Ashanti, and Accra as SDs from WHO median, 1988–2003.[21]

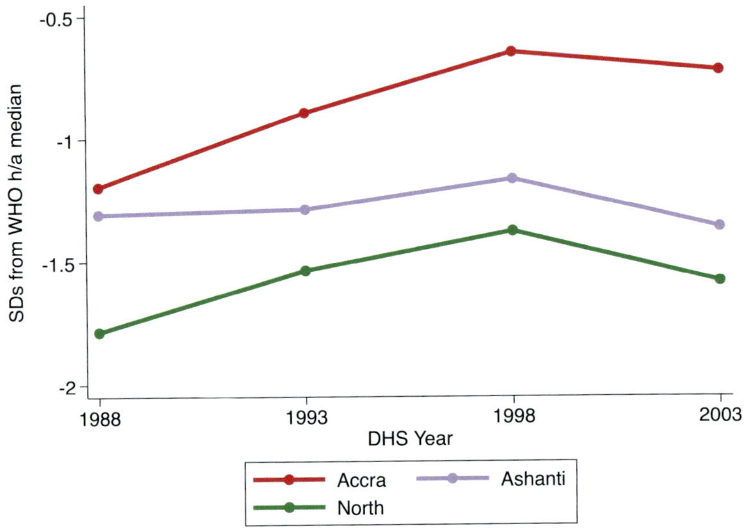

Figure 8.4 Average height-for-age figures for children <36 months as mean SDs from WHO median, 1988–2003.[22]

Using the four DHS surveys undertaken between 1993 and 2008, one 2013 study concluded that the decline in child malnutrition in Ghana was statistically significant, albeit with some demographic peculiarities.[23] Although not precisely matching this survey selection, the figures presented here give no reason to doubt these conclusions. However, a longer view of Ghana's anthropometric history allows more pressing questions to emerge. In the 1950s and 1960s, years of fairly consistent economic growth, Ghanaian heights also increased, and largely in parallel with the economy (see Figure 6.1). Yet between 1988 and 2003, a period which saw GDP per capita increase by nearly 50 per cent, there was only modest improvement in average infant growth rates (see Figure 8.5). Although the adult heights of women born during these years did increase, increases were not as sharp as in previous periods of macroeconomic growth. This might suggest that GDP per capita is not as accurate a bellwether for standards of living as it had once been, perhaps also pointing to new dislocations between macroeconomy and nutritional status. These years also saw marked changes in other national health indicators. Under-five mortality for instance dropped from 138 per thousand in 1988 to 91 per thousand in 2003, yet the incidence of clinical malnutrition remained remarkably flat (see Figure 8.6).[24]

An essential question for the spatial history of nutrition detailed here, as well as for the epidemiological potential of cross-sectional

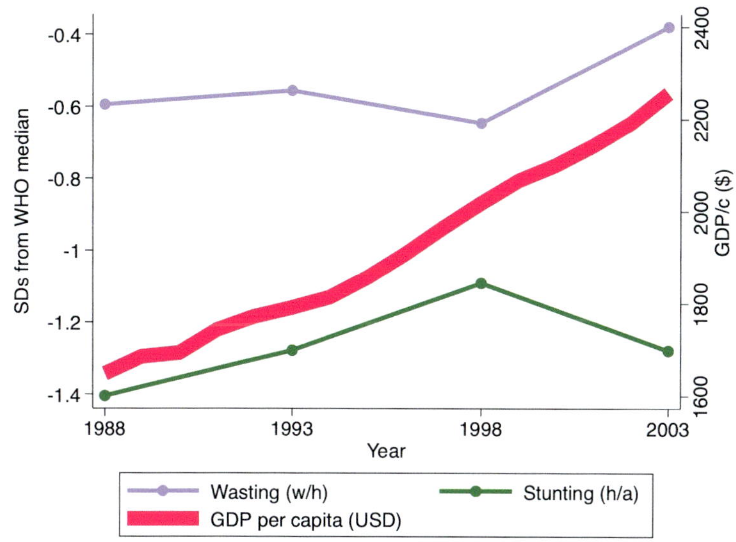

Figure 8.5 Average all-Ghana growth figures (as mean SDs from WHO medians) for children <36 months as compared to GDP/capita, 1988–2003.[25]

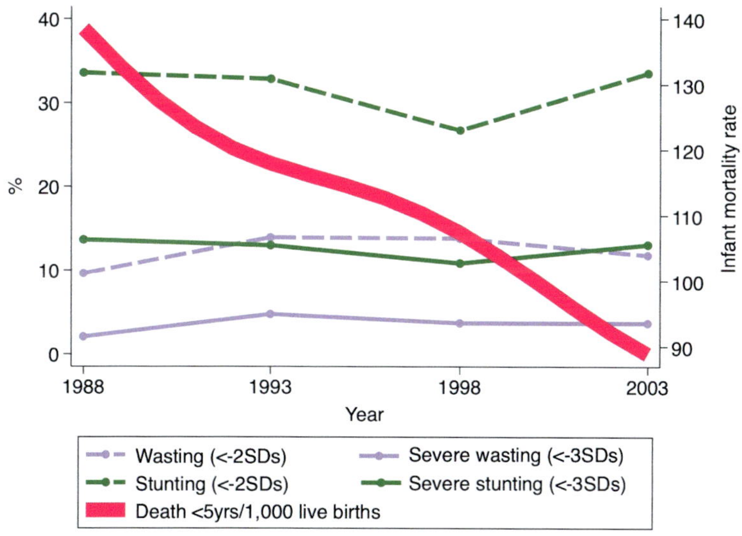

Figure 8.6 Incidence of stunting (height-for-age) and wasting (weight-for-height) for children <36 months across Ghana as compared to under five-year mortality rate, 1988–2003.[26]

surveillance, is the degree to which such data can accurately suggest the incidence of malnutrition in a given population. Here, sample sizes represent a key problem. In the 1998 GDHS, for instance, the three northernmost regions accounted for 74 of the 400 clusters surveyed. On average, in each cluster, anthropometric data was collected for only 11 children under the age of three. However, anthropometric studies require large sample sizes to accurately estimate the population mean; a sample of a thousand will, generally, lie closer to the real average than a sample of 10. In order to judge the relative adequacy of GDHS samples at a given degree of geospatial detail, we need to estimate the number of observations (*n*) necessary to achieve a 95 per cent confidence interval (CI) of length (*l*) at, for instance, 0.5 cm, 1 cm, or 2 cm deviations from either side of the mean. If we were to run repeated samples at a 95 per cent CIs, our sample would contain the population mean 95 per cent of the time. As children are exposed to more heterogeneous environments in the weeks and months after birth, the range of anthropometric measurements grows quickly. Due to the limited variation in the measurements of full-term newborns, SDs and requisite sample sizes are also small, with, for example, an SD of only 1.91 cm for newborn girls according to the WHO MGRS standard. For these children, with normally distributed heights, CIs can be calculated as:

$$n = \left[1.96\left(\frac{1.91}{l}\right)\right]^2$$

This means that to have 95 per cent confidence in our sample's accuracy at SDs of 0.5 cm, 1 cm, and 2 cm, we need samples of 56, 14, and 4 children respectively.[27] By the time girls reach 36 months of age, SDs are larger (4.04 cm by WHO standards), and we need larger sample sizes in order to accurately estimate the population mean – in this case, 251, 63, and 16 for the same degree of accuracy. For the entire age group, 0–36 months, we can split the difference. A 2 cm deviation from the average population height is significant even in adults – it took three decades for such an increase in twentieth-century Europe – for children, 2 cm is a much more significant deviation. With this in mind, cross-sectional anthropometry has to be approached with caution. In the 1998 GDHS, the average number of anthropometric observations per region was only 166; in 2003, it was 191. These sample sizes may be adequate to explain regional trends but are clearly insufficient for more granular analyses.[28]

Since the WHO adjusted for skewness in their weight-for-height standard, estimating sample sizes requisite for specific CIs at specific ages is more difficult.[29] Despite this, wasting statistics are more reliable with small samples, since, although wasting is pegged to variations in height, there is less genetic variation in weight. Cluster-level data is then more likely to represent the true incidence of wasting in the surrounding population. At least one study has suggested that clinical wasting is more likely to appear repeatedly in individual clusters than stunting, which, in comparison with other common anthropometric measures, shows the least association within individual rural villages.[30] Another study has, however, suggested that the contrary is true, and that stunting is more prone to geographic clustering, although the lower incidence of wasting means that the geographic targeting of wasting would be slightly more effective.[31] A further study found no significant anthropometric clustering in either Abidjan or Accra and questioned the place of the urban environment in this regard.[32] What all of these studies agree on, however, is the fallibility of geographical targeting for malnutrition and the potential for resource leakage should such data inform action. What they highlight for us is how difficult it is to trace the granular geographic incidence of malnutrition, even when armed with such a wealth of data.

Part of the problem is the multifaceted aetiology of malnutrition. Over the course of dozens of cross-sectional studies, childhood malnutrition has been linked with maternal education, paternal employment, maternal employment, breastfeeding practices, the prevalence of disease, or clean water supply, or sanitation. Demographic characteristics, such as mother's age at childbirth, the child's sex and age at time of survey, and the length of birth spacing have also all proved statistically significant.[33] Correlating nutrition indicators with such explanatory factors is clearly not straightforward. Information which intersects with infant anthropometry, such as details of previous illnesses or of present childcare practices, is derived from interviews with parents and is susceptible to recall errors.[34] For instance, literate mothers have been found to report the incidence of child morbidity more readily than illiterate mothers.[35] A higher-order problem is that such surveys generally work with rigid definitions and cannot account for more flexible realities. For instance, 'households' are generally defined as a closed unit in both the DHS and living standards surveys. Yet this definition precludes the cross-household entitlements which are often central to the mitigation of poverty, food insecurity, and the burdens of childrearing.[36]

Perhaps more importantly, the many factors which subtly dictate growth can prove both spatially isolated and temporally transient. As a representation of acute malnutrition, a high local incidence of wasting may, for instance, reflect a bout of infectious disease.[37] In the savannah, where undernutrition can follow a poor harvest, bumper crop and breadline can be separated by a dozen miles or a few more able bodies on the farm (see Chapter 5). Sanitation, water supply, and health provisioning are less transitory but cluster locally, determined by infrastructure at a very local level.[38] At the same time, the uptake of best practice has been seen to mitigate environmental problems but also varies from person to person.[39] As an indicator of chronic malnutrition, stunting is influenced by these same spatial determinants but is a better reflection of less transient, perennial problems which can be seen to concentrate along broad spatial differences in climate or economy. However, as an indicator of inadequate feeding over the long term, stunting in non-crisis environments generally results from a familial-level failure to provide. Though the most practical and cost-effective method of assessing malnutrition and its determinants, cross-sectional data can only capture a partial, fleeting snapshot of the sufferers, their families, their burdens, and their resources.[40]

At a more fundamental level, basing research on the analysis of anthropometric standards also leaves nutritional science overly reliant on a social construction of normalcy.[41] This potentially reductive understanding of malnutrition forms part of a biomedical framework which is 'increasingly oriented towards bringing about the normal, confusing a statistical construct with true wellbeing'.[42] Although recognising that anthropometric indices are valuable indicators of nutritional stress, anthropometric data cannot be used in isolation. Instead, empirical approaches to malnutrition should be considered in view of precise historical and geographical contexts, and in conjunction with small-scale studies which incorporate complementary methodologies and the narrative accounts which can better speak to lived experience.

Although the value of nutrition surveys should not be understated, it is also important to remember that their value derives from a context of retrenched healthcare, small governments, and internationalist involvement in health policy. Ghana's mid-century experience suggests that economic growth, unaccompanied by rapidly rising inequality, was associated with broad improvements in community nutrition. By contrast, the global ascendency of nutrition surveying, as well as targeted interventions determined by the notional precision of such surveys, must be seen as part of a potentially troubling process which promotes efficiency, cost-effectiveness, and individual agency in healthcare over its visibility or accessibility. As a system of passive surveillance, the DHS forms part of a new culture of hyper-efficient nutrition care which, like CMAM and RUTFs (see Chapter 7), normalises the prevalence of malnutrition, as well as the state's inability to confront it.[43] Nutrition surveillance is, then, part of a larger trend, a shifting of biopower from the national to the international and from the reactive paternalism of statist governments to a more passive faith in the individual and the market.

Defining a place for poverty

The collection of nutrition indicators was only one part of the drive to explain worsening nutrition in the period following Structural Adjustment. These data were complemented by social and economic metrics against which anthropometry might be correlated. Although research invariably notes the complex social aetiology of malnutrition, poverty is usually seen as a persistent contributor to poor nutrition, with studies from Ghana and elsewhere in Africa emphasising poverty as the most important determinant of malnutrition.[44] Controlling for a range of geographical, environmental, and demographic factors contained in the 2003 GDHS survey, one study found that Ghanaian children living in the poorest 60 per cent of households were more than twice as likely to be chronically undernourished as those born in the wealthiest 20 per cent of households.[45] So, can enduring poverty account for the endurance of malnutrition following adjustment?

Most of the literature regarding poverty over these years is drawn from the GLSS, run in conjunction with the World Bank. The first GLSS, undertaken in 1987/8, found that nearly 80 per cent of poverty was in rural areas, where 43 per cent of people lived below the defined national poverty line, as compared with 27 per cent of non-Accra urban residents, and only 4 per cent of Accra residents.[46] The savannah zone accounted for most of this poverty, followed by the forest, and finally the coast. These conclusions correlate closely with the general patterns seen in anthropometry data from the 1988 GDHS. However, the significant nationwide decline in poverty – from 36.9 per cent in 1987/8 to 31.5 per cent at the 1991/2 third round of the GLSS – belies the only modest improvements in anthropometric indicators as well as the increase in severe stunting and wasting (see Figures 8.5 and 8.6). Even more striking is that, between these two surveys, the proportion of rural people living below the poverty line decreased from 41.9 to 33.9 per cent at the same time as the incidence of clinical wasting increased in the countryside from 9.8 per cent to 15.5 per cent, with clinical stunting rising from 34.8 per cent to 37.2 per cent too.[47] At the end of the 1990s, the Ghana Statistical Service concluded from GLSS data that the general trend was one of significant poverty decline, from 52 to 40 per cent, as well as a significant decline in extreme poverty, from 37 to 27 per cent.[48] The greatest declines in poverty were concentrated in Accra and the rural forest. However, these conclusions were not reflected in infant anthropometry. Average nutritional status and the incidence of clinical malnutrition did not see 10 per cent declines. In fact, severe acute malnutrition became more common in Accra and Ashanti, the apparent centres of poverty reduction (see Figures 8.1 to 8.4). If poverty is truly the primary determinant of malnutrition, then why did it endure in the face of these considerable poverty reductions?

Malnutrition, asset-poverty, and the political economy of poverty reduction

Part of the problem is that the quantification of poverty is imperfect and relies on subjective, politically sensitive definitions. Most cross-sectional surveys, such as the GLSS, conceptualise poverty in the sense of horizontal disparities in assets, income, or consumption. Often this is explained in terms of interregional or urban/rural differences.[49] However, if poverty can also be understood as an inability to meet the various necessities of life in any given society, this approach relativises poverty across spaces which cannot be plainly compared. In much the same way that cross-sectional analyses of the determinants of malnutrition can never fully capture the subtle epidemiology of nutrition, the quantification of poverty downplays the geographical and temporal contexts which define the social dimensions of wealth. The relative value of social support is difficult to quantify, for instance, as are the costs of aspirational living and social participation.[50]

As we have already seen, the association between affluence and good nutrition is rarely linear but is instead refracted by the cultural, social, and economic conditions of a given time and place. This is clearly true of post-ERP Ghana and is especially apparent in the Ashanti Region, where affluence, as defined by the GDHS's wealth quintiles, was fairly evenly distributed. In Ashanti, compiled data for 1993–2003 show that economic estimations of wealth *are* a sensitive indicator of average nutritional status. However, this example also suggests that wealth, by this standard at least, does not necessarily prevent or precede extreme deviations away from anthropometric standards or the onset of clinical deficiency (see Figure 8.7). In their study of Ghanaian malnutrition, Van de Poel et al. conclude that variations in wealth were responsible for about one-third of the socioeconomic inequality in malnutrition and recognise that poorer children are more likely to live in regions with

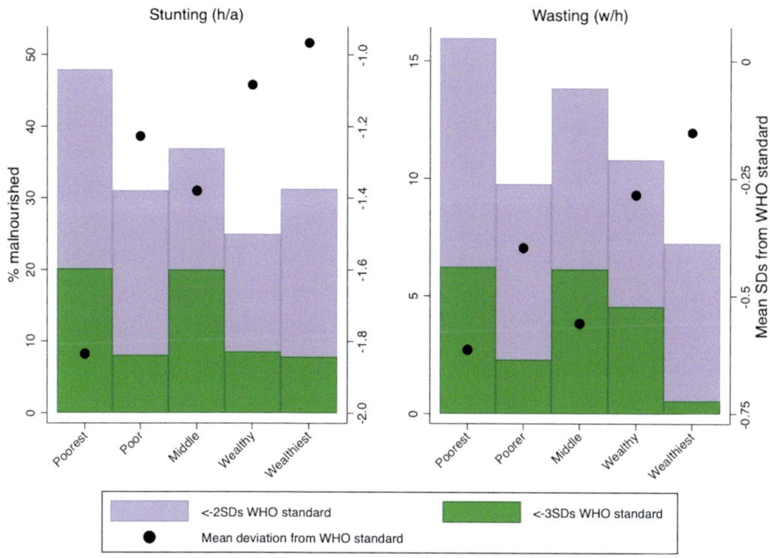

Figure 8.7 Incidence of malnutrition and average deviation from WHO growth standards by wealth quintiles, Ashanti Region, 1993–2003 combined.[51]

disadvantageous characteristics. However, they also emphasise that, 'given the strong regional associations with malnutrition, after controlling for a broad range of socioeconomic and demographic covariates, there must be other important regional aspects'.[52] Elsewhere, such as in Côte d'Ivoire, research has shown that neither stunting nor wasting correlates with economic indicators of poverty, concluding that 'malnourishment is only one of many negative consequences of poverty'.[53]

Despite these shortcomings, asset-based definitions of poverty came to dictate poverty alleviation programmes and, by extension, direct the debate on the relationship between poverty and nutrition. Yet international concentration on income poverty is suggestive of a more fundamental politics of poverty. By using narrow, asset-based definitions, the World Bank's poverty reduction strategy simply reflects a broader international development programme which focused on proletarianisation and increasing the productive capacity of the poor in the global market.[54] In this respect, the definitions and discourses regarding poverty, and its attendant social ills, were at least partially constructed with reference to the neoliberal consensus from which they emerged. Indeed, in post-adjustment Ghana, these were definitions of poverty which helped focus poverty relief on the 'soft poor', not necessarily the structural poor, or those most likely to suffer from food insecurity or malnutrition.

Sparked initially by the work of UNICEF, the World Bank's acknowledgement of the rise of malnutrition in the late 1980s was part of its broader acknowledgement that adjustment policies had led to increases in poverty. In Ghana, as elsewhere, these increases were concentrated among the most vulnerable groups, the structural poor, those with the least social capital, or those least able to readily modify their incomes. Female-headed households, pregnant and nursing women, children, the elderly, and the disabled were seen to be the worst affected.[55] Although, for most Ghanaians, standards of living after restructuring were not worse than in the early 1980s, they had not improved much either. It was widely understood that adjustment had strengthened the economy but, and unlike economic growth in the 1960s and 1970s, growth under the ERP conferred little in the way of social security. For Rawlings' fragile government, and for the World Bank's nascent African adjustment experiment, this juncture presented a problem.

Informed by both economic reality and political pragmatism, adjustment programmes around the world began to include 'pro-poor' policies as part of 'adjustment with a human face'.[56] Over the course of the 1980s and 1990s, existing programmes were adapted to address the long-term economic integration of the poor, as well as the short-term amelioration of the more immediate effects of adjustment. With monetarist Western sponsors reluctant to encourage direct transfers of capital or food, pro-poor policies prioritised investments in human and productive capital, with direct spending to be tightly targeted, highly visible, and cost-effective or, ideally, revenue-generating. This allowed for the prioritisation of a certain type of 'deserving poor' or, in World Bank parlance, a 'new poor, who had been in higher socio-economic categories before the economic crisis and subsequent adjustment, but who have fallen into poverty as a result'.[57] Often, the 'new poor' was made up of young or low-grade public servants who had been recently retrenched. Skilled and educated, as well as politically articulate, they were both a potential boon and a potential threat to the process of adjustment.

Built around what might be considered a cynical approach to poverty, in 1987 Ghana's Programme of Actions to Mitigate the Social Costs of Adjustment (PAMSCAD) became the World Bank's first short-term, pro-poor intervention in Africa. However, as a poor-relief programme, PAMSCAD proved largely ineffectual.[58] Set back by modest funding, complicated donor arrangements, and inter-ministerial competition, projects, when they were eventually implemented, were poorly targeted, inefficiently orchestrated, and failed to incorporate local actors.[59] Yet poor relief was not necessarily the Bank's or the PNDC's primary rationale for the implementation of PAMSCAD. Instead, policy documentation lamented the 'plight of the poor' but focused on how the poor might undermine the 'very sustainability of the economic reforms being pursued if inadequate attention is paid to their plight'.[60] Described by one World Bank official in Accra as nothing more than 'a big public relations exercise', officially PAMSCAD was built to ensure the 'sustainability and acceptability of the ERP', the PNDC, and the economics of adjustment.[61] Some funding found its way to high-visibility projects which addressed the needs of the chronic poor, but much more was spent on the mollification of political capital. Investments concentrated on the redeployment of retrenched civil servants and the low rate of loan repayments speaks to the use of credit as a political sop rather than an economic salve. Among the political elite, the administration of PAMSCAD dispersed prestige and the (mis)direction of funds curried favour for a fragile dictatorship.[62]

Inequality and malnutrition

The 'smoke and mirrors' politicking of PAMSCAD ultimately reflects the same politics of poverty which can be found in the cross-sectional surveys. By emphasising poverty as an absolute absence of assets or income, these definitions deny poverty as a relative phenomenon and ignore the import of vertical or class-based variations in consumption.[63] However, increasing intra- and interregional inequality was a prominent feature of the post-ERP economy, and was an important driver of malnutrition.[64]

In terms of interregional inequality, the national-level decline in income poverty over the course of the 1990s was driven by sizeable poverty declines only in Accra and the rural forest. These reinvigorated centres of capital production housed all the fastest-growing industries during these years: cocoa, mining, forestry, and services.[65] However, even in these specific locales, the profits deriving from economic growth were not equitably distributed. For instance, rural poverty decline between the late 1980s and early 1990s was concentrated among traders enjoying the newly liberalised market, something confirmed by parallel improvements in the wealth of female-headed households.[66] In Accra too, between 1992 and 1999, the average income of the highest-paid 10 per cent of workers increased by 6,000 per cent. For the poorest 10 per cent, the increase was only 38 per cent.[67] There was little political or economic interest in addressing the rise of inequality, either. Heavy taxation was considered an assault on entrepreneurship and redistributive transfers a potential precursor of fiscal destabilisation and growth reduction. Instead, income stratification was explicitly encouraged as an incentive for hard work. International consultants suggested that salary ratios between senior and junior civil servants should increase from 2:1, as was the case in the early 1980s, to 13:1. By 1991, senior civil servants earned 10 times as much as their junior colleagues.[68] It was only in the later 1990s that economists brought the general study of wealth distribution 'in from the cold', with a number of important papers highlighting inequality as an impediment to poverty reduction.[69] More recently, researchers even within the IMF have begun to question whether the entire neoliberal project has been 'oversold' in respect of its contribution to national and international inequality.[70]

It was this growing inequality which most impacted the Ghanaian poor. Income rose, health improved (at least in terms of longevity), ownership of consumer durables increased everywhere and for most people. However, since the benefits of economic growth were concentrated among the wealthy, reductions in absolute poverty did not necessarily represent an experiential improvement.[71] At the turn of the millennium, and counter to the story detailed in the statistics, one narrative study concluded that 'all the sites and groups interviewed felt that their problems have become more severe over the last decade and that if current conditions prevail the problems will worsen in the future. In fact, a gloomy picture of the future has been painted by all.'[72] Although concerns varied across the country, they all presented a view of poverty which extends over time and space, an understanding which accounts for current wellbeing with an eye to the past and to the future. This is because increasing inequality relativises poverty along a broader scale. The accumulation of wealth and the diversification of consumption at the top emphasises the absence of wealth and constraints on consumption at the bottom.

From the late 1980s, liberalised markets once again filled shops and streets with Western goods, but the devaluation of the cedi meant that fewer people could afford them. By 1995, those in the formal economy found real wages were half what they had been in 1970.[73] In the rural forest, declining purchasing power and the falling value of most crops drove migration and the readoption of cocoa.[74] According to one researcher working in the savannah, by the early 2000s, 'it looked like a mockery to mothers when I asked them if they give complementary foods, such as baby formula, fresh milk, powdered milk, juice, fruits and other things ... [they] lamented that they even find it very hard buying the basic ingredients such as dawadawa, salt and pepper.'[75] Even into the 1990s it was said that 'many people wonder what has happened to money since the late 1970s'. Travel had become prohibitively expensive, due to the 200 per cent increase in the price of petrol between 1989 and 1994, and a larger proportion of household budgets had to be spent on the same medicines and school fees.[76] The spread of film and television only fed desires which could not be readily satisfied, and the struggle to earn and the desire to spend seeped into Ghanaian popular culture, modifying moral codes and religious mores.[77] Although income inequality was actually greatest in the North, the Northern elite were small and their affluence far less visible.[78] Here, it was found that 'well-being is described more in abstract forms, such as being comfortable'; in Accra, where conspicuous wealth tended to concentrate, the 'poor base their criteria of well-being mostly on ownership of property such as cars, houses, good dresses and money'.[79]

Recently, increased social differentiation has been highlighted as an important determinant of international patterns of disease, with high relative poverty seen as a driver of anxiety, unhappiness, detrimental health behaviours, and social dysfunction.[80] In Ghana's Upper West Region, relative deprivation was primarily the concern of recently returned male migrants. Divided between urban and rural yet unable to fulfil the responsibilities of either, one woman explained that men were prone to drinking the prophetically named local gin, '"kill me quick", get drunk and come and beat you on top'.[81] In 1989, in an address to the University of Ghana, the historian and then opposition politician Albert Adu Boahen highlighted the economic contradictions which were growing so acutely in Accra: 'it is true that not only the shops but even the streets are full of goods of all sorts, but how many of us can afford them ... how many of us have three square meals, or even two, a day today?'[82] It seems likely that there is some relationship here. Given that individual diet and the diets of dependants can be sacrificed in the face of more pressing needs, it is reasonable to assume that open markets and diversifying demands had an impact on nutrition in view of a broadened scale of relative wealth. New cultures of aspiration, especially in the South, directed expenditure away from food and towards other commodities.

Expenditure surveys suggest that this was in fact the case. Food expenditure in the late 1980s and early 1990s presented a similar pattern to that which was seen in the 1950s and 1960s, with Engel's law – the assumption that, as income rises, the proportion of income spent on food falls – still failing to hold true.[83] The result being, as the economic anthropologist Jane Guyer's re-examination of the problem concludes, that 'the poor person lives a diminished, but otherwise similarly balanced, version of the good life to the better off'.[84] Although the wealthiest urban quintile from across Ghana enjoyed an income nearly three-times as large as the poorest fifth, food still accounted for 66 per cent and 63 per cent of respective monthly expenditures. Most of this difference was made up by disparities in spending on meat or fish, which, even here, were fairly negligible.[85] However, by 1998, one study of food security in Accra found that the poorest fifth spent 61 per cent of their income on food and the wealthiest only 41 per cent. That the income differential between the richest and poorest quintiles had more than doubled in the interceding years probably accounts for most of this difference. This disparity also readily translated into diet, with average caloric intakes ranging from 1,786 calories per day for the poorest fifth to 3,309 for the wealthiest.[86] By the late 1990s, inequalities in income had diverged to the extent that Accra's rich were no longer bound to the food economy in the same way as their forebears. This suggests a social removal from hunger and speaks to a gulf which was growing between those who had benefited from adjustment and those who had suffered under it.

In 1987, *South Magazine* wrote that 'Ghana has come a long way since 1983, the year of hunger, when people queued to buy kenkey and rationed petrol. Protruding collar bones, known as Rawlings chains, have been replaced by protruding stomachs, now known as Rawlings coats.'[87] But Rawlings did not have coats for everyone. Throughout the 1990s, mounting economic inequality was seen in anthropometric data, with the range and distribution of BMIs continuing to grow well into the 2000s (see Figure 8.8). Although this trend reflects Ghana's 'double burden of disease' – the growing incidence of obesity and non-communicable disease, and a growing reliance on cheap, innutritious, or highly processed foods – it is also a striking indication of the fundamental changes adjustment has wrought on nutrition in Ghana.[88] While the globalised economy has encouraged dietary inequality, inflexible definitions of poverty as absolute have worked to obscure the relationship between diet and wealth distribution. The spread and scale of inequality under adjustment may even come to represent a landmark in the history of African poverty. Jack Goody notably explained that poverty in precolonial Africa was exceptional because unproductive agriculture facilitated a relative absence of wealth. This, he suggested, precipitated undiversified class structures defined by dietary homogeneity and the universal impact of famine.[89] By the turn of the twenty-first century, these conclusions had never been less true.

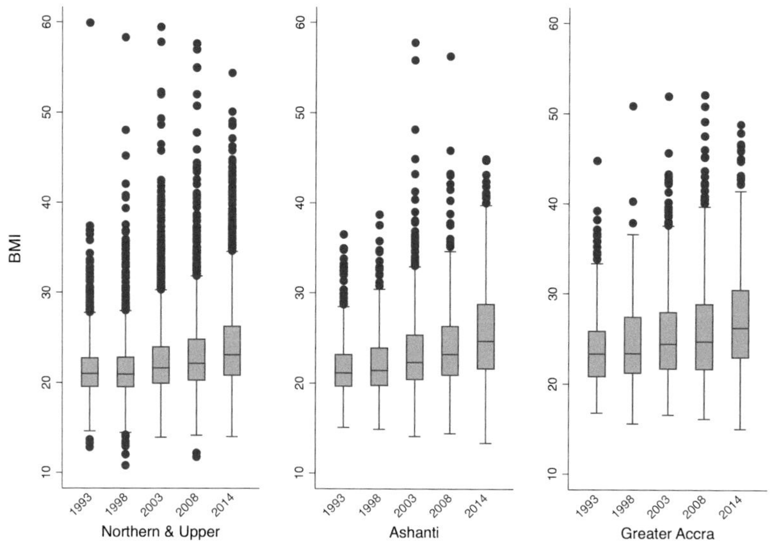

Figure 8.8 Women's BMI distribution by location, 1993–2014.[90]

Food acquisition and family maintenance in the adjustment economy

In Europe and North America, historians have suggested that elites promoted collective solutions to inequality over the course of centuries, slowly creating welfarist social contracts in a piecemeal, self-interested, and cost-effective solution to the threats which were posed by the poor, as well as the opportunities which could be derived from their labour.[91] But if the poor present neither a threat nor an opportunity, then the fortunes of the rich are no longer tangled up with those of the poor. The spread of infectious disease, the physical imposition of migrants, and the threat of crime were less pressing concerns for wealthy Ghanaians in the late twentieth century than they had been in nineteenth-century Europe. Unlike in other times and places, wealthy individuals were able to remove themselves from the social effects of poverty via inoculations and individualised healthcare, and through physical segregation and access to elite spaces, such as private transport and distinct professional and commercial environments. At the same time, investments in the lives of the poor offered less economic value. With fewer people in government service and little impetus to invest in forward linkages, Ghana's agricultural and light industrial base required limited skill or education and could be staffed by an almost inexhaustible army of workers.[92]

The ascendency of neoliberal hegemony in the years after the ERP further freed the Ghanaian elite from the social restraints of poverty. Faith in free market solutions cemented elite removal from the pains of hunger and the pressures of food acquisition, while simultaneously alleviating communal responsibility for the health effects of poverty. By succumbing to market forces, the social insurances which had previously ensured physical wellbeing and healthy social reproduction were progressively denied their worth. The pointed dismantling of statist forms of social security, such as centralised healthcare, education, and agricultural extension, undermined the processes which had helped prevent malnutrition and assuage the weight of childrearing during Ghana's halting capitalist transformation. At the same time, the communalism and socialised understandings of medicine which had traditionally provided some insurance against malnutrition were progressively undone by a more insidious culture of neoliberalism. The social and spiritual conflation of wealth and health posed that economic security should instead derive from cash-earning, hard work, and the largesse of the rich. Under adjustment, state and society, the dual pillars of nutrition security, progressively wore away. Rude health and good food instead became commodities secured by individual success in the dynamic global market.

Strained domesticities and government withdrawal

Success in the dynamic global market was, however, not available to everyone. Opportunity was not distributed equitably across the country or within individual communities. Opportunity instead collected around long-established centres of capital creation and reflected long-established patterns of discrimination. For instance, the absence of protection for or encouragement of local food production undermined the value of agriculture in areas reliant on the sale of surplus subsistence produce. Without fertiliser subsidies, the profitability and productivity of peasant farming dropped considerably in comparison with globally engaged export agriculture. Outcompeted by foreign imports, stymied by their distance from the market and by the environmental limitations on savannah agriculture, it was Northern peasant producers that were the hardest hit by adjustment.[93] In this environment, Northern food farmers wistfully recalled the Acheampong regime as a halcyon 'time of Agric'.[94] The devaluation of subsistence agriculture drove monetisation, economic migration, and the more general process of proletarianisation. It would, however, be wrong to assume that this was a passive or unpolitical process, a result of the 'invisible hand'. Even in the late 1980s, price incentives, the extension of easy credit, and the physical presence of agricultural extension officers complemented declining real incomes in order to induce the switch from food to cocoa-cropping.[95]

That the process of proletarianisation can lead to the devaluation of reproductive labour was seen with the Gold Coast's transition to colonial capitalism in the first half of the twentieth century (see Chapters 3 to 5). Since domestic reproduction is usually unpaid, monetarist economics denies it any value. However, it is with reproductive labour that children are born, fed, and educated. By extension, the bearing, feeding, and education of children is also devalued. Ghana's shift to market fundamentalism in the years following the ERP reinvigorated this earlier trend by demanding deep cuts in public services. Since these responsibilities have historically been ascribed to women, the onset of adjustment shifted burdens of social reproduction onto 'a quiet army' of wives, co-wives, mothers, grandmothers, and aunts. Though female traders and wealthy female family heads enjoyed the newly profitable market, for most women adjustment created new room for gendered exploitation and preceded an increase in sexual conflict.[96]

The position of rural women quickly worsened following the onset of adjustment. The promotion of export crops and increasing competition from imports devalued food-cropping and led to declining terms of trade in traditionally female-led industries.[97] In the late 1980s, in the Akan forest, Dei found that men were often removing their labour from food farms in order to concentrate on cash-earning, the profits from which might be concentrated in non-food expenses, such as house-building, clothing, or marriage. By contrast, the GLSS suggest that female-headed households prioritised health, education, and food.[98] Dei concludes that 'on the average, therefore, female spouses in male-headed households tend to be economically worse off than female heads of households'.[99] Nutrition surveys in the late 1980s suggest that women had borne the weight of recent changes. Women were said to be working harder during pregnancy and breastfeeding than before, with clinical signs of malnutrition 50 per cent higher among pregnant than non-pregnant women of reproductive age. By 1987, 69 per cent of pregnant women tested at antenatal clinics were anaemic by WHO standards. In Northern Ghana, one study classified 36 per cent of women as severely underweight in the lean season, as compared with 19 per cent the rest of the year. For men, the figures were 23 and 3 per cent respectively.[100] Although not necessarily comparable, the 1961 nutrition survey found that malnutrition in the savannah was lower and less gendered. The average incidence of 'gross underweightedness' was 11 per cent for women and 6 per cent for men.[101] The large increase in wasting seen in the North and in rural areas throughout the country between 1988 and 1993 might speak to a swift decline in female standing into the 1990s (see Figures 8.1 and 8.2). Indeed, a notable narrative study of malnutrition in Nandom, Upper West Region, found that 'the problem goes back as far as November 1993, when as many as three hundred children were found to be malnourished … there was the need for resources to be mobilized to meet the apparently great increase in child malnutrition'.[102] This was generally seen as a decline in traditional communal support and it was 'common to hear people say – *yɛb bɛ kyaa bei* – meaning there is no more brother'.[103] The 'unprecedented seasonal outmigration of husbands and grownup sons' in search of cash concentrated the demands of farm and family on those left behind, leading to an 'alarming increase in the workload of the already overburdened Dàgàrà [Dagaaba] mothers'.[104]

Since formal employment was also concentrated away from women, male outmigration in search of work increased de facto female headship to over half of all rural households. This conferred the burdens of rural survival squarely on women.[105] However, female headship granted greater agency over land, labour, and capital use. Following the initial shock of adjustment, a tradition of flexibility, alongside new forms of collective action, allowed women in Bawku's shea nut trade to actively mitigate their insecurity while also manipulating the market for their own advantage.[106] Perhaps prompted by the ERP's further marginalisation of women, or by the spread of female agency at home, the years after adjustment saw more women directly reject the status quo. Female dissatisfaction with rural life in Upper West Region, for instance, led to the growing feminisation of migration. With the more regular remittances from female children propping up families at home, one Dagaaba man explained that now, 'if you have only sons, you are dead'.[107] Throughout rural Ghana, consistent remittances did much to assuage the loss of rural labour and the declining value of trade in food. By 1999, only 14 per cent of female-headed households were not receiving remittances.[108] In the rural forest, remitted income actively drove poverty reduction over the course of the 1990s, increasing from 11.2 to 24.7 per cent of all income between 1991 and 1999. Although asset poverty did not improve in Northern Ghana, remittances increased from 4.8 per cent of income to 12.2 per cent, with this cash income probably also providing a degree of food security.[109] By the end of the twentieth century, the practice of remitting home led to some households actively compelling outmigration among their youth.[110] Perhaps because of these changes, Destombes' 2000 restudy of Hunter's late 1960s survey found very little seasonal variation in women's weights in Upper East Region, concluding, in stark contrast to even the 1980s, that women were the 'prime beneficiaries' of an 'escape from seasonal hunger'.[111]

In urban areas, on the other hand, retrenched civil servants and large numbers of the recently unemployed flooded the informal commercial sectors which had been traditionally dominated by women. Fewer constraints on time and energy at home, as well as readier access to capital, meant that men were often able to outcompete women in trade. In what has been described as a pattern of 'failed masculinities' and 'strained femininities', declining male household contributions intensified the domestic effects of competition in traditionally female economies, leaving women and their children to suffer this 'double burden' of urban adjustment.[112] The structural violence habitually endured by Ghanaian women has only increased in these years, concentrating among the most marginal women as well as their dependants. For instance, although the prevalence of human immunodeficiency virus (HIV) remains relatively low for sub-Saharan Africa, economic migrants and sex workers are especially at risk and have been seen to 'drive HIV dynamics' in Accra.[113] HIV itself partly drives malnutrition figures too. Recent epidemiological studies have found that as many as 20 per cent of severely malnourished children at Princess Marie Louise Children's Hospital in Accra are HIV-positive.[114] Given the increasing marginalisation of urban women, it is perhaps unsurprising that the incidence of acute malnutrition climbed in Accra and other urban spaces in the 2000s (see Figures 8.1 to 8.4).

For the growing numbers of urban poor, the pervasive decline in food and economic security was accentuated by ideological attacks on urban survival mechanisms. In the mid-1990s, it was generally assumed that 'rural communities saw far more opportunities for action at the level of the community to increase livelihood security than their counterparts in the urban sector'.[115] Indeed, in the countryside, economic incentives to divest from the subsistence economy were heeded with caution, and cash-crops were produced 'in addition to' rather than 'instead of' food crops.[116] Urban agriculture also became an important survival tool after adjustment. Over the course of the 1990s, income from urban agriculture rose from zero to 5.3 per cent of total income in Accra and from 2.4 to 9.8 per cent in other urban areas.[117] Whether via agriculture, street-hawking, or slum housing, urban survival was increasingly dependent upon the creation of an urban commons and urban communality predicated upon the decommodification of food, shelter, and economic opportunity.[118] However, municipal governments have progressively encroached upon these freedoms by harassing street traders, levelling slums, and claiming land tended by urban farmers for building works.[119] The privatisation of common property haunted the rural poor too. Tax breaks and liberalised land concessions encouraged large-scale, multinational ventures in high-growth industries like forestry and mining, marginalising artisanal production and promoting proletarianisation.[120] At the same time, population growth and privatisation inhibited access to inelastic necessities sometimes required for appropriate feeding, often useful for supplementary food security and previously thought to be common property. For instance, an upward trend in the sale of firewood and an increase in prosecutions for stealing firewood led to a 'rural energy crisis' by the late 1980s and, by the early 2000s, to an environment where it was 'as expensive in money or time to put the fuel under the pot as to put the food into the pot'.[121] These, again, were burdens largely borne by women.

Defined by David Harvey as 'accumulation by dispossession', or primitive accumulation driven by the privatisation of previously common property, this trend has become a prominent feature of neoliberal governance.[122] Though often more forceful in the 'global city', many of the more malign impacts are environmental, and affect the longer-term deterioration of nutrition and food security in rural areas. For instance, the government's leasing of forestry contracts to foreign firms and the promotion of cocoa farming have facilitated deforestation and biodiversity decline.[123] At the same time, foreign ownership of leases undercuts the social and spiritual responsibility which had previously ensured a degree of environmental sustainability.[124] Combined with piecemeal environmental legislation, pollution from mining has contributed to adverse health effects and soil degeneration.[125] With a considerable proportion of these growth industries concentrated in Asante, adjustment policies further devalued the 'broad forest rent' which had provided relative equity in terms of food, health, and livelihood security. In the North, desertification and increasingly unpredictable rainfall have had a far greater direct effect on food, nutrition, and water security, as well as upon the mechanisms which insure these concerns.[126] Although less directly related to in-country policy, growing hardships in the savannah reflect the global effects of accumulation by dispossession and the often unrestrained commodification of natural resources. Sadly, the worst of these environmental effects have still not been fully realised.

The government's more pointed divestment from infrastructural insurances only accentuated strains in domestic economies. Using GLSS data, one study found that average anthropometric measures often reflected access to health infrastructure. For instance, height-for-age was significantly higher in the presence of well-stocked health clinics, while a reduction in distance from the rural mean (4.8 km) to the urban mean (0.6 km) would reduce the gap between rural and urban weight-for-height by almost 50 per cent.[127] However, infrastructural improvements rarely grew up in response to the greatest need, but were instead built to support centres of capital accumulation. This ultimately aped the colonial pattern, which saw the urban South accruing most of the benefit. In 1989, urban areas with one-third of the population received 42 per cent of the Public Investment Programme (PIP) spending; by 1992 the figure had risen to 48.7 per cent. Of the 62 PIP education projects in the North, Tamale absorbed 62 per cent. By 1997, there was an excess of 7,000 teachers in urban areas, with 21,000 positions left to be filled around the country. Health spending followed a similar pattern. In 1985, the government implemented health-user fees, initiating a massive and immediate drop in hospital usage and a cultural shift away from biomedicine, especially among the rural poor.[128] By 1991, Accra enjoyed nearly 600 per cent more per capita health investment than any other region, with 60 per cent of equipment and vehicles too.[129] Access to the remaining public services and the ability to employ best nutrition practice were also dictated by more fundamental access to transport, sanitation, and electrification infrastructure. The market forces behind extractive economics encouraged road building and infrastructural advantage in centres of capital accumulation, compounding public spending and concentrating health advantage in these areas.[130] A good example of this is AngloGold Ashanti's pioneering anti-malarial spraying operation undertaken around Obuasi, then home to Ghana's largest gold mine and its greatest single source of foreign exchange. At the end of the project, in 2013, AngloGold Ashanti concluded that 'the mine has reported an 84 percent reduction in new cases over the past three years and a 94 percent reduction in the Malaria Lost Time Frequency Rate (MLTIFR)'.[131] In neoliberal Ghana, even worthwhile and ostensibly civic-minded public health improvements came not as a reasoned reaction to public need but in response to the specific demands of capital formation.

Filling gaps in the market: church, charity, and civil society as social insurance

With the state in retreat and domestic reproduction in crisis, good health and freedom from physical want became increasingly reliant upon new forms of security. The social insurances which emerged did not necessarily grow up in defence of neoliberal dominance, but were all formed in response to the economic realities of the post-ERP period and reflect the social anxieties which developed in the years after adjustment. Two prominent forms of social security which were invigorated by adjustment are particularly illuminating and speak to important shifts in the relationship between social change and societal support: the (re) emergence of church-based support and the growing importance of NGOs and foreign aid, especially with regard to the promotion of civil society, suggest a pervasive and insidious cultural shift. In the Weberian tradition of 'Protestant work ethics' and the 'spirit of capitalism', this 'spirit of neoliberalism' appoints the wealthy as arbiters of social survival and grants the individual accumulation of capital a degree of moral authority.

The primary foreign financiers of Ghanaian development projects largely followed the direction set by the World Bank, with the priorities of the UK's Department for International Development (DFID) and USAID's client NGOs generally pursuing a common mandate to bring Ghana more fully into the global fold.[132] Though generalising the NGO sector's wide range of often antagonistic standpoints, NGO distributions of aid and expertise have been central to the functioning of Ghana's neoliberal economy.[133] Yet, as the adjustment programme moved out of the initial stabilisation stages – overseen by a small group of technocrats and ministerial advisors – the number of actors required to implement and consolidate economic liberalisation grew significantly. This next stage required consensus building and a notional community ownership of the development trajectory. Billed as representing grass-roots support for liberalisation, the nascent civil society which came to participate in the country's economic reforms was largely built from the elite beneficiaries of adjustment.[134] Pointed at as a means to reinforce democracy, populist rule, and moral accountability, civil society has been touted as an effective recourse against the worst excesses of political accumulation and kleptocratic governments.[135] Indeed, 1995 saw the largest protest since the 1948 riots; here oppositional political parties, a lively independent media, and organised professional associations provided successful opposition to the PNDC's attempt to implement a value-added tax.[136] However, by opposing state involvement in the economy, an NGO-led civil society instead exalts the freedom of the market as the cornerstone of political liberty. As was the case with PAMSCAD in the 1980s, NGOs accumulate foreign capital to further these ends, building patronage by extending social security for the poor and employment for the elite.[137] We are now not far from Bayart's original conceptualisation of civil society as part of the 'reciprocal assimilation of elites'; micro-credit effortlessly replaced the paternalism of previous years as a means to build a culture of market-led solutions to poverty and hunger.[138] Into the 2000s, NGOs operating in the Northern savannah (then familiar enough to be termed 'n-joos') underwrote the sort of affordable fertiliser and agricultural extension which had defined Acheampong's OFY programme in the 1970s.[139] Nutrition security was also attended to by the *noblesse oblige* of donor governments and their client NGOs. In the late 1980s, attendance at health centres without food was half that at those with CRS take-home rations.[140] By providing security outside of the state but within the market, the internationalist promotion of a poorly defined civil society has provided a panacea for the ills of neoliberalism. It suggests a meaningful social existence in a time of declining social support, mitigating the threat of the Smithian 'society of strangers'.[141]

These same processes are perhaps more evident in Ghana's rapidly growing Pentecostal and Charismatic churches. Here, both spiritual and terrestrial insurances are underwritten by the economic success and spiritual authority of wealthy church leaders.[142] As has been explained with reference to the Pentecostal movement, these churches flourish where 'neoliberal forces have eroded the capacity of liberal democratic states to provide education, health and welfare'.[143] In these spaces, popular churches can quickly establish, fund, and run schools, employment services, and their own forms of healthcare.[144] In this respect, Pentecostal churches provide a new community, characterised by mutual trust and mutual aid. However, in a time of increasing healthcare costs, some observers question whether Pentecostal churches have oriented health-seeking behaviours towards faith-based medicine.[145] Religious support is also not always so tangible. Instead, some churches extol the ideas that, with personal endeavour in a free market and under the guidance of the 'prosperity gospel', born-again Christians may be blessed with the same prosperity that has benefited the church's primary evangelists. In the Volta Region, Pentecostal churches have been seen to provide spiritual protection for commercialism while also justifying individualism and allowing community decay.[146]

Whereas NGOs promote civil society as a protection against the mores of state accumulation, Pentecostal churches provide spiritual justification for faith in the free market alternative. In valorising their success in this environment, church leaders and the heads of secular civil society are exalted as spiritually sanctified or politically significant. Their station validates the same 'spirit of neoliberalism' which brought them to that position. Although we should not overstate the value of NGOs or

Pentecostal churches for everyday survival for most people, proselytising from either the pulpit or the credit union works to reproduce the ideas upon which they are based, compounding the inequality and communal strain which was already cheapening domestic reproduction.

Expensive children and cheap childhoods

Often the social and medical pressures which accompanied Ghana's transition to market fundamentalism were felt most acutely by children. The strained domestic economy and the rising cost of living made childrearing more expensive, cheapening childhood in view of a growing need for children to become more directly productive assets. The growing cost of dependants was both sharply realised and frankly addressed during these years. By the late 1980s, UNICEF reported on the alarming increase in child pawning.[147] In the mid-1990s, Christine Oppong explained that this formed part of a growing reaction to unwanted fertility which also included 'escalating evidence of … abortion, child neglect, abandonment and abuse'.[148] Also beginning in the 1990s, a rash of articles began to call attention to the same 'spirit children' which had impaired family survival around Kassena-Nankani District in the Upper East Region during the colonial period (see Chapter 5).[149] One 2001 study suggests that perhaps 15 per cent of mortality in children under three months was due to infanticide relating to spirit children.[150] Elsewhere, older children were quickly incorporated into the labour force, with the familial production of cocoa or 'artisanal' production of gold increasingly reliant on child labour.[151] The educational reforms introduced in 1987 did little to prevent the ready commodification of children, their primary objectives being 'increasing access to first cycle education and increasing its practical and vocational content so that its products are more easily absorbed into productive activities'.[152]

Although infant healthcare was ostensibly free, the rising cost of transport, alongside constraints on maternal time and energy, proved a significant impediment to its use. In the years following the ERP, but before the advent of CMAM or Plumpy'nut, the languorous 43-day nutrition rehabilitation programme was financially impossible for working mothers or for families living far away from nutrition clinics.[153] Attendance was sporadic and drop-out rates were extremely high. Into the early 2000s, only 22 per cent of children were officially discharged from one programme in Accra.[154] Even with a good understanding of nutritional best practice, these same mechanisms impede the employment of this knowledge. In order to stem the use of *koko* and thin cereal porridges for weaning, in 1987 the government began to encourage the uptake of Weanimix, a cereal–legume mixture. However, one mother at an Accra rehabilitation centre explained that 'if someone doesn't have money she can't cook like they did at the NRC [Nutrition Rehabilitation Centre]'.[155] Instead, many mothers continued to buy *koko* and other innutritious street foods as time- and cost-effective solutions to the pressures of domestic reproduction in adjustment Accra.

The informed nutritional compromises undertaken by Accra mothers reflect more fundamental shifts in Ghana's food culture and the broader growth of dietary inequality. Liberalisation pressured women into working longer hours, and unaffordable housing pushed poor people out of city centres, where they arrived home too late or too tired to cook *fufu* or the other staples which had, even recently, been a central aspect of ethnic identity. In one study of urban food security, published in 2000, households in the poorest expenditure quintile spent nearly 40 per cent of their entire food budget on snacks and meals away from home, as compared with only 25 per cent in the highest group.[156] By the 1990s, and in a significant break from the past, families began to relegate *fufu* to Sundays alone.[157] As the anthropologist Gracia Clark explains, 'shrinking access of ordinary households to high-status traditional foods ... suggests that their routine consumption may eventually signal exclusive elite status in the same way that wearing hand-woven *kente* cloth to ordinary events already does'.[158]

Diet and the new processes of food acquisition in global Ghana

New food cultures have flourished, and new foodstuffs have sustained Ghana's new economic trajectory. Today, in both Ghana and Nigeria, millennials brought up on a diet of instant noodles are sometimes derisively referred to as the 'Indomie generation'. If you are what you eat, then at least some older Ghanaians would say that children today lack substance, just like their food. But the ascendency of Indomie – an omnipresent night-time street food, usually complemented by the addition of egg, tinned fish, and vegetables – is part of the same phenomenon which has caused the steady disappearance of *fufu* from Southern diets. The umami-allure and affordability of Indomie only complemented its convenience among the expanding, time-poor working class.

As was also the case with earlier trends, globalisation and neoliberal governance influence nutrition through the dual mechanisms of food and feeding. Changes in Ghana's food economy since the onset of the ERP have influenced the availability of particular foods at the same time as shifts in domestic life have changed which foods caregivers provide and how and when they provide them. These are the economic drivers of what has been described as the 'nutrition transition' from fruit and vegetable-heavy, cereal-based diets to high-fat, high-sugar, high-animal protein 'Western' diets.[159]

As we have just seen, a common theme in the post-adjustment food culture is that dietary compromise can garner economic efficiency at the household level. This is true at the national level too, leaving adjustment at least partially built on dietary compromise, especially for the poor. That the process of proletarianisation is facilitated by the displacement of peasant agriculture in favour of capitalist agriculture is something which has long been recognised in Marxist circles as a basal feature of primitive accumulation.[160] More recently, this has been explained as a process in which international corporate food regimes 'dispossess farmers as a condition for the consolidation of corporate agriculture' – that is to say, as an element of 'accumulation by dispossession'.[161] The correlate of this is that the transition to wage labour is secured by cheap food. Here we are reminded of the same ideas which cultured colonial dietetics, of William Ormsby-Gore's 1926 visit to the Gold Coast, and his argument that 'the capacity of labour ... is bound up with the question of food'.[162] Although this myopic attention to bodily efficiency (and its dietary determinants) has always been problematic, in the years following adjustment, these logics have been extended across a truly global market. The promotion of export agriculture, the abolition of import tariffs, the absence of subsidies or other protection for domestic produce, and a quickly growing national population all precipitated an increased dependence on food imports.[163] In order to rebuff overseas competition, the response which was forwarded for domestic agriculture was the increased production of innutritious but easily produced local staples, such as cassava.[164]

The problem with economically efficient diets is that they generally promote long-lasting and energy-dense foodstuffs at the expense of those with a more holistic nutritional value. Fresh fruit, vegetables, and animal produce are more difficult to pack and transport and more likely to spoil than processed foods. Elsewhere, the proliferation of heavily constructed foods has been forwarded as a feature of a neoliberal food economy, where diminished governmental control over the use of agricultural surpluses has led to an increase in the consumption of energy-dense 'pseudo-foods' and a commensurate increase in cardiovascular and metabolic disorders, the incidence of which is often concentrated among the poor.[165] The spread of similar foods in Ghana has prompted concerns regarding a similar rise of chronic, food-related illnesses.[166] Of course, this problem is by no means new, but it is exacerbated by increased globalisation and the neoliberal turn. The breastmilk substitutes which initially hampered infant nutrition in the mid-twentieth century – then interacting with the domestic pressures brought about by the onset of colonial capitalism – became even more widely available, and still present problems. These early imports have since been joined by products which help to further cheapen domestic reproduction. Rice, vegetable oil, and instant noodles all contribute to quick, affordable, and popular meals, but bring their own health hazards. Nestlé's Maggi noodles, for instance – one of several brands generically referred to as Indomie – were found to contain so much lead, and later ash, that their sale was banned in India.[167] If the neoliberal period can be considered a 'race to the bottom', then its food economy often reflects this. In the truly global food economy, it is cheap and innutritious food which props up increasingly strained domestic economies, plays out along income inequities, and concentrates the malign effects of poor nutrition among the poorest people.

Given that misinformation and opacity still characterise the science of nutrition, it is as difficult as ever to parse out the health effects of dietary change since the late 1980s. Neither academics nor consumers have the tools to fully identify the risks. As a conscious concern, hunger is what makes food such an inelastic commodity. However, since good nutrition is essentially a subconscious, physiological want, nutritious food can be extremely income-elastic. This is especially problematic in an era of globalised and processed food, where cheap fats, sugars, and salt are used to play on innate, hedonic preferences for these food elements.[168] In places like Accra, the entrepôt of a successful globalised economy, nutrition insecurity did not necessarily manifest in malnutrition, as it had in previous decades. In view of Ghana's quickly shifting food culture and food economy, the growth of anthropometric inequality (see Figure 8.8) casts doubt on the degree to which anthropometric indicators can speak to nutritional health in a more holistic sense. Can we assume that increasing average weight-for-height is beneficial or even benign? There is, for instance, certainly evidence to suggest that, even if they outgrow their peers, non-breastfed babies are in danger of obesity, diabetes, and associated risks later in life.[169] Contemporary nutritional science cannot account for these changes without qualitative research which gives greater credence to economic, cultural, and historical contexts.

What is clear, however, is that globalised food markets and strained domesticities have radically altered Ghanaian nutrition in a remarkably short space of time. Although concentrating in Accra and other urban areas, diets are changing everywhere in response to market integration on a global scale. It is reasonable to assume that the free market doctrines which bore these changes have had some effect on both foodways and childrearing. One of the defining characteristics of the neoliberal political economy is the promotion of the individual. This was felt in Ghana from the late 1980s, when the communal support structures, labour partnerships, and cottage industries which had sustained rural forest communities during the crisis years started to collapse.[170] Households were, instead, 'reintegrating fully into the market economy' and encountered a new and 'marked dependence on available imported goods'.[171] Perhaps it is this individualisation which explains why a 1999 study of nutrition in Accra found that malnutrition does not cluster because of 'any lack of variation between clusters, but from a surprisingly large degree of variation within clusters'.[172] This, as similar studies have also shown, suggests that the unfavourable environmental conditions which might reasonably promote a high local incidence of malnutrition can be offset by the practices and resources employed by an increasingly nucleated family unit.[173] At least by 2008, household nucleation was found to be a reliable predictor of good infant growth.[174] Increasingly, individualised nutrition is also suggested by the growing polarisation of heights and especially weights (see Figure 8.8). Although most obvious in Accra, but increasingly relevant to nutritional health elsewhere, we cannot discount the possibility that these changes 'are concrete, historically specific outworkings of millennial capitalism and the culture of neoliberalism'.[175]

Notes

1 Quoted in Anna Davin, 'Imperialism and Motherhood', *History Workshop Journal*, 5 (1978), 9–65 (p. 29).
2 See Chapter 1; Foucault, *History of Sexuality*; Searle, *Quest*.
3 Quoted in Deborah M. Valenze, *Milk: A Local and Global History* (New Haven, CT: Yale University Press, 2011), p. 254.
4 This was for children over seven. Free milk for secondary school pupils had already ended, in 1968, under a Labour government already bowing to a dawning neoliberal consensus. But this does rather ruin the metaphor.
5 Berg, *Accelerated Development*.
6 For the history of neoliberalism, see David Harvey, *A Brief History of Neoliberalism* (Oxford: Oxford University Press, 2005).
7 The best account of adjustment in Ghana is Eboe Hutchful, *Ghana's Adjustment Experience: The Paradox of Reform* (Oxford: James Currey, 2002).

8 Eboe Hutchful, 'Why Regimes Adjust: The World Bank Ponders Its "Star Pupil"', *Canadian Journal of African Studies*, 29.2 (1995), 303–17.

9 Kwadwo Konadu-Agyemang, 'The Best of Times and the Worst of Times: Structural Adjustment Programs and Uneven Development in Africa: The Case Of Ghana', *The Professional Geographer*, 52.3 (2000), 469–83.

10 CRS figures quoted in Lavy et al., *Quality of Health Care*, p. 3.

11 World Bank, *Ghana: Population, Health and Nutrition* (Washington, D.C.: World Bank, 1989), p. 53.

12 As during colonial rule, the accounts of anthropologists provide essential evidence for these changes. See, among many others, Jean Comaroff and John L. Comaroff, 'Millennial Capitalism: First Thoughts on a Second Coming', *Public Culture*, 12.2 (2000), 291–343; James Ferguson, *Global Shadows: Africa in the Neoliberal World Order* (Durham, NC: Duke University Press, 2006). On the relationship between economic adjustment, health and food, see, for instance, James Pfeiffer and Rachel Chapman, 'Anthropological Perspectives on Structural Adjustment and Public Health', *Annual Review of Anthropology*, 39.1 (2010), 149–65; Gracia Clark, 'From Fasting to Fast Food in Kumasi, Ghana', in *Food Consumption in Global Perspective: Essays in the Anthropology of Food in Honour of Jack Goody*, ed. by Jakob Klein and Anne Murcott (Basingstoke: Palgrave Macmillan, 2014), pp. 45–64 (p. 57).

13 Cris Shore and Susan Wright, 'Governing by Numbers: Audit Culture, Rankings and the New World Order', *Social Anthropology*, 23.1 (2015), 22–8. See also Adams, *Metrics*; Bandola-Gill, Grek, and Tichenor, *Governing*.

14 On the troubling history of BMI and obesity metrics, see, for instance, Sabrina Strings, *Fearing the Black Body: The Racial Origins of Fat Phobia* (New York: NYU Press, 2019), pp. 197–203. For some history of infant anthropometry, see M. de Onis and R. Yip, 'The WHO Growth Chart: Historical Considerations and Current Scientific Issues', *Bibliotheca Nutritio Et Dieta*, 53 (1996), 74–89.

15 Vincanne Adams, 'Introduction', in Adams (ed.), *Metrics*, pp. 1–18 (p. 6).

16 Some of these issues have been detailed, with reference to non-communicable disease, in Olutobi Sanuade, 'Estimating and Monitoring the Burden of Non-Communicable and Chronic Diseases in Ghana', in *Epidemiological Change and Chronic Disease in Sub-Saharan Africa: Historical and Anthropological Perspectives*, ed. by Megan Vaughan, Kafui Adjaye-Gbewonyo, and Marissa Mika (London: UCL Press, 2021), pp. 212–30.

17 On the political complicity and social construction of data, see, for instance, Crystal Biruk, *Cooking Data: Culture and Politics in an African Research World* (Durham, NC: Duke University Press Books, 2018); *'Raw Data' Is an Oxymoron*, ed. by Lisa Gitelman (Cambridge, MA: MIT Press, 2013).

18 Adams, 'Introduction', p. 9.

19 GDHS, 1988–2003.

20 GDHS, 1988–2003.

21 GDHS, 1988–2003.

22 GDHS, 1988–2003.

23 Dickson A. Amugsi, Maurice B. Mittelmark, and Anna Lartey, 'An Analysis of Socio-Demographic Patterns in Child Malnutrition Trends Using Ghana Demographic and Health Survey Data in the Period 1993–2008', *BMC Public Health*, 13 (2013), 960.

24 The GDHS gives contrary figures which actually suggest a slight rise in infant and child mortality between 1998 and 2003; despite this, under-five mortality fell from 155 to 111 between 1988 and 2003.

25 GDHS, 1988–2003; GDP/c from Bolt and van Zanden.

26 GDHS, 1988–2003; mortality data from <https://data.worldbank.org> [accessed 4 January 2016].

27 1.96 is used because 95 per cent of the area under a normal distribution lies within 1.96 SDs of the mean.

28 I must thank Alexander Moradi for his advice here. WHO MGRS height means taken from M. de Onis, 'Assessment of Differences in Linear Growth among Populations in the WHO Multicentre Growth Reference Study', *Acta Pædiatrica*, 95 (2006), 56–65.

29 World Health Organization, *WHO Child Growth Standards: Methods and Development* (Geneva: World Health Organization, 2006).

30 Joanne Katz, 'Sample-Size Implications for Population-Based Cluster Surveys of Nutritional Status', *The American Journal of Clinical Nutrition*, 61.1 (1995), 155–60.
31 Bridget Fenn, Saul S. Morris, and Chris Frost, 'Do Childhood Growth Indicators in Developing Countries Cluster? Implications for Intervention Strategies', *Public Health Nutrition*, 7.7 (2004), 829–34.
32 Saul S. Morris et al., 'Does Geographic Targeting of Nutrition Interventions Make Sense in Cities? Evidence from Abidjan and Accra', *World Development*, 27.11 (1999), 2011–19.
33 See, among very many other papers, Harold Alderman, *Nutritional Status in Ghana and Its Determinants*, Social Dimensions of Adjustment (Washington, D.C.: World Bank, 1990), pp. 1–52; Lisa C. Smith and Lawrence J. Haddad, *Explaining Child Malnutrition in Developing Countries: A Cross-Country Analysis*, FCND Discussion Paper (Washington, D.C.: International Food Policy Research Institute, 1999); Venanzio Vella et al., 'Determinants of Nutritional Status in South-West Uganda', *Journal of Tropical Pediatrics*, 41.2 (1995), 89–98; S.A. Esrey et al., 'Drinking Water Source, Diarrheal Morbidity, and Child Growth in Villages with Both Traditional and Improved Water Supplies in Rural Lesotho, Southern Africa', *American Journal of Public Health*, 78.11 (1988), 1451–5; E.A. Frongillo, M. de Onis, and K.M. Hanson, 'Socioeconomic and Demographic Factors Are Associated with Worldwide Patterns of Stunting and Wasting of Children', *The Journal of Nutrition*, 127.12 (1997), 2302–9.
34 For a technical analysis of these issues, see Sian L. Curtis, *Assessment of the Quality of Data Used for Direct Estimation of Infant and Child Mortality in DHS-II Surveys*, DHS Occasional Papers (Calverton, MD: Macro International, 1995).
35 Alireza Olyaee Manesh et al., 'Accuracy of Child Morbidity Data in Demographic and Health Surveys', *International Journal of Epidemiology*, 37.1 (2008), 194–200.
36 Sara Randall and Ernestina Coast, 'Poverty in African Households: The Limits of Survey and Census Representations', *The Journal of Development Studies*, 51.2 (2015), 162–77.
37 See, for instance, Joanne Katz et al., 'Estimation of Design Effects and Diarrhea Clustering within Households and Villages', *American Journal of Epidemiology*, 138.11 (1993), 994–1006.
38 G. Benneh et al., *Environmental Problems and the Urban Household in the Greater Accra Metropolitan Area* (Stockholm: Stockholm Environment Institute, 1993); Kwasi Owusu Boadi and Markku Kuitunen, 'Environment, Wealth, Inequality and the Burden of Disease in the Accra Metropolitan Area, Ghana', *International Journal of Environmental Health Research*, 15.3 (2005), 193–206.
39 Marie T. Ruel et al., 'Good Care Practices Can Mitigate the Negative Effects of Poverty and Low Maternal Schooling on Children's Nutritional Status: Evidence from Accra', *World Development*, 27.11 (1999), 1993–2009.
40 Randall and Coast, 'Poverty in African Households', p. 173.
41 de Onis and Yip, 'WHO Growth Chart'.
42 Margaret M. Lock and Vinh-Kim Nguyen, *An Anthropology of Biomedicine* (Oxford: Wiley-Blackwell, 2010), p. 45.
43 Redfield, 'Bioexpectations', p. 170.
44 Ellen Van de Poel et al., 'Malnutrition and the Disproportional Burden on the Poor: The Case of Ghana', *International Journal for Equity in Health*, 6 (2007), 1–12; Rathavuth Hong, 'Effect of Economic Inequality on Chronic Childhood Undernutrition in Ghana', *Public Health Nutrition*, 10.4 (2007), 371–8; Nguyen Minh Thang and Barry M. Popkin, 'In an Era of Economic Growth, Is Inequity Holding Back Reductions in Child Malnutrition in Vietnam?', *Asia Pacific Journal of Clinical Nutrition*, 12.4 (2003), 405–10.
45 Hong, 'Economic Inequality', p. 375.
46 E. Oti-Boateng et al., *A Poverty Profile for Ghana, 1987–88*, Social Dimensions of Adjustment in Sub-Saharan Africa Working Paper, 5 (Washington, D.C.: World Bank, 1990).
47 Hutchful, *Adjustment Experience*, pp. 124–5.
48 Ghana Government, *Poverty Trends in Ghana in the 1990s* (Accra: Ghana Statistical Service, 2000).
49 Hutchful, *Adjustment Experience*, pp. 120–4; Ghana Government, *Poverty Trends*.
50 Howard White, 'Combining Quantitative and Qualitative Approaches in Poverty Analysis', *World Development*, 30.3 (2002), 511–22; Randall and Coast, 'Poverty in African Households', p. 164.
51 GDHS, 1993–2014.

52 Van de Poel et al., 'Malnutrition', p. 9.
53 Paul Glewwe and Jacques van der Gaag, 'Identifying the Poor in Developing Countries: Do Different Definitions Matter?', *World Development*, 18.6 (1990), 803–14 (pp. 807, 812).
54 Paul Cammack, 'What the World Bank Means by Poverty Reduction, and Why It Matters', *New Political Economy*, 9.2 (2004), 189–211 (p. 206).
55 UNICEF, 'Adjustment Policies and Programmes to Protect Children and Other Vulnerable Groups in Ghana', in *Adjustment with a Human Face: Country Case Studies*, ed. by Giovanni Andrea Cornia, Richard Jolly, and Frances Stewart, 2 vols (Oxford: Clarendon Press, 1987), ii, 93–125; UNICEF and Ghana Government, *Children and Women of Ghana: A Situation Analysis 1989–90* (Accra: UNICEF, 1990).
56 See, for instance, Frances Stewart, 'The Many Faces of Adjustment', *World Development*, 19.12 (1991), 1847–64.
57 World Bank, *The Social Dimensions of Adjustment in Africa: A Policy Agenda* (Washington, D.C.: World Bank, 31 March 1990), pp. 1–34 (p. 5).
58 Eboe Hutchful, '"Smoke and Mirrors": The World Bank's Social Dimensions of Adjustment (SDA) Programme', *Review of African Political Economy*, 21.62 (1994), 569–84; Samuel K. Gayi, 'Adjusting to the Social Costs of Adjustment in Ghana: Problems and Prospects', *The European Journal of Development Research*, 7.1 (1995), 77–100.
59 Gayi, 'Adjusting', pp. 84–93.
60 Ghana Government, *Programme of Actions to Mitigate the Social Costs of Adjustment* (Accra: Government Printer, 1987), p. 7.
61 Quoted in Gayi, 'Adjusting', p. 97; Ghana Government, *Programme*, p. 8.
62 Gayi, 'Adjusting', pp. 93–4.
63 Hutchful, *Adjustment Experience*, pp. 120–4.
64 Franklin Obeng-Odoom, 'Neoliberalism and the Urban Economy in Ghana: Urban Employment, Inequality, and Poverty', *Growth and Change*, 43.1 (2012), 85–109; Ernest Aryeetey and Andrew McKay, 'Growth with Poverty Reduction, but Increased Spatial Inequality: Ghana over the 1990s', in *Determinants of Pro Poor Growth: Analytical Issues and Findings from Country Cases*, ed. by Michael Grimm, Stephen Klasen, and Andrew McKay (Basingstoke: Palgrave Macmillan, 2007), pp. 57–80.
65 Ernest Aryeetey and Andrew McKay, *Operationalizing Pro-Poor Growth: A Country Case Study on Ghana* (Washington, D.C.: World Bank, 1 October 2004), pp. 1–72 (p. 17).
66 Hutchful, *Adjustment Experience*, p. 125.
67 Obeng-Odoom, 'Neoliberalism', p. 101.
68 Joseph R.A. Ayee, 'Civil Service Reform in Ghana: A Case Study of Contemporary Reform Problems in Africa', *African Journal of Political Science*, 6.1 (2004), 1–41 (p. 13).
69 A.B. Atkinson, 'Bringing Income Distribution in From the Cold', *The Economic Journal*, 107.441 (1997), 297–321; Nancy Birdsall and Juan Luis Londoño, 'Asset Inequality Matters: An Assessment of the World Bank's Approach to Poverty Reduction', *The American Economic Review*, 87.2 (1997), 32–7; Howard White and Edward Anderson, 'Growth versus Distribution: Does the Pattern of Growth Matter?', *Development Policy Review*, 19.3 (2001), 267–89.
70 Jonathan D. Ostry, Prakash Loungani, and Davide Furceri, 'Neoliberalism: Oversold?', *Finance & Development*, 53.2 (2016), 38–41.
71 Harold Coulombe and Andrew McKay, 'Growth with Selective Poverty Reduction – Ghana in the 1990s', in *Growth and Poverty Reduction: Case Studies from West Africa*, ed. by Quentin Wodon (Washington, D.C.: World Bank Publications, 2007), pp. 9–94.
72 Ernest Y. Kunfaa, *Consultations with the Poor: Ghana Country Synthesis Report* (Kumasi: CEDEP on behalf of the World Bank, 1999), pp. 1–89 (p. 74).
73 Ben Fine and Kwabia Boateng, 'Labour and Employment under Structural Adjustment', in *Economic Reforms in Ghana: The Miracle and the Mirage*, ed. by Ernest Aryeetey, Jane Harrigan, and Machiko Nissanke (Oxford: James Currey, 2000), pp. 227–45 (p. 230).
74 George J.S. Dei, 'The Renewal of a Ghanaian Rural Economy', *Canadian Journal of African Studies*, 26.1 (1992), 24–53 (p. 32).
75 Cuthbert Baataar, *Malnourished Infants in Nandom Rehabilitation Centre: A Case Study of Deficits in Care* (Legon, Accra: University of Ghana, 2005), p. 52.
76 Lynne Brydon and Karen Legge, *Adjusting Society: The World Bank, the IMF and Ghana* (London: Tauris Academic Studies, 1996), pp. 83–4; Konadu-Agyemang, 'Best of Times', p. 474.

77 Birgit Meyer, 'Commodities and the Power of Prayer: Pentecostalist Attitudes Towards Consumption in Contemporary Ghana', *Development and Change*, 29.4 (1998), 751–76; Birgit Meyer, 'Visions of Blood, Sex and Money: Fantasy Spaces in Popular Ghanaian Cinema', *Visual Anthropology*, 16.1 (2003), 15–41.

78 Paul Glewwe and Kwaku A. Twum-Baah, *The Distribution of Welfare in Ghana, 1987–88* (Washington, D.C.: World Bank, 1991), pp. 1–108 (pp. 59–60).

79 Kunfaa, *Consultations*, p. 23.

80 See, for a survey of literature to this end, Richard G. Wilkinson and Kate E. Pickett, 'Income Inequality and Social Dysfunction', *Annual Review of Sociology*, 35 (2009), 493–511.

81 Quoted in Abdul-Korah, '"Only Sons"', p. 398.

82 Boahen, *Ghanaian Sphinx*, p. 51.

83 This received some lively discussion through the late 1950s and early 1960s but little again until recently. See Polly Hill, 'Some Puzzling Spending Habits in Ghana', *Economic Bulletin of Ghana*, 1.10 (1957), 3–11; Thomas Poleman, *The Food Economies of Urban Middle Africa: The Case of Ghana* (Stanford, CA: Food Research Institute, Stanford University, 1961); Rowena M. Lawson, 'Engel's Law and Its Application to Ghana', *Economic Bulletin of Ghana*, 6.4 (1962), 334–46; P.L.H. Davey, 'Some Puzzling Spending Habits in Ghana', *Economic Bulletin of Ghana*, 7.1 (1963), 17–28.

84 Jane I. Guyer, *Marginal Gains: Monetary Transactions in Atlantic Africa* (Chicago, IL: University of Chicago Press, 2004), p. 146.

85 Alderman, *Nutritional Status*, pp. 21–2; Glewwe and Twum-Baah, *Distribution of Welfare*, p. 64.

86 Daniel G. Maxwell et al., *Urban Livelihoods and Food and Nutrition Security in Greater Accra, Ghana* (Washington, D.C.: International Food Policy Research Institute, 2000), pp. 54–7.

87 Quoted in Boahen, *Ghanaian Sphinx*, p. 41.

88 Agyei-Mensah and Aikins, 'Epidemiological Transition'.

89 Goody, *Cooking*.

90 GDHS, 1993–2014. Women with BMI over 60 (i.e. 1.5 times the WHO's start point for 'clinical obesity') were excluded from this data. This accounted for 21 women of the 18,845 surveyed (0.1 per cent). Bottom and top bands of box represents first and third quartiles, and the band inside shows the median. Whiskers extend to 1.5 times the interquartile range.

91 Abram de Swaan, *In Care of the State: Health Care, Education and Welfare in Europe and the USA in the Modern Era* (Cambridge: Polity, 1988).

92 Abram de Swaan, 'Elite Perceptions of the Poor: Reflections on a Comparative Research Project', in *Elite Perceptions of Poverty and Inequality*, ed. by Elisa Pereira Reis and Mick Moore (London: ZED Books, 2005), pp. 182–94.

93 See, for instance, Alexander Sarris and Hadi Shams, *Ghana under Structural Adjustment: The Impact on Agriculture and the Rural Poor* (New York: New York University Press for IFAD, 1991); V.K. Nyanteng and A. Wayo Seini, 'Agricultural Policy and the Impact on Growth and Productivity 1970–95', in *Economic Reforms in Ghana: The Miracle and the Mirage*, ed. by Ernest Aryeetey, Jane Harrigan, and Machiko Nissanke (Oxford: James Curry, 2000), pp. 267–83.

94 Alice Wiemers, 'A "Time of Agric": Rethinking the "Failure" of Agricultural Programs in 1970s Ghana', *World Development*, 66 (2015), 104–17.

95 George J.S. Dei, 'A Ghanaian Town Revisited: Changes and Continuities in Local Adaptive Strategies', *African Affairs*, 91.362 (1992), 95–120 (pp. 105–6); Dei, 'Renewal', pp. 42–3.

96 An excellent introduction to this point is Pamela Sparr, 'Feminist Critiques of Structural Adjustment', in *Mortgaging Women's Lives: Feminist Critiques of Structural Adjustment*, ed. by Pamela Sparr (London: ZED Books, 1994), pp. 13–39; or, in the same collection but with a focus on Ghana, Manu Takyiwaa, 'Ghana: Women in the Public and Informal Sectors under the Economic Recovery Programme', in *Mortgaging Women's Lives: Feminist Critiques of Structural Adjustment*, ed. by Pamela Sparr (London: ZED Books, 1994), pp. 61–77.

97 Takyiwaa, 'Ghana', p. 70.

98 Juan Carlos Guzmán, Andrew R. Morrison, and Mirja Sjöblom, 'The Impact of Remittances and Gender on Household Expenditure Patterns: Evidence from Ghana', in *The International Migration of Women*, ed. by Andrew R. Morrison, Maurice Schiff, and Mirja Sjöblom (Washington, D.C.: World Bank, 2008), pp. 125–52.

99 Dei, 'Renewal', p. 38.

100 World Bank, *Ghana: Population*, pp. 53–4.
101 Ghana Government, *The Nutrition of Adults in Northern Ghana: A Report of the National Nutrition Survey of the National Food and Nutrition Board* (Accra: Mimeo., 1962).
102 Baataar, *Malnourished Infants*, p. 14.
103 Baataar, *Malnourished Infants*, p. 35.
104 Baataar, *Malnourished Infants*, p. 60.
105 Elizabeth Ardayfio-Schandorf, 'Household Headship and Women's Earning in Ghana', in *Family and Development in Ghana*, ed. by Elizabeth Ardayfio-Schandorf (Legon, Accra: Ghana Universities Press, 1994), pp. 30–47.
106 Brenda Chalfin, 'Risky Business: Economic Uncertainty, Market Reforms and Female Livelihoods in Northeast Ghana', *Development and Change*, 31.5 (2000), 987–1008.
107 Abdul-Korah, '"Only Sons"', p. 396.
108 Guzmán, Morrison, and Sjöblom, 'Impact of Remittances', p. 130.
109 Aryeetey and McKay, 'Poverty Reduction', p. 74; Coulombe and McKay, 'Growth', p. 34.
110 Kunfaa, *Consultations*, p. 36.
111 Destombes, 'Long-Term', p. 205.
112 Overå, 'When Men Do Women's Work'.
113 Anne-Marie Côté et al., 'Transactional Sex Is the Driving Force in the Dynamics of HIV in Accra, Ghana', *AIDS*, 18.6 (2004), 917–25.
114 Edem M.A. Tette et al., 'Changing Patterns of Disease and Mortality at the Children's Hospital, Accra: Are Infections Rising?', *PLOS ONE*, 11.4 (2016), 1–12; Edem M.A. Tette et al., 'Maternal Profiles and Social Determinants of Malnutrition and the MDGs: What Have We Learnt?', *BMC Public Health*, 16 (2016), 214.
115 Andy Norton et al., *Poverty Assessment in Ghana – Using Qualitative and Participatory Research Methods*, PSP Discussion Paper (Washington, D.C.: The World Bank, 1995), p. v.
116 Brydon and Legge, *Adjusting Society*, p. 83.
117 Coulombe and McKay, 'Growth', p. 34.
118 Tom Gillespie, 'Accumulation by Urban Dispossession: Struggles over Urban Space in Accra, Ghana', *Transactions of the Institute of British Geographers*, 41.1 (2016), 66–77.
119 Franklin Obeng-Odoom, 'The Informal Sector in Ghana under Siege', *Journal of Developing Societies*, 27.3–4 (2011), 355–92; Alex B. Asiedu and Samuel Agyei-Mensah, 'Traders on the Run: Activities of Street Vendors in the Accra Metropolitan Area, Ghana', *Norwegian Journal of Geography*, 62.3 (2008), 191–202.
120 See, for instance, Gavin Hilson and Clive Potter, 'Structural Adjustment and Subsistence Industry: Artisanal Gold Mining in Ghana', *Development and Change*, 36.1 (2005), 103–31 (pp. 121–4).
121 Baataar, *Malnourished Infants*, p. 66; Elizabeth Ardayfio-Schandorf, *Rural Energy Crisis in Ghana: Its Implications for Women's Work and Household Survival* (Geneva: International Labour Organization, 1986).
122 David Harvey, 'The "New" Imperialism: Accumulation by Dispossession', *Socialist Register*, 40.40 (2009), 63–87.
123 Samuel Nii Ardey Codjoe and Fred M. Dzanku, 'Long-Term Determinants of Deforestation in Ghana: The Role of Structural Adjustment Policies', *African Development Review*, 21.3 (2009), 558–88.
124 George J.S. Dei, 'A Forest beyond the Trees: Tree Cutting in Rural Ghana', *Human Ecology*, 20.1 (1992), 57–88.
125 Hilson and Potter, 'Structural Adjustment', pp. 121–4.
126 Frederick A. Armah et al., 'Food Security and Climate Change in Drought-Sensitive Savanna Zones of Ghana', *Mitigation and Adaptation Strategies for Global Change*, 16.3 (2010), 291–306; Joseph Awetori Yaro, 'Is Deagrarianisation Real? A Study of Livelihood Activities in Rural Northern Ghana', *The Journal of Modern African Studies*, 44.1 (2006), 125–56.
127 Lavy et al., *Quality of Health Care*, p. 21.
128 C.J. Waddington and K.A. Enyimayew, 'A Price to Pay: The Impact of User Charges in Ashanti-Akim District, Ghana', *The International Journal of Health Planning and Management*, 4.1 (1989), 17–47; Lavy et al., *Quality of Health Care*, p. 10.
129 Konadu-Agyemang, 'Best of Times', p. 479; Hutchful, *Adjustment Experience*, pp. 119, 130. For similar patterns in the spread of doctors and attempts to resist centralisation, see Nott 'Material History'.

130 C.A. Anyinam, 'Spatial Implications of Structural Adjustment Programmes in Ghana', *Tijdschrift Voor Economische En Sociale Geografie*, 85.5 (1994), 446–60.

131 AngloGold Ashanti, 'Case Study: Creating a Sustainable Solution for Malaria in Continental Africa Region', 2013 <http://www.aga-reports.com/13/os/case-study/car-malaria> [accessed 3 August 2016].

132 Paul Cammack, 'Making the Poor Work for Globalisation?', *New Political Economy*, 6.3 (2001), 397–408.

133 See, for instance, Ian Gary, 'Confrontation, Co-operation or Co-optation: NGOs and the Ghanaian State during Structural Adjustment', *Review of African Political Economy*, 23.68 (1996), 149–68; Tina Wallace, 'NGO Dilemmas: Trojan Horses for Global Neoliberalism?', *Socialist Register*, 40 (2009), 202–19.

134 Julie Hearn, 'The "Uses and Abuses" of Civil Society in Africa', *Review of African Political Economy*, 28.87 (2001), 43–53 (pp. 45–7).

135 See Bayart, *The State in Africa*.

136 Philip D. Osei, 'Political Liberalisation and the Implementation of Value Added Tax in Ghana', *The Journal of Modern African Studies*, 38.2 (2000), 255–78.

137 Jean-Pascal Daloz, '"Big Men" in Sub-Saharan Africa: How Elites Accumulate Positions and Resources', *Comparative Sociology*, 2.1 (2003), 271–85 (pp. 279–80).

138 Bayart, *The State in Africa*, pp. 155–63.

139 Wiemers, '"Time of Agric"', p. 108.

140 World Bank, *Ghana: Population*, pp. 54–5.

141 Comaroff and Comaroff, 'Millennial Capitalism', pp. 330–4.

142 Paul Gifford, 'Ghana's Charismatic Churches', *Journal of Religion in Africa*, 24.3 (1994), 241–65.

143 Jean Comaroff and John L. Comaroff, 'Second Comings: Neo-Protestant Ethics and Millennial Capitalism in Africa, and Elsewhere', in *2000 Years and Beyond: Faith, Identity, and the 'Common Era'*, ed. by Paul Gifford (London: Routledge, 2003), pp. 291–343 (p. 121).

144 Joel Robbins, 'The Globalization of Pentecostal and Charismatic Christianity', *Annual Review of Anthropology*, 33.1 (2004), 117–43 (p. 131).

145 Isaac Addai, 'Determinants of Use of Maternal-Child Health Services in Rural Ghana', *Journal of Biosocial Science*, 32.1 (2000), 1–15 (p. 14).

146 Meyer, 'Commodities and the Power of Prayer', pp. 762–6.

147 UNICEF, 'Adjustment Policies', II, p. 106.

148 Christine Oppong, 'Some Roles of Women: What Do We Know?', in *Family and Development in Ghana*, ed. by Elizabeth Ardayfio-Schandorf (Legon, Accra: Ghana Universities Press, 1994), pp. 57–94 (p. 63).

149 Aaron R. Denham et al., 'Chasing Spirits: Clarifying the Spirit Child Phenomenon and Infanticide in Northern Ghana', *Social Science & Medicine*, 71.3 (2010), 608–15.

150 P. Allotey and D. Reidpath, 'Establishing the Causes of Childhood Mortality in Ghana: The "Spirit Child"', *Social Science & Medicine*, 52.7 (2001), 1007–12.

151 Hilson and Potter, 'Structural Adjustment'; Gavin Hilson, 'Child Labour in African Artisanal Mining Communities: Experiences from Northern Ghana', *Development and Change*, 41.3 (2010), 445–73.

152 Ghana Government, *Enhancing the Human Impact of the Adjustment Programme: Report Prepared by the Government of Ghana for the Sixth Meeting of the Consultative Group for Ghana, Paris, 14–15 May 1991* (Accra: Government Printer, 1991), p. 28.

153 World Bank, *Ghana: Population*, pp. 54–5.

154 Esi K. Colecraft et al., 'A Longitudinal Assessment of the Diet and Growth of Malnourished Children Participating in Nutrition Rehabilitation Centres in Accra, Ghana', *Public Health Nutrition*, 7.4 (2004), 487–94 (p. 490).

155 Colecraft et al., 'Longitudinal Assessment', p. 491.

156 Maxwell et al., *Urban Livelihoods*, p. 61.

157 Clark, 'Fasting', p. 57.

158 Clark, 'Fasting', p. 47.

159 See, for instance, Popkin, 'Nutrition Transition'.

160 Henry Bernstein, *Class Dynamics of Agrarian Change* (Halifax, NS: Fernwood, 2010), pp. 25–37.

161 Philip McMichael, 'Reframing Development: Global Peasant Movements and the New Agrarian Question', *Canadian Journal of Development Studies*, 27.4 (2006), 471–83 (p. 476); Harvey, 'The "New" Imperialism'.

162 Quoted in Metcalfe, *Great Britain and Ghana*, p. 613.

163 A similar destruction of Mexican foodways is detailed in Alyshia Gálvez, *Eating NAFTA: Trade, Food Policies, and the Destruction of Mexico* (Oakland, CA: University of California Press, 2018).

164 See, for instance, Harold Alderman and Paul A. Higgins, *Food and Nutritional Adequacy in Ghana* (Ithaca, NY: Cornell Food and Nutrition Policy Program, 1992), pp. 1–61.

165 Gerardo Otero et al., 'The Neoliberal Diet and Inequality in the United States', *Social Science & Medicine*, 142 (2015), 47–55.

166 Agyei-Mensah and Aikins, 'Epidemiological Transition'.

167 Preetika Rana, 'Nestlé's Noodles Face More Scrutiny in India', *Wall Street Journal*, 31 March 2016 <http://www.wsj.com/articles/nestles-noodles-face-more-scrutiny-in-india-1459428231> [accessed 10 August 2016].

168 A. Drewnowski, 'Taste Preferences and Food Intake', *Annual Review of Nutrition*, 17.1 (1997), 237–53.

169 Ricardo Uauy, Cecilia Albala, and Juliana Kain, 'Obesity Trends in Latin America: Transiting from Under- to Overweight', *The Journal of Nutrition*, 131.3 (2001), 893S–899S; Christopher G. Owen et al., 'Effect of Infant Feeding on the Risk of Obesity across the Life Course: A Quantitative Review of Published Evidence', *Pediatrics*, 115.5 (2005), 1367–77; Christopher G. Owen et al., 'Does Breastfeeding Influence Risk of Type 2 Diabetes in Later Life? A Quantitative Analysis of Published Evidence', *The American Journal of Clinical Nutrition*, 84.5 (2006), 1043–54.

170 Posnansky, 'How Ghana's Crisis Affects a Village'.

171 Dei, 'Renewal', pp. 32–3.

172 Morris et al., 'Geographic Targeting'.

173 For the influence of household composition, see Ruel et al., 'Good Care Practices'. For increasing nucleation, see Samuel Kobina Annim, Kofi Awusabo-Asare, and Joshua Amo-Adjei, 'Household Nucleation, Dependency and Child Health Outcomes in Ghana', *Journal of Biosocial Science*, 47.5 (2015), 565–92.

174 Annim, Awusabo-Asare, and Amo-Adjei, 'Household Nucleation'.

175 Comaroff and Comaroff, 'Millennial Capitalism', p. 334.

9
Space, time, and the nature of nutrition in the twenty-first century

History is repeating itself today at the Tamale Teaching Hospital (TTH). Extensively modernised and refurbished since it was upgraded from a regional hospital in the early 2000s, its old buildings have been renovated and added to. The number of beds has doubled, and several new units have been established, including a high-tech neonatal intensive care unit. With external runways and awnings sculpted into long metallic waves, the new, main building is an imposing presence in the low-lying city. Throughout much of the hospital, the signage is rendered in a uniform red and yellow. The text for 'Consulting Room 1', 'Maternity Ward', 'Blood Bank', and 'Diet Therapy' appears in bright red on a bright yellow background (see Figure 9.1). On the left side of these signs is a photograph of a Lucozade bottle, overlaid with the words 'fast acting glucose energy'. In order to emphasise its biomedical effect, the line which underscores these words spirals into a heart-rate monitor. This is not only the case in Tamale: Lucozade sponsors public hospital and polyclinic signage across Ghana. The promotion of a carbonated, sugary drink as a healthful source of energy derives from Lucozade's earlier history in Britain, where it was initially sold through pharmacies, advertised in medical journals, and often brought, alongside grapes and flowers, to friends and relatives in hospital.[1] In Britain, however, by the 1980s, and amid slowly emerging concerns about the health effects of sugar, Lucozade pivoted from health drink to sports drink, a market position which it still vigorously maintains.[2] Its continued promotion in Ghanaian hospitals, despite even firmer understandings of the relationship between sugar and ill-health, has the faint echo of Nestlé nurses and their hawkish promotion of breastmilk substitutes in the mid-twentieth century. As with the epidemic infant malnutrition which resulted in part

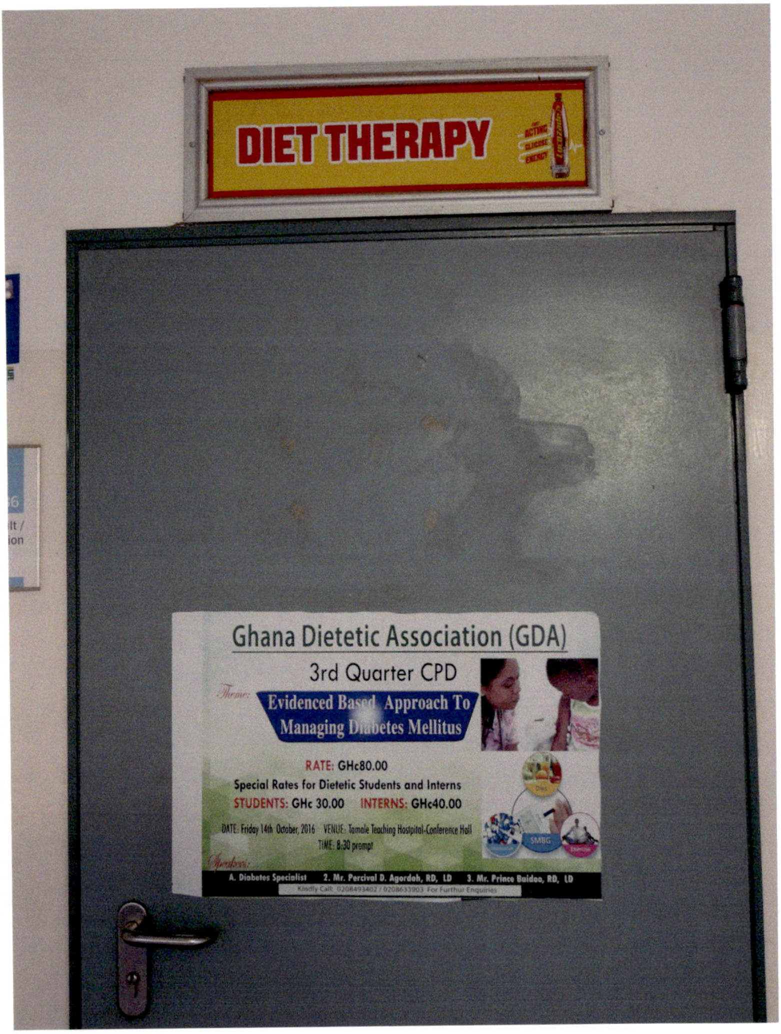

Figure 9.1 Diet therapy room at Tamale Teaching Hospital, 2019. Photo: author's own.

from these marketing practices, cause and effect manifest in the patients treated at TTH too. Posted on the door of the Diet Therapy room is an advert for a Ghana Dietetic Association conference on the management of diabetes.

Capitalism's innate drive to create new tastes and new needs has long been a central tenet of both food history and pharmaceutical history.[3] The epidemiology of dietary disease is shaped by the development of these new tastes – tastes for foods and for ways of eating. Emerging medical and nutritional demands are also increasingly addressed via increasingly marketised solutions to disease management – through health foods, nutrition supplements, or the long-term prescription of pharmaceuticals for chronic illness. This symbiotic relationship is evidenced in the close association between food and pharmaceutical industries. GlaxoSmithKline, for instance, produces drugs which are commonly used to treat diabetes and, until 2013, also produced Lucozade. Although codified as non-communicable diseases, both infant malnutrition and chronic diseases of adulthood, such as type 2 diabetes, have been seen to spread quickly in periods of market liberalisation. Ghana's economic transformation under British-colonial government saw the devaluation of domestic labour, the promotion of breastmilk substitutes, and epidemics of childhood malnutrition. As with these earlier epidemics, the incidence of chronic disease in the period following Structural Adjustment can only be understood with reference to the political economy of food, feeding, and public-service provision.

However, if infant malnutrition proved a riddle for physicians in the mid-twentieth century, the relationship between diet and chronic disease is even more obstruse. Diet is certainly not the only driver of chronic disease; physical activity, drug use (broadly defined), psychological and emotional stress, and exposure to pollution have also all been found to play some role. Older age, and simply living longer amid any such detrimental exposures, also increases the likelihood of developing a chronic health condition. In Ghana, life expectancy has increased steadily throughout the early twenty-first century. In 2000, around 51 per cent of men and 56 per cent of women lived until 65; by 2019 it was 61 and 67 per cent respectively.[4] Food, in terms of its availability and affordability, will have played some role in this increase. There have also been consistent reductions in infant mortality over these years and, as detailed in the previous two chapters, remarkable advances in the treatment of severe malnutrition have saved many young lives. Despite the imprecise aetiology of chronic illness, diet is still often touted as their principal cause and a key means of protection against their emergence later in life. The increasing incidence of chronic illness in Ghana – at rates far outpacing increases in life expectancy – must, then, suggest some recent change in the relationship between food and health.

Take diabetes, again, as the example. In 1958, the pioneering Ghanaian physician Silas Dodu found that 0.4 per cent of outpatients attending Accra hospitals were clinically diabetic.[5] Two years later, in a community survey conducted in Ho, the provincial capital of the Volta Region, Dodu and de Heer reported a diabetes prevalence of

0.2 per cent.[6] By the late 1960s, however, Dodu noted that diabetes was 'being diagnosed with increasing frequency', and that the 'sugar disease' was well-known among urban communities.[7] By 2002, a prevalence study conducted in Accra suggested that perhaps 6.3 per cent of the population were clinically diabetic.[8] Although diabetes diagnoses were clearly increasing during the second half of the twentieth century, a review of hospital data from Kumasi's Komfo Anokye Teaching Hospital suggests that the rate of increase has been more significant in the past few decades. Between 1983 and 2014, diabetes admissions increased from 2.36 per thousand to 14.94 per thousand, a rise of more than 600 per cent. Inpatient deaths from diabetes likewise increased from 7.6 per thousand in 1983 to 30 per thousand in 2014.[9] Similar increases in hypertension, stroke, and cancer have also all been suggested by population-level studies, and there are both spatial and gendered dimensions to the epidemiology of chronic disease, with urban and Southern communities, and also men, usually found with higher prevalence rates.[10] Research suggests that the relationship between diet and chronic disease is well understood by the patient public. However, and as was also found in the 1990s, among the mothers of children attending nutrition rehabilitation centres, knowledge of nutritional best practice is not necessarily enough to resist the structural determinants of diet.[11]

Despite the increasing incidence of chronic conditions all across Africa, epidemics of non-communicable disease have not been treated with the same urgency as infectious disease. This point is made clear in Amy Moran-Thomas's telling anthropological vignette, which compares a Tamale diabetes clinic in 2009 with the office of the Guinea-worm eradication programme just across town. Struggling to track the final few cases of Guinea worm, the eradication office housed several dozen campaign staff, Ministry of Health officials and consultants from The Carter Center, a US NGO. The public hospital's once-weekly diabetes clinic was, by contrast, attended by upwards of 30 patients, some of whom had travelled for hours, and all of whom were waiting outside for the one doctor. Called away on another emergency, the doctor never arrived. A painful and visually dramatic parasitic disease, Guinea worms are rarely fatal, and is often not considered nearly as urgent by its hosts as by 'the foreign photographers taking pictures of them'. Yet, as Moran-Thomas notes, 'a diabetes ulcer becoming infected had been categorised as nobody's emergency, even though a resulting amputation could result in searing pains and patterned disability for a lifetime'.[12] Because of the chronic nature of diabetes, the targeted approaches to treatment which have developed for infectious disease, as well as for clinical manifestations of malnutrition, are less possible. Instead, chronic illnesses require the sort of expensive, long-term care which hollowed-out, neoliberal medical systems have limited capacity to provide.

Ghana has been certified as Guinea-worm-free since 2015, but the eradication campaign is still a visible feature of Ghanaian public health, driven by the attractive logic of infectious disease eradication and the international philanthropy which has sustained such an expensive crusade. Epidemic diabetes has, by contrast, been somewhat overlooked, in part because of its ready classification as a 'lifestyle disease', the onus for which is placed with the individual patient.[13] As 'lifestyle diseases', or a consequence of 'overconsumption', epidemics of diabetes or heart disease also do not wield the same political capital as 'malnutrition' or 'undernutrition'. Instead, as fat studies scholars and activists have most prominently argued, the onset of chronic diseases, and proneness to chronic disease, is often portrayed as a failure to comply with the 'healthist' expectations of 'biocitizenship'. A failure to be thin enough, exercise enough, or eat well enough to avoid such diagnoses later in life.[14]

Other narratives naturalise the spread of chronic disease as part of an 'epidemiological transition', itself the result of a 'nutrition transition'. Here, the shift from coarse cereals, fruits, and vegetables to highly processed, energy-dense foods is said to drive the incidence of non-communicable disease.[15] However, as the historian Simon Szreter has recently argued, 'the intellectual work that all "transitions" do is to deal ahistorically with the problem of time'. Theorising epidemiological or nutritional change as part of a transition offers social scientists and policymakers a reassuring, linear link between past, present, and future, allowing for the acknowledgement 'that they live and work in historical time … without having to engage with the complexity of the history'.[16] Ahistorical and also largely apolitical, transition theories pave over the undulating political economy of health, instead coding epidemics of chronic disease as inevitable, or even positive – the teleological endpoint of social and economic development. This logic, however, also assumes that social and economic development will also be broadly equitable with the European or North American experience, and that infrastructures have a similar capacity to provide long-term care to the chronically ill. In Ghana's case, as with many of her continental neighbours, the emergence of chronic disease alongside enduring burdens of infectious disease and infant malnutrition has been seen to stretch transition models 'beyond plausibility'.[17] This slippage between health transitions which are seen to work in Europe and fail in Africa, the 'double burden' being the most enduring of these, is perhaps better understood as one of many stilted or partial transformations in African economic history, the subordinate, extractive version of colonial capitalism being the prime example of this.[18] Hospital signage is a rather small thing by comparison, but the continued promotion of high-sugar products in healthcare settings struggling under the weight of chronic illness speaks to precisely this sort of partial transformation.

Throughout the later twentieth century, epidemiological research into the relative absence of cardiovascular and metabolic disease in Africa provided the West with the conceptual foundations for preventive public health campaigns, for legislation around food marketing, and for the endless, ongoing debates about the relative influence of carbohydrates and fats in the aetiology of chronic disease.[19] In Ghana, however, it is only recently, some decades later, that similar forms of preventive dietetics have become a visible aspect of medical discourse. Here, in the post-adjustment economy, these ideas are loudly promoted from inside the rapidly diversifying market for foods. Today, if you travel a few miles along Liberation Road – say, from the University of Ghana campus in Legon and towards the centre of Accra – you will pass billboards for rice and tomato paste, both advertised as being 'fortified' with various vitamins; adverts for sunflower oil, which is 'naturally low in cholesterol'; and for condensed milk, which has the protein and calcium necessary for 'a good start to the day'. Driven by the threat of chronic disease, as well as individual responsibility for its prevention, these adverts trade on the blurring distinction between food and drug, eating and medicating.[20] This, an increasingly commercial and industrial form of nutritionist dietetics, is also actively promoted by the state. In what is the first significant government interruption of the free market for foodstuffs since the onset of the ERP – and emerging as part of Ghana's diverse and increasingly organised food sovereignty movement – even the flagship Planting for Food and Jobs (PFJ) programme, which began in 2017, has provided large subsidies in pursuit of crop diversity and biofortification.[21]

Although the production of and market for enhanced foods and nutraceuticals initially flourished in the neoliberal political economy, it draws credibility from evolving scientific understandings of the relationship between chronic illness and the environments in which we live. This, the science of epigenetics, or the study of how behaviours and environments can effect changes in gene expression, has transformed the foods we eat into one of a number of environmental 'exposures' which our bodies 'metabolise', 'absorb', or 'weather', and which will ultimately shape our future health.[22] Research into the 'developmental origins of health and disease (DOHaD)' takes that the epigenomes of foetuses and infants are especially plastic, and that adverse food environments in early life can contribute to an increased propensity for chronic diseases in adulthood. More strikingly, epidemiological research into the descendants of European famine survivors suggests that genetic predisposition to chronic disease is at least partially heritable.[23] Epigenetics, in this respect, produces a body that is 'heavily impregnated by its own past and by the social and material environment within which it dwells. It is a body that is imprinted by evolutionary and transgenerational time, by "early-life," and a body that is highly susceptible to changes in its social and material environment.'[24] Hastened by the 'great acceleration' of anthropogenic climate change, and correlating the rise of adulterants in our food, water, and air with recent constraints on market regulation, epigenetics is a 'post-industrial' addendum to the science of nutrition.[25] As Hannah Landecker's work has most notably explained, today more than ever before, 'metabolism is *in* history: the material of the bodies fed by an industrialized agriculture and food-processing systems'.[26]

As case histories of maternal and infant malnutrition begin to threaten health in the present, the long social history of food and feeding gathers some scientific import. These histories have new potential to direct, or to misdirect, debates within contemporary medicine. For instance, some of the earliest antecedents of epigenetics argued that there were 'thrifty genes' which slowed metabolisation among African populations, both on the continent and in the Americas, whose ancestors were assumed to have been regularly exposed to hunger.[27] This stereotyping of Africa's past – via narratives which are held up neither by genomic research nor in the historical accounting detailed in the first chapters of this book and in other recent work – have been used to naturalise high rates of chronic disease in racialised populations and postcolonial spaces.[28] Despite the lack of evidence, these histories have retained some cachet in contemporary medicine, informing discourses which emphasise an inherited and inherently African 'maladaption' to new lifestyles, and which put forward the industrial enhancement of food as a solution.[29]

If, today, epigenetics means that health is indeed '*in* history', then it is also in the practice of history. Histories considerate of the structural determinants of epidemiological pasts – inclusive of both medical preoccupation and the political economies of health – offer a means to critique epidemiological presents and challenge epidemiological futures. When drawing from more explicitly critical histories of nutrition, epigenetics actively agitates against the foodways and food practices which cheapen domestic reproduction in capitalist modernity: against the overuse of RUTFs, or the (even appropriate) use of breastmilk substitutes, practices which have both been shown to increase the likelihood of chronic disease in later life.[30]

Of course, the necessity of RUTFs and other technical solutions to hunger in contemporary Ghana is itself proof of the persistence of childhood deficiency. As a powerful epigenetic exposure, high rates of chronic disease in twenty-first century Ghana are, at least in part, evidence of a more recent history of malnutrition. There is, however, good reason to hope that high rates of endemic malnutrition, the other side of the 'double burden', may be starting to fade. Unlike the relatively staid changes seen between 1983 and 2003, and detailed in the last chapter, the period between the 2008 and 2014 DHS surveys saw marked improvements in terms of infant anthropometry; for the country as a whole, the incidence of both clinical stunting and wasting halved in between the two surveys. Although these dramatic advances deserve celebration, these numbers still mean that around 20 per cent of children surveyed in 2014 were stunted by international standards. By contrast, the period between the 2014 and 2022 DHS surveys saw very little change, with a small decline in stunting and a small rise in wasting. The obstinate nature of childhood malnutrition is indicative of another partial macroeconomic transformation, Ghana's escape from famine.

For the most part, the European escape from famine had, by the early twentieth century, also provided relative freedom from endemic malnutrition. Indeed, this is one of the reasons why colonial service physicians were so fascinated by kwashiorkor. For many other parts of the world, including Ghana, this has not been the case. The history of this partial escape from hunger has to be traced over the long term, and with particular reference to the spatial and structural impositions of colonial economic development. In some respects, the formalisation of the Gold Coast as a new and unified polity alleviated the threat of famine in the savannah and among communities more prone to climatic shocks. The development of a countrywide market for labour during the first part of the twentieth century facilitated migration, urbanisation, and economic diversification, and provided new avenues for the exertion of economic agency in spaces which had been made marginal over the course of centuries.[31] Yet these same processes have also reinforced the economic marginality of the savannah, concentrating the means of production in historical and emerging centres of power – in Asante, Accra, and Britain – and encouraging the growth of an insecure labouring class which was initially made up of Northern migrants. Although the forest economies were the initial beneficiaries of the cash-crop transition, the continued primacy of export agriculture progressively undermined food production and food sovereignty everywhere, as well as eroding the moral economies and social insurances which had previously assuaged the threat of food insecurity and childhood malnutrition.[32] Integration into a more global economy has, instead, tended to demand sacrifices in terms of social reproduction and, for the ever-growing numbers of market-dependent poor, led to an increased propensity for nutritional illness, especially at times of local or personal crisis.[33]

When widespread, such crises have been important agents of change in Ghana. In 1948, rising food prices led to peaceful protests in Accra, to the killing of three protesting ex-servicemen by colonial police, to widespread rioting, and, ultimately, to the galvanisation of the independence movement and the national experiment with socialism.[34] The final end to this experiment came a few decades later when, in 1983, political turmoil and climatic bad fortune led to the collapse of the food market and widespread hunger, an IMF bailout, and the onset of Structural Adjustment. During this period, it was those reliant on the market and with limited access to the traditional-agrarian world – a population which had swelled enormously in the intervening decades – that were the most prone to hunger. Although stabilising the economy and providing new avenues for macroeconomic growth, the ERP did nothing to address these fundamental insecurities. If anything, Structural Adjustment reinforced and reemphasised the earlier, colonial-era emphasis on capital extraction at the expense of social reproduction. However, by encouraging and facilitating the spread of new foods and new ways of eating, some of which have been linked with the spread of chronic disease, Structural Adjustment has also bolstered food and nutrition security, albeit perhaps at the expense of future health.

There is, then, still a certain brittleness to the Ghanaian food economy. The threat of hunger has endured, even if infrastructures and technologies – inclusive of food aid, RUTFs, and cheap, energy-dense foods – mitigate any associated increase in mortality. This is a feature of many, or perhaps most, contemporary economies.[35] The near doubling of grain prices in 2008, for instance, did not lead to a significant increase in mortality anywhere in the world, but the number of malnourished people was estimated to have grown from 100 million to perhaps one billion.[36] More recently still, the Covid-19 pandemic led to renewed questions about Ghana's capacity to absorb similar economic shocks. As in most countries, the government heeded WHO advice and implemented lockdowns in cities with high rates of infection, including Accra, Kumasi, Tema, and Kasoa. Unlike many other countries, restrictions were lifted after only three weeks, and before any significant reduction in infection. As President Nana Akufo-Addo explained at the time, 'I cannot ignore the impact that this lockdown is having on several constituencies of our nation, especially the informal workers … who need to have a day out in the market or otherwise in order to provide for their families.'[37] Although the ascendency of an unequal, perhaps unhealthy, but undeniably robust global marketplace for food has softened the impact of economic insecurity, free market foodways cannot entirely moderate the threat of market contraction and the resulting loss of income, no matter how cheap food becomes.

Notes

1 'They like Lucozade … and They Keep It Down', *Proceedings of the Royal Society of Medicine*, 50.2 (1957), ii.

2 On the history of sugar in nutritional medicine, see Rachel Meach, 'From John Yudkin to Jamie Oliver: A Short but Sweet History on the War against Sugar', in *Proteins, Pathologies and Politics: Dietary Innovation and Disease from the Nineteenth Century*, ed. by David C. Gentilcore and Matthew Smith (London: Bloomsbury Academic, 2018), pp. 95–108.

3 This was one of Sidney Mintz's driving arguments in his seminal history of sugar: Mintz, *Sweetness and Power*; for the pharmaceutical history, see Joseph Dumit, *Drugs for Life: How Pharmaceutical Companies Define Our Health* (Durham, NC: Duke University Press, 2012).

4 Taken from United Nations Population Division, <https://data.worldbank.org> [accessed 9 May 2022].

5 Silas R.A. Dodu, 'The Incidence of Diabetes Mellitus in Accra (Ghana); A Study of 4,000 Patients', *The West African Medical Journal*, 7.3 (1958), 129–34.

6 Silas R.A. Dodu and N. De Heer, 'A Diabetes Case-Finding Survey in Ho, Ghana', *Ghana Medical Journal*, 3 (1964), 75–80.

7 Silas R.A. Dodu, 'Diabetes in the Tropics', *The British Medical Journal*, 2.5554 (1967), 747–50 (p. 747).

8 Albert G.B. Amoah, Samuel K. Owusu, and Samuel Adjei, 'Diabetes in Ghana: A Community Based Prevalence Study in Greater Accra', *Diabetes Research and Clinical Practice*, 56.3 (2002), 197–205.

9 Osei Sarfo-Kantanka et al., 'Secular Trends in Admissions and Mortality Rates from Diabetes Mellitus in the Central Belt of Ghana: A 31-Year Review', *PLOS ONE*, 11.11 (2016), 1–14.

10 A thorough review of NCDs in Ghana can be found in *Chronic Non-Communicable Diseases in Ghana: Multidisciplinary Perspectives*, ed. by Ama de-Graft Aikens, Samuel Agyei-Mensah, and Charles Agyemang (Accra: Sub-Saharan Publishers, 2013).

11 Charlotte Wrigley-Asante, Samuel Agyei-Mensah, and Faustina Adomaa Obeng, 'It's Not All about Wealth and Beauty: Changing Perceptions of Fatness among Makola Market Women of Accra, Ghana', *Singapore Journal of Tropical Geography*, 3.38 (2017), 414–28.

12 Amy Moran-Thomas, 'The Para-Communicable: Living between Infectious and Non-Communicable Conditions', in *Epidemiological Change and Chronic Disease in Sub-Saharan Africa: Historical and Anthropological Perspectives*, ed. by Megan Vaughan, Kafui Adjaye-Gbewonyo, and Marissa Mika (London: UCL Press, 2021), pp. 233–51 (pp. 233–6).

13 Megan Vaughan, 'Conceptualising Metabolic Disorder in Southern Africa: Biology, History and Global Health', *BioSocieties*, 14.1 (2019), 123–42; Sara Glasgow and Ted Schrecker, 'The Double Burden of Neoliberalism? Noncommunicable Disease Policies and the Global Political Economy of Risk', *Health & Place*, 34 (2015), 279–86.

14 See, for instance, Strings, *Fearing the Black Body*; Susan Greenhalgh, *Fat-Talk Nation* (Ithaca, NY: Cornell University Press, 2015); Deborah Lupton, *Fat* (New York: Routledge, 2013). For a fine analysis of fatness in Accra, see Wrigley-Asante, Agyei-Mensah, and Obeng, 'Not All about Wealth'.

15 See Popkin, 'Nutrition Transition'. The conceptual origin of the epidemiological transition theory can be found in Abdel R. Omran, 'The Epidemiologic Transition: A Theory of the Epidemiology of Population Change', *The Milbank Memorial Fund Quarterly*, 49.4 (1971), 509–38.

16 Simon Szreter, 'The Epidemiologic Transition Turned Upside Down: Britain's Mortality History as an Imaginative Resource for Africa', in *Epidemiological Change and Chronic Disease in Sub-Saharan Africa: Historical and Anthropological Perspectives*, ed. by Megan Vaughan, Kafui Adjaye-Gbewonyo, and Marissa Mika (London: UCL Press, 2021), pp. 39–79 (p. 71).

17 Vaughan, 'Conceptualising Metabolic Disorder', p. 130.

18 See, for instance, Ha-Joon Chang, *Kicking Away the Ladder: Development Strategy in Historical Perspective* (London: Anthem, 2002).

19 It is interesting to note that some of this research was driven by the very same nutritionists that had focused on kwashiorkor in previous decades. See, for instance, *Western Diseases: Their Emergence and Prevention*, ed. by H.C. Trowell and D.P. Burkitt (Cambridge, MA: Harvard University Press, 1981).

20 Hannah Landecker, 'Food as Exposure: Nutritional Epigenetics and the New Metabolism', *BioSocieties*, 6.2 (2011), 167–94 (p. 185).

21 Ghana Government, *Investing for Food and Jobs (IFJ): An Agenda for Transforming Ghana's Agriculture (2018–2021)* (Accra: Ministry of Food and Agriculture, 2018). These developments can be seen as a notable softening of neoliberal agricultural policy. Early analyses of PFJ have been positive, and may prove to be a boon for Ghanaian food sovereignty and for food-crop areas. See, Mohammed Tanko, Salifu Ismaila, and Saeed Abu Sadiq, 'Planting for Food and Jobs (PFJ): A Panacea for Productivity and Welfare of Rice Farmers in Northern Ghana', *Cogent Economics & Finance*, 7.1 (2019), 1693121. Approaches to nutrition among the diverse actors involved in growing demands for food sovereignty are deserving of greater investigation. For an ethnographic account of the Ghanaian food sovereignty movement between 2012 and 2021, see Joeva Sean Rock, *We Are Not Starving: The Struggle for Food Sovereignty in Ghana* (East Lansing, MI: Michigan State University Press, 2022).

22 For social scientific analysis of this fascinating field, see, for instance, Jörg Niewöhner, 'Epigenetics: Embedded Bodies and the Molecularisation of Biography and Milieu', *BioSocieties*, 6.3 (2011), 279–98; Landecker, 'Food as Exposure'; Margaret Lock, 'Comprehending the Body in the Era of the Epigenome', *Current Anthropology*, 56.2 (2015), 151–77; Harris Solomon, *Metabolic Living: Food, Fat and the Absorption of Illness in India* (Durham, NC: Duke University Press, 2016); Jörg Niewöhner and Margaret Lock, 'Situating Local Biologies: Anthropological Perspectives on Environment/Human Entanglements', *BioSocieties*, 13.4 (2018), 681–97.

23 Landecker, 'Food as Exposure', pp. 177–8.

24 Niewöhner, 'Epigenetics', pp. 289–90.

25 Landecker, 'Postindustrial Metabolism'; for an overview of the history of anthropogenic climate change in Africa, see Gareth Austin, 'Africa and the Anthropocene', in *Economic Development and Environmental History in the Anthropocene: Perspectives on Asia and Africa*, ed. by Gareth Austin (London: Bloomsbury Publishing, 2017), pp. 95–118.

26 Landecker, 'Postindustrial Metabolism', p. 497.

27 James V. Neel, 'Diabetes Mellitus: A "Thrifty" Genotype Rendered Detrimental by "Progress"?', *American Journal of Human Genetics*, 14.4 (1962), 353–62.

28 See, for instance, Logan, *The Scarcity Slot*; Nott, 'Malnutrition in a Modernising Economy'; Amy Moran-Thomas, *Traveling with Sugar: Chronicles of a Global Epidemic* (Oakland, CA: University of California Press, 2019); Margery Fee, 'Racializing Narratives: Obesity, Diabetes and the "Aboriginal" Thrifty Genotype', *Social Science & Medicine*, 62.12 (2006), 2988–97.

29 Susan Reynolds Whyte, 'Knowing Hypertension and Diabetes: Conditions of Treatability in Uganda', *Health & Place*, 39 (2016), 219–25; Vaughan, 'Conceptualising Metabolic Disorder'.

30 See, for instance, Owen et al., 'Does Breastfeeding Influence Risk of Type 2 Diabetes in Later Life?'; Natasha Lelijveld et al., 'Chronic Disease Outcomes after Severe Acute Malnutrition in Malawian Children (ChroSAM): A Cohort Study', *The Lancet. Global Health*, 4.9 (2016), e654–662.

31 This echoes something of Iliffe's argument regarding famine in Zimbabwe: see Iliffe, *Famine in Zimbabwe*.

32 This is much the same as Watts found in Northern Nigeria: see Watts, *Silent Violence*. In this respect, considering the history of nutrition in Ghana as a whole and over the long term – as a kaleidoscope of individual but interdependent histories – rehabilitates some of the historiographical debates around food, hunger, and colonisation.

33 This can be understood as a widespread decline in 'entitlement'. See Sen, *Poverty*. Similar processes were seen elsewhere – in Uganda, for instance. See Nott, 'Malnutrition in a Modernising Economy'.

34 Brandi Simpson Miller, 'Food and Nationalism in an Independent Ghana', in *The Emergence of National Food: The Dynamics of Food and Nationalism*, ed. by Atsuko Ichijo, Venetia Johannes, and Ronald Ranta (London: Bloomsbury Publishing, 2019), pp. 61–70 (p. 61).

35 The recent return and continuing rise of food banks in Western Europe and North America suggests that food security is not assured, even in ostensibly advanced economies with ostensibly sophisticated systems of social security.

36 Ó Gráda, *Eating People*, p. 205.

37 Kojo Emmanuel, 'Nana Addo Gives Reasons and Factors That Led to Lifting of Lockdown', *Pulse Ghana*, 2020 <https://www.pulse.com.gh/news/local/nana-addo-gives-reasons-and-factors-that-led-to-lifting-of-lockdown/br9hwsz> [accessed 1 April 2022].

References

Archival sources

Ghana

Public Records and Archives Administration Department (PRAAD), Accra

A/ADM/5/3/99, Report of the Select Committee on Federal System of Government and Second Chamber for the Gold Coast, 1955
ADM/5/4/62, Welfare and mass education in the Gold Coast, 1946–51
ADM/11/1/1294, Report of the standing committee to study the important question of human nutrition
ADM/56/1/128, Report on food supply in Frafra, 1911
CSO/8/1/12, Food supplies in the Northern Territories, 1930–1
CSO/11/1/337, Index to the Literature of Food Investigation, 1933
CSO/11/1/355, Deaths following injections, 1934
CSO/11/5/1, Maternal mortality and morbidity in the Gold Coast, 1932
CSO/11/6/4, Infant welfare centres – Principles, 1931–2
CSO/11/6/10, IWC Tamale, 1932
CSO/11/16/79, Anti-trypanosomiasis injections – deaths following, 1942
CSO/11/19/12, Anti-trypanosomiasis injections – deaths at Navrongo following, 1936–8
CSO/20/6/4, Northern Territories Welfare Committee, 1944–5
RG 3/5/600, Meat Supply Survey, Gold Coast, 1940

Public Records and Archives Administration Department (PRAAD), Kumasi

ARG/2/1/9, Price controls, general, 1948–53
ARG/2/1/61, Cost of living enquiry, 1960–1
ARG/2/8/69, Ministry of Health, 1964–75
ARG/2/8/111, Ministry of Agriculture, 1973–4
ARG/2/8/118, Food Distribution Corporation, 1974–7
ARG/2/12/17, Operation Feed Yourself, First Phase (Vol. 1), 1972–3
ARG/2/12/25, Operation Feed Yourself, Second Phase (Vol. 1), 1973
ARG/2/12/27, Operation Feed Yourself, Third Phase (Vol. 4), 1973–7
ARG/6/14/7, Diet and Nutrition Surveys, 1940–7
ARG/13/3/12, Annual Report MOH, 1957–8
ARG/13/4/37, Child Welfare Clinics (Midwives' Returns)

Public Records and Archives Administration Department (PRAAD), Tamale

NRG/8/3/204, Economic Surveys and Reports, 1955–60
NRG/8/2/209, Cattle in Frafra, 1950
NRG/8/6/57, Ghana Food and Nutrition Board, 1964–8
NRG/8/9/58, Mass Education General, 1964–75
NRG/8/11/66, Food Production Drive [Urban Allotments] Including Food Shortages, 1958–62
NRG/8/13/29, Child Welfare Clinic, Tamale, 1954–63
NRG/8/13/40, Health Education, 1959–65
NRG/8/17/8, Migrant Labour, 1952–3
NRG/8/37/4, Food Shortage and Storage in the Northern Region 1959–62
NRG/8/37/5, Food Storage in Northern Region, 1962–6
NRG/9/4/68, Ghana Food Distribution Corporation, 1972–3
NRG/9/19/1, Food shortage in the Upper Region, 1964–9
NRG/9/19/2, Food shortage in the Upper Region, 1969–70

NRG/18/1/5, Monthly Food Production Reports, 1952–7
NRG/18/8/1, Diet and nutrition, 1930–57

Council for Scientific and Industrial Research Library (CSIR), Accra
Boone, S.A., *Survey of Contemporary Ghana: Nutrition in Ghana* (Accra: Nutrition Research Unit, undated, c.1965)
Dovlo, Florence E., *A Study of Infant Feeding Practices in Accra*, FRI Research Bulletin (Accra: Food Research Institute, CSIR, 1968)

United Kingdom

Bodleian Library of Commonwealth and African Studies at Rhodes House (RH), University of Oxford
Gold Coast Government, *Medical Department Annual Reports* [*MDAR*], 1902–55 (Accra: Government Printer)
RH/MSS.Afr.S.1872 Box XX, J.N.P. Davies, Personal Reminiscences
RH/MSS.Afr.S.1872 Box XXXV, H.C. Trowell, Interview, 1982
RH/MSS.Afr.S.2003, Yvonne P. Fox, 'Three chapters of memoirs on life in the Northern Territories of the Gold Coast', c.1930s

The British Library, London
Gold Coast Government, *Agricultural Department Annual Reports* [*ADAR*], 1900–55 (Accra: Government Printer), various microfilms
Gold Coast Government, *Education Department Annual Reports* [*EDAR*], 1900–56 (Accra: Government Printer), various microfilms

The London School of Hygiene and Tropical Medicine (LSHTM), London
0809/Nutrition/03, Volta River Project – Ghana

The National Archives (TNA), Kew
CO/96/751/14, C.W. Lynn, *Agriculture in North Mamprusi* (Accra: Department of Agriculture, 1937)
CO/323/1570/7, Committee on Nutrition in the Colonial Empire, Economic Advisory Council: papers circulated, 1938
CO/323/1571/5, Nutrition in the British Colonial Empire, summary of replies to circular dispatch of 18 April 1936, November 1937
CO/859/14/6, Report on Nutrition in the Colonial Empire, 1939
CO/859/68/1, Nutrition research survey: Gold Coast, 1941–3
CO/859/115/3, Gold Coast: Extracts from informal colonial medical reports, development plans and other papers [pertaining to nutrition], 1944–6
CO/927/2/3, Series of reports by Miss P. Ady relating to wages and standards of living in Accra, 1945–6
FD/12/273, Medical Research Council, Child Nutrition Research Unit (Formerly Infantile Malnutrition Research Unit), Kampala, Uganda, 1961

Wellcome Library (WL), London
PP/CDW, Cicely Williams's Papers

Datasets
Bolt, Jutta, and Jan Luiten van Zanden, 'The First Update of the Maddison Project: Re-Estimating Growth before 1820', 2013 <https://www.clio-infra.eu/datasets/select/indictorr/288/> [accessed 16 November 2014]
Ghana Statistical Service and ICF, 'Ghana Demographic and Health Survey [GDHS] 2022'
Ghana Statistical Service and Institute for Resource Development/Macro Systems, Inc., 'Ghana Demographic and Health Survey [GDHS], 1988'
Ghana Statistical Service, Ghana Health Service, and ICF International, 'Ghana Demographic and Health Survey [GDHS], 2014'
Ghana Statistical Service, Ghana Health Service, and ICF Macro., 'Ghana Demographic and Health Survey [GDHS], 2008'

Ghana Statistical Service and Macro International Inc., 'Ghana Demographic and Health Survey [GDHS], 1993'
Ghana Statistical Service and Macro International Inc., 'Ghana Demographic and Health Survey [GDHS], 1998'
Ghana Statistical Service, Noguchi Memorial Institute for Medical Research, and ORC Macro., 'Ghana Demographic and Health Survey [GDHS], 2003'
Moradi, Alexander, 'Men under Arms in Colonial Africa: Gold Coast Regiment', 2009. Anthropometric data provided by the author
Natural Earth, open-source GIS data <http://www.naturalearthdata.com> [accessed 3 December 2015]
World Bank, various data <https://data.worldbank.org> [accessed 9 May 2022]
United States Geological Survey (USGS), Shuttle Radar Topography Mission (SRTM) data <http://www.opendem.info/download_contours.html> [accessed 9 May 2016]

Governmental sources

Censuses

Ghana Government, *1960 Population Census of Ghana* (Accra: Census Office, 1962)
Gold Coast Government, *Report on the Census of the Gold Coast Colony for the Year 1891* (Accra: Census Committee, 1892)
Gold Coast Government, *Report on the Census for the Year 1901* (Accra: Census Committee, 1902)
Gold Coast Government, *The Gold Coast Appendices, Containing Comparative Returns and General Statistics of the 1931 Census* (Accra: Government Printer, 1932)
Gold Coast Government, *Census of Population 1948, Report and Tables* (Accra: Government Printer, 1950)

Expenditure reports

Ghana Government, *Survey of Cocoa Producing Families in Ashanti, 1956–1957* (Accra: Office of the Government Statistician, 1956)
Gold Coast Government, *Agricultural Statistical Survey of South-East Akim Abuakwa 1952–3* (Accra: Office of the Government Statistician, 1953)
Gold Coast Government, *1953 Accra Survey of Household Budgets* (Accra: Office of the Government Statistician, 1953)
Gold Coast Government, *Kumasi Survey of Population and Household Budgets, 1955* (Accra: Office of the Government Statistician, 1956)
Gold Coast Government, *Sekondi-Takoradi Survey of Population and Household Budgets, 1955* (Accra: Office of the Government Statistician, 1956)

Other Gold Coast Government publications

Brown du Sautoy, Marjorie, *Some Gold Coast Foods or What to Eat for a Balanced Diet* (Accra: Government Printing Department, 1953)
Cardinall, A.W., *The Gold Coast, 1931: A Review of Conditions in the Gold Coast in 1931 as Compared with Those of 1921 Based on Figures and Facts Collected by the Chief Census Officer of 1931, Together with a Historical, Ethnographical and Sociological Survey of the People of That Country* (Accra: Government Printer, 1932)
Fortes, Meyer, *Marriage Law among the Tallensi* (Accra: Government Printer, 1937)
Gold Coast Government, *Gold Coast Nutrition and Cookery* (Edinburgh: Published for the Gold Coast Government by T. Nelson and Sons, 1953)
Gold Coast Government, *Report of the Commission of Enquiry into the Health Needs of the Gold Coast* (Accra: Government Printer, 1952)
Gold Coast Government, *The Development Plan, 1951: Being a Plan for the Economic and Social Development of the Gold Coast as Approved by the Legislative Assembly, September 1951* (Accra: Government Printer, 1951)
Guggisberg, Frederick Gordon, *The Gold Coast: A Review of the Events of 1920–1926 and the Prospects of 1927–1928* (Accra: Government Printer, 1927)
Labi, Adame, and B. Selormey, *Report on the Enquiry into Begging and Destitution in the Gold Coast, 1954* (Accra: Government Printer, 1955)
Lewis, W. Arthur, *Report on Industrialisation and the Gold Coast* (Accra: Government Printer, 1953)

Seers, Dudley, and Claud Richard Ross, *Report on Financial and Physical Problems of Development in the Gold Coast* (Accra: Office of the Government Statistician, 1952)

Tooth, Geoffrey, *A Survey of Juvenile Delinquency in the Gold Coast* (Accra: Government Printer, 1946)

Tudhope, W.S., *Enquiry into the Gold Coast Cocoa Industry: Final Report, 1918–1919* (Accra: Government Printer, 1919)

Other Ghana Government publications

Acheampong, I.K., *Two Years in Office of Colonel Ignatius Kutu Acheampong, 13th January 1972–12th January 1974* (Accra: Office of the Press Secretary to the National Redemption Council, 1974)

Ghana Government, *Economic Survey, 1968* (Accra: Government Printer, 1969)

Ghana Government, *Enhancing the Human Impact of the Adjustment Programme: Report Prepared by the Government of Ghana for the Sixth Meeting of the Consultative Group for Ghana, Paris, 14–15 May 1991* (Accra: Government Printer, 1991)

Ghana Government, *Investing for Food and Jobs (IFJ): An Agenda for Transforming Ghana's Agriculture (2018–2021)* (Accra: Ministry of Food and Agriculture, 2018)

Ghana Government, *Poverty Trends in Ghana in the 1990s* (Accra: Ghana Statistical Service, 2000)

Ghana Government, *Programme of Actions to Mitigate the Social Costs of Adjustment* (Accra: Government Printer, 1987)

Ghana Government, *Report of the Commission of Enquiry into Trade Malpractices in Ghana* (Ghana: Ministry of Information, 1965)

Ghana Government, *Seven-Year Plan for National Reconstruction and Development: Financial Years 1963/64–1969/70* (Accra: Office of the Planning Commission, 1964)

Ghana Government, *The Nutrition of Adults in Northern Ghana: A Report of the National Nutrition Survey of the National Food and Nutrition Board* (Accra: Mimeo., 1962)

Konotey-Ahulu, F.I.D., *Report of the Committee Appointed to Investigate Hospital Fees, 1970* (Accra: Government Printer, 1973)

British Government and Colonial Office publications

Callwell, C.E., *Small Wars: Their Principles and Practice* (London: HMSO, 1896)

Dow, Hugh, *East Africa Royal Commission 1953–1955 Report* (London: HMSO, 1955)

McCance, R.A., 'The History, Significance and Aetiology of Hunger Oedema', in *Studies of Undernutrition, Wuppertal 1946–9: Medical Research Council Special Report Series, No. 275*, ed. by Department of Experimental Medicine University of Cambridge (London: HMSO, 1951), pp. 21–82

McCulloch, W.E., *An Inquiry into the Dietaries of the Hausas and Town Fulani of Northern Nigeria, with Some Observations of the Effects on the National Health, with Recommendations Arising Therefrom* (Lagos: Government Printer, 1930)

Orr, J.B., and J.L. Gilks, *Studies of Nutrition: The Physique and Health of Two African Tribes* (London: HMSO, 1931)

Uganda Government, *Review of Nutrition in Uganda: A Summary of Previous Work and An Appreciation of the Present Position* (Entebbe: Government Printer, 1945)

Watson, Andrew Aiken, *Statement by His Majesty's Government on the Report of the Commission of Enquiry into Disturbances in the Gold Coast, 1948* (London: HMSO, 1948)

Non-governmental sources

Newspapers and magazines

'Colonies and Calories', *West African Review*, March 1946, 255–6

Drennan, William, 'To Ireland', in *The Monthly Magazine*, ed. by John Aikin and Benson Earle Hill (London: R. Phillips, 1796), p. 404

Emmanuel, Kojo, 'Nana Addo Gives Reasons and Factors That Led to Lifting of Lockdown', *Pulse Ghana*, 21 April 2020 <https://www.pulse.com.gh/news/local/nana-addo-gives-reasons-and-factors-that-led-to-lifting-of-lockdown/br9hwsz> [accessed 1 April 2022]

Freeman, T.B., 'Life and Travels on the Gold Coast', *The Western Echo* (Cape Coast, 6 March 1886), p. 8

Freeman, T.B., 'Life and Travels on the Gold Coast', *The Western Echo* (Cape Coast, 24 February 1886), p. 8

Hailey, Malcolm, 'Nutrition in the Colonies', *The Times* (London, England, 26 July 1939), p. 15
'Labour Problems of the Gold Coast Are Being Faced', *West African Review*, December 1942, p. 18
Motavalli, Jim, 'Let Them Eat Plumpy'Nut', *Foreign Policy*, 8 October 2009 <https://foreignpolicy.com/2009/10/08/let-them-eat-plumpynut/> [accessed 15 June 2016]
'Nutrition in West Africa', *West African Review*, June 1946, 618–19
Posnansky, Merrick, 'How Ghana's Crisis Affects a Village', *West Africa*, 1 December 1980, pp. 2418–40
Purcell, F.M., 'The Gold Coast Government, the Colonial Office, and Nutrition: Facts of an Astonishing Colonial Episode, Letters to the Editor', *West Africa*, 4 December 1943, p. 1095
Rana, Preetika, 'Nestlé's Noodles Face More Scrutiny in India', *Wall Street Journal*, 31 March 2016 <http://www.wsj.com/articles/nestles-noodles-face-more-scrutiny-in-india-1459428231> [accessed 9 August 2016]
'They like Lucozade … and They Keep It Down', *Proceedings of the Royal Society of Medicine*, 50.2 (1957), ii

Unpublished PhDs and conference papers

Bening, R. Bagulo, 'The Evolution of the Administrative Boundaries of Northern Ghana, 1898–1965' (unpublished PhD, University of London, 1971)
Destombes, Jérôme, 'Nutrition and Chronic Deprivation in the West African Savanna: North-Eastern Ghana, c. 1930–2000' (unpublished PhD, London School of Economics, 2001)
Lipscomb, Margaret Mary, 'Changing Meanings of Development: Dudley Seers – An Intellectual Biography' (unpublished PhD, University of Southampton, 1993)
van der Mei, Jeltje, '26 Years of Paediatric Practice in Rural Ghana: Child Health in Ashanti-Akim District, Working towards a Comprehensive Approach' (unpublished PhD, University of Groningen, 2005)
Merchant, Emily K., 'Prediction and Control: Global Population, Population Science, and Population Politics in the Twentieth Century' (unpublished PhD, University of Michigan, 2015)
Merchant, Emily K., 'The Imperial Politics of (Mal)Nutrition in Colonial Gold Coast' (Unpublished working paper, University of Michigan, 2005)
Scott-Smith, Tom, 'Defining Hunger, Redefining Food: Humanitarianism in the Twentieth Century' (unpublished DPhil, University of Oxford, 2014)
Serra, Gerardo, 'From Scattered Data to Ideological Education: Economics, Statistics and the State in Ghana, 1948–1966' (unpublished PhD, London School of Economics, 2015)
Serra, Gerardo, 'Towards a Political Economy of Statistics: A Study of Household Budget Surveys in the Gold Coast, 1945–1957' (presented at the African Economic Development: Measuring Success and Failure conference, Simon Fraser University, Vancouver, 2013)
Tappan, Jennifer, '"A Healthy Child Comes from a Healthy Mother": Mwanamugimu and Nutritional Science in Uganda, 1935–1973' (unpublished PhD, Columbia University, 2010)
Williams, Cicely D., 'The Mortality and Morbidity of the Children of the Gold Coast' (unpublished MD, University of Oxford, 1936)

Books and reports

Acquah, Ioné, *Accra Survey: A Social Survey of the Capital of Ghana, Formerly Called the Gold Coast, Undertaken for the West Africa Institute of Social and Economic Research, 1953–1956* (London: University of London Press, 1958)
Adams, Vincanne (ed.), *Metrics: What Counts in Global Health* (Durham, NC: Duke University Press, 2016)
Addae, Stephen, *The Evolution of Modern Medicine in a Developing Country: Ghana 1880–1960* (Bishop Auckland: Durham Academic Press, 1996)
Addo, Nelson Otu, Margaret Peil, and A.K. Quarcoo, *Madina Survey: A Study of the Structure and Development of a Contemporary Sub-Urban Settlement* (Legon, Accra: University of Ghana, 1967)
Agarwal, Seema, *Bearing the Weight: The Kayayoo, Ghana's Working Girl Child* (Legon, Accra: University of Ghana, 1997)
Ahmad, Naseem, *Deficit Financing, Inflation and Capital Formation: The Ghanaian Experience 1960–65* (Munich: Weltforum Verlag, 1970)
Aikens, Ama de-Graft, Samuel Agyei-Mensah, and Charles Agyemang (eds), *Chronic Non-Communicable Diseases in Ghana: Multidisciplinary Perspectives* (Accra: Sub-Saharan Publishers, 2013)

Ainsworth, Mary D. Salter, *Infancy in Uganda: Infant Care and the Growth of Love* (Baltimore, MD: Johns Hopkins Press, 1967)
Akon, Samuel, Adam Anaba, David Spratt, and Tony Naden, *Kusaas Siilima: Kusaasi Proverbs* (Tamale: Ghana Institute of Linguistics, 1980)
Alderman, Harold, *Nutritional Status in Ghana and Its Determinants*, Social Dimensions of Adjustment (Washington, D.C.: World Bank, 1990)
Alderman, Harold, and Paul A. Higgins, *Food and Nutritional Adequacy in Ghana* (Ithaca, NY: Cornell Food and Nutrition Policy Program, 1992)
Allan, William, *The African Husbandman* (Edinburgh: Oliver & Boyd, 1967)
Allman, Jean, *The Quills of the Porcupine: Asante Nationalism in an Emergent Ghana* (Madison, WI: University of Wisconsin Press, 1993)
Allman, Jean, and Victoria Tashjian, *'I Will Not Eat Stone': A Women's History of Colonial Asante*, Social History of Africa (Oxford: James Currey, 2000)
Amadiume, Ifi, *Male Daughters, Female Husbands: Gender and Sex in African Society* (London: ZED Books, 1987)
Amin, Samir, *Unequal Development: An Essay on the Social Formations of Peripheral Capitalism* (Hassocks, Sussex: Harvester Press, 1976)
Anderson, Warwick, *Colonial Pathologies: American Tropical Medicine, Race, and Hygiene in the Philippines* (Durham, NC: Duke University Press, 2006)
AngloGold Ashanti, 'Case Study: Creating a Sustainable Solution for Malaria in Continental Africa Region', 2013 <http://www.aga-reports.com/13/os/case-study/car-malaria> [accessed 3 August 2016]
Ardayfio-Schandorf, Elizabeth, *Rural Energy Crisis in Ghana: Its Implications for Women's Work and Household Survival* (Geneva: International Labour Organization, 1986)
Armstrong, George, *An Essay on the Diseases Most Fatal to Infants* (London: T. Cadell, 1771)
Aryeetey, Ernest, and Andrew McKay, *Operationalizing Pro-Poor Growth: A Country Case Study on Ghana* (Washington, D.C.: World Bank, 1 October 2004)
Austin, Dennis, *Politics in Ghana, 1946–1960* (Oxford: Oxford University Press, 1970)
Austin, Gareth, *Labour, Land, and Capital in Ghana: From Slavery to Free Labour in Asante, 1807–1956* (Rochester, NY: University of Rochester Press, 2005)
Autret, M., and M. Behar, *Síndrome Policarencial Infantil (Kwashiorkor) and Its Prevention in Central America* (Rome: FAO Nutritional Studies, no. 13, 1954)
Awedoba, A.K., *An Introduction to Kasena Society and Culture through Their Proverbs* (Lanham, MD: University Press of America, 2000)
Baataar, Cuthbert, *Malnourished Infants in Nandom Rehabilitation Centre: A Case Study of Deficits in Care* (Legon, Accra: University of Ghana, 2005)
Bandola-Gill, Justyna, Sotiria Grek, and Marlee Tichenor, *Governing the Sustainable Development Goals: Quantification in Global Public Policy* (Cham: Springer International Publishing, 2022).
Bashford, Alison, *Global Population: History, Geopolitics, and Life on Earth* (New York: Columbia University Press, 2014)
Bayart, Jean-François, *The State in Africa: The Politics of the Belly* (London: Longman, 1993)
Beckett, W.H., *Akokoaso: A Survey of a Gold Coast Village* (London: P. Lund, Humphries & Co., 1944)
Bemille, Sebastian K., *Dàgàrà Proverbs* (Berlin: Dietrich Reimer, 2010)
Bening, R. Bagulo, *A History of Education in Northern Ghana, 1907–1976* (Accra: Ghana Universities Press, 1990)
Bening, R. Bagulo, *Ghana: Administrative Areas and Boundaries, 1874–2009* (Accra: Ghana Universities Press, 2010)
Bening, R. Bagulo, *Ghana: Regional Boundaries and National Integration* (Accra: Ghana Universities Press, 1999)
Benneh, G., J. Songsore, J.S. Nabila, A.T. Amuzu, K.A. Tutu, Y. Yangyuoru, and G. McGranahan, *Environmental Problems and the Urban Household in the Greater Accra Metropolitan Area* (Stockholm: Stockholm Environment Institute, 1993)
Berg, Elliot, *Accelerated Development in Sub-Saharan Africa: An Agenda for Action* (Washington, D.C.: World Bank, 1981)
Bernstein, Henry, *Class Dynamics of Agrarian Change* (Halifax, NS: Fernwood, 2010)
Bledsoe, Caroline, *Contingent Lives: Fertility, Time, and Aging in West Africa* (Chicago, IL: University of Chicago Press, 2002)

Biruk, Crystal, *Cooking Data: Culture and Politics in an African Research World* (Durham, NC: Duke University Press Books, 2018)

Boahen, Albert Adu, *The Ghanaian Sphinx: Reflections on the Contemporary History of Ghana 1972–1987* (Accra: Ghana Academy of Arts and Sciences, 1989)

Boateng, E.A., *A Geography of Ghana* (Cambridge: Cambridge University Press, 1966)

Boserup, Ester, *Women's Role in Economic Development* (London: George Allen & Unwin, 1971)

Bowdich, T.E., *Mission from Cape Coast Castle to Ashantee: With a Statistical Account of That Kingdom and Geographical Notices of Other Parts of the Interior of Africa* (London: John Murray, 1819)

Bowdich, T.E., *The British and French Expeditions to Teembo: With Remarks on Civilization in Africa* (Paris: J. Smith, 1821)

Brantley, Cynthia, *Feeding Families: African Realities and British Ideas of Nutrition and Development in Early Colonial Africa* (Portsmouth, NH: Heinemann, 2002)

Brock, J.F., and M. Autret, *Kwashiorkor in Africa* (Rome: FAO, Nutritional Studies, no. 8, 1952)

Brydon, Lynne, and Karen Legge, *Adjusting Society: The World Bank, the IMF and Ghana* (London: Tauris Academic Studies, 1996)

Burton, Richard Francis, and Verney Lovett Cameron, *To the Gold Coast for Gold: A Personal Narrative* (London: Chatto and Windus, 1883)

Busia, K.A., *Report on a Social Survey of Sekondi-Takoradi* (London: Crown Agents for the Colonies on behalf of the Govt of the Gold Coast, 1950)

Busia, K.A., *The Position of the Chief in the Modern Political System of Ashanti: A Study of the Influence of Contemporary Social Changes on Ashanti Political Institutions* (London: Published for the International African Institute by Oxford University Press, 1951)

Caldwell, John C., *African Rural-Urban Migration: The Movement to Ghana's Towns* (Canberra: Australian National University Press, 1969)

Cardinall, A.W., *In Ashanti and Beyond* (London: Seeley, Service & Co., 1927)

Cardinall, A.W., *The Natives of the Northern Territories of the Gold Coast: Their Customs, Religion and Folklore* (London: George Routledge & Sons, 1920)

Carpenter, Kenneth J., *Beriberi, White Rice, and Vitamin B: A Disease, a Cause, and a Cure* (Berkeley, CA: University of California Press, 2000)

Carpenter, Kenneth J., *Protein and Energy* (Cambridge: Cambridge University Press, 1994)

Castro, Josué de, *The Geography of Hunger* (Boston, MA: Little, Brown, 1952)

Chang, Ha-Joon, *Kicking Away the Ladder: Development Strategy in Historical Perspective* (London: Anthem, 2002)

Chazan, Naomi, *An Anatomy of Ghanaian Politics: Managing Political Recession 1969–1982* (Boulder, CO: Westview Press, 1983)

Chetley, Andrew, *The Politics of Baby Foods* (London: F. Pinter, 1986)

Christaller, Johann Gottlieb, *A Dictionary of the Asante and Fante Language Called Tshi (Chwee, Twi)* (Basel: Evangelical Missionary Society, 1881)

Clapp, Jennifer, *Hunger in the Balance: The New Politics of International Food Aid* (Ithaca, NY: Cornell University Press, 2012)

Clark, Gracia, *Onions Are My Husband: Survival and Accumulation by West African Market Women* (Chicago, IL: University of Chicago Press, 1994)

Coghe, Samuël, *Population Politics in the Tropics: Demography, Health and Transimperialism in Colonial Angola* (Cambridge: Cambridge University Press, 2022)

Cornia, Giovanni Andrea, Richard Jolly, and Frances Stewart (eds), *Adjustment with a Human Face*, 2 vols (Oxford: Clarendon Press, 1987)

Craddock, Sally, *Retired Except on Demand: The Life of Doctor Cicely Williams* (Oxford: Green College, 1983)

Crisp, Jeff, *The Story of an African Working Class: Ghanaian Miners' Struggles, 1870–1980* (London: ZED Books, 1984)

Curtin, Philip D., *Death by Migration: Europe's Encounter with the Tropical World in the Nineteenth Century* (Cambridge: Cambridge University Press, 1989)

Curtis, Sian L., *Assessment of the Quality of Data Used for Direct Estimation of Infant and Child Mortality in DHS-II Surveys*, DHS Occasional Papers (Calverton, MD: Macro International, 1995)

Czerny, A., and A. Keller, *Des Kindes Ernährung, Ernährungsstörungen Und Ernährungstherapie* (Leipzig: Franz Deuticke, 1906)

Danquah, J.B., *Gold Coast: Akan Laws and Customs and the Akim Abuakwa Constitution* (London: G. Routledge & Sons, 1928)
Davies, J.N.P., *Pestilence and Disease in the History of Africa* (Johannesburg: Witwatersrand University Press, 1979)
Davis, Mike, *Late Victorian Holocausts: El Niño Famines and the Making of the Third World* (London: Verso, 2002)
Der, Benedict G., *The Slave Trade in Northern Ghana* (Accra: Woeli, 1998)
Destombes, Jerôme, *Nutrition and Economic Destitution in Northern Ghana, 1930–1957: A Historical Perspective on Nutritional Economics*, Economic History Working Papers (London: Department of Economic History, LSE, 1999)
de Waal, Alex, *Famine Crimes: Politics and the Disaster Relief Industry in Africa* (Oxford: James Currey, 1997)
Doku, E.V., *Cassava in Ghana* (Accra: Ghana Universities Press, 1969)
Dumit, Joseph, *Drugs for Life: How Pharmaceutical Companies Define Our Health* (Durham, NC: Duke University Press, 2012)
Dupuis, Joseph, *Journal of a Residence in Ashantee: Comprising Notes and Researches Relative to the Gold Coast and the Interior of Western Africa; Chiefly Collected from Arabic Mss. and Information Communicated by the Moslems of Guinea; to Which Is Prefixed an Account of the Origin and Causes of the Present War* (London: H. Colburn, 1824)
Dzorgbo, Dan-Bright S., *Ghana in Search of Development: The Challenge of Governance, Economic Management and Institution Building* (Aldershot: Ashgate, 2001)
Elkins, Caroline, *Britain's Gulag: The Brutal End of Empire in Kenya* (London: Jonathan Cape, 2005)
Ewusi, Kodwo, *Economic Inequality in Ghana* (Legon, Accra: University of Ghana, 1977)
Ewusi, Kodwo, *The Distribution of Monetary Incomes in Ghana* (Legon, Accra: University of Ghana, 1971)
FAO, *FAO Production Yearbook* (Rome: FAO, 1980)
FAO Committee on Protein Requirements, *Protein Requirements* (Rome: FAO Nutritional Studies, no. 16, 1957)
FAO/WHO Expert Group, *Protein Requirements* (Geneva: WHO Technical Report, no. 301, 1965)
FAO/WHO/UNICEF Protein Advisory Group, *Lives in Peril: Protein and the Child* (Rome: FAO, World Food Problems, no. 12, 1970)
Feierman, Steven, and John M. Janzen (eds), *The Social Basis of Health and Healing in Africa* (Berkeley, CA: University of California Press, 1992)
Ferguson, James, *Global Shadows: Africa in the Neoliberal World Order* (Durham, NC: Duke University Press, 2006)
Field, M.J., *Religion and Medicine of the Gã People* (Oxford: Oxford University Press, 1937)
Field, M.J., *Search for Security: An Ethno-Psychiatric Study of Rural Ghana* (London: Faber and Faber, 1960)
Fildes, Valerie A., *Breasts, Bottles and Babies: A History of Infant Feeding* (Edinburgh: Edinburgh University Press, 1985)
Firmin-Sellers, Kathryn, *The Transformation of Property Rights in the Gold Coast: An Empirical Analysis Applying Rational Choice Theory* (Cambridge: Cambridge University Press, 1996)
Fisher, Kate, *Birth Control, Sex, and Marriage in Britain 1918–1960* (Oxford: Oxford University Press, 2006)
Fitch, Robert Beck, and Mary Oppenheimer, *Ghana: End of an Illusion* (London: Monthly Review Press, 1968)
Fortes, Meyer, *The Dynamics of Clanship among the Tallensi: Being the First Part of an Analysis of the Social Structure of a Trans-Volta Tribe* (Oxford: Oxford University Press, 1945)
Fortes, Meyer, *The Web of Kinship among the Tallensi: The Second Part of an Analysis of the Social Structure of a Trans-Volta Tribe* (Oxford: Oxford University Press, 1949)
Foster, Philip, *Education and Social Change in Ghana* (London: Routledge & Kegan Paul, 1965)
Foucault, Michel, *The History of Sexuality. Vol. 1: The Will to Knowledge* (London: Penguin, 1979)
Frank, André Gunder, *Capitalism and Underdevelopment in Latin America: Historical Studies of Chile and Brazil* (London: Monthly Review, 1967)
Freeman, R. Austin, *Travels and Life in Ashanti and Jaman* (London: A. Constable & Co., 1898)

Frimpong-Ansah, J.H., *The Vampire State in Africa: The Political Economy of Decline in Ghana* (London: James Currey, 1991)

Galen, *Galen on Food and Diet, Translation and Notes by Mark Grant* (London: Routledge, 2000)

Gálvez, Alyshia, *Eating NAFTA: Trade, Food Policies, and the Destruction of Mexico* (Oakland, CA: University of California Press, 2018)

van der Geest, Kees, *We're Managing!: Climate Change and Livelihood Vulnerability in Northwest Ghana* (Leiden: African Studies Centre, 2004)

Gitelman, Lisa (ed.), *'Raw Data' Is an Oxymoron* (Cambridge, MA: MIT Press, 2013)

Glewwe, Paul, and Kwaku A. Twum-Baah, *The Distribution of Welfare in Ghana, 1987–88* (Washington, D.C.: World Bank, 1991)

Goody, Esther, *Parenthood and Social Reproduction: Fostering and Occupational Roles in West Africa* (Cambridge: Cambridge University Press, 1982)

Goody, Jack, *Cooking, Cuisine and Class: A Study in Comparative Sociology* (Cambridge: Cambridge University Press, 1982)

Gordon, Linda Perlman, *Woman's Body, Woman's Right: Birth Control in America* (New York: Penguin, 1990)

Gould, Peter R., *The Development of the Transportation Pattern in Ghana* (Evanston, IL: Department of Geography, Northwestern University, 1960)

Grant, Faye Woodard, *The Nutrition and Health of Children in the Gold Coast* (Chicago, IL: University of Chicago, 1955)

Graunt, John, *Natural and Political Observations Mentioned in a Following Index, and Made upon the Bills of Mortality* (London: Thomas Roycroft, 1662).

Greenhalgh, Susan, *Fat-Talk Nation* (Ithaca, NY: Cornell University Press, 2015)

Grischow, Jeff D., *Globalisation, Development and Disease in Colonial Northern Ghana, 1906–1960*, WOPAG – Working Paper on Ghana: Historical and Contemporary Studies (Helsinki: Institute of Asian and African Studies, University of Helsinki, 2006)

Grischow, Jeff D., *Shaping Tradition: Civil Society, Community and Development in Colonial Northern Ghana, 1899–1957* (Leiden: Brill, 2006)

Grischow, Jeff D., *Tsetse and Trypanosomiasis in the Gold Coast, 1924–1954*, WOPAG – Working Paper on Ghana: Historical and Contemporary Studies (Helsinki: Institute of Asian and African Studies, University of Helsinki, 2005), pp. 1–22

Guyer, Jane I., *Marginal Gains: Monetary Transactions in Atlantic Africa* (Chicago, IL: University of Chicago Press, 2004)

Harrison, Paul, *The Greening of Africa: Breaking through in the Battle for Land and Food* (London: Paladin, 1987)

Harvey, David, *A Brief History of Neoliberalism* (Oxford: Oxford University Press, 2005)

Haushofer, Lisa, *Wonder Foods: The Science and Commerce of Nutrition* (Berkeley, CA: University of California Press, 2022).

Hawkins, Sean, *Writing and Colonialism in Northern Ghana: The Encounter Between the LoDagaa and 'the World on Paper'* (Toronto: University of Toronto Press, 2002)

Haynes, Douglas M., *Imperial Medicine: Patrick Manson and the Conquest of Tropical Disease* (Philadelphia, PA: University of Pennsylvania Press, 2001)

Hill, Polly, *The Gold Coast Cocoa Farmer: A Preliminary Survey* (Oxford: Oxford University Press, 1956)

Hill, Polly, *The Migrant Cocoa-Farmers of Southern Ghana: A Study in Rural Capitalism* (Cambridge: Cambridge University Press, 1963)

Hilton, T.E., *Ghana Population Atlas: The Distribution and Density of Population in the Gold Coast and Togoland under United Kingdom Trusteeship* (Edinburgh: Thomas Nelson & Sons for the University of Ghana, 1960)

Hoorweg, Jan, and Ian McDowell, *Evaluation of Nutrition Education in Africa: Community Research in Uganda, 1971–1972* (The Hague: Mouton, 1979)

Hopkins, A.G., *An Economic History of West Africa* (London: Longman, 1973)

Howard, Mary, and Ann V. Millard, *Hunger and Shame: Poverty and Child Malnutrition on Mount Kilimanjaro* (London: Routledge, 1997)

Howard, Rhoda E., *Colonialism and Underdevelopment in Ghana* (London: Croom Helm, 1978)

Howard, Richard Baron, *An Inquiry into the Morbid Effects of Deficiency of Food, Chiefly with Reference to Their Occurrence amongst the Destitute Poor* (London: Simpkin, Marshall and Co., 1839)

Hunt, Nancy Rose, *A Colonial Lexicon of Birth Ritual, Medicalization, and Mobility in the Congo* (Durham, NC: Duke University Press, 1999)
Hunter, Monica, *Reaction to Conquest: Effects of Contact with Europeans on the Pondo of South Africa* (Oxford: Oxford University Press, 1936)
Hutchful, Eboe, *Ghana's Adjustment Experience: The Paradox of Reform* (Oxford: James Currey, 2002)
Hutchful, Eboe, *The IMF and Ghana: The Confidential Record* (London: ZED Books, 1987)
Iliffe, John, *Africans: The History of a Continent* (Cambridge: Cambridge University Press, 1995)
Iliffe, John, *East African Doctors: A History of the Modern Profession* (Cambridge: Cambridge University Press, 2002)
Iliffe, John, *Famine in Zimbabwe, 1890–1960* (Gweru, Zimbabwe: Mambo Press, 1990)
Iliffe, John, *The African Poor: A History* (Cambridge: Cambridge University Press, 1987)
Ittmann, Karl, *A Problem of Great Importance: Population, Race, and Power in the British Empire, 1918–1973* (Berkeley, CA: University of California Press, 2014)
Janzen, John M., *The Quest for Therapy in Lower Zaire* (Berkeley: University of California Press, 1978)
Johnson, Marion (ed.), *Salaga Papers* (Legon, Accra: University of Ghana, 1965)
Johnson-Hanks, Jennifer, *Uncertain Honor: Modern Motherhood in an African Crisis* (Chicago, IL: University of Chicago Press, 2006)
Kakwani, N., *On Measuring Undernutrition* (Helsinki: WIDER, 1986)
Kamminga, Harmke, and Andrew Cunningham (eds), *The Science and Culture of Nutrition, 1840–1940* (Amsterdam: Brill Rodopi, 1995)
Kay, Geoffrey Barry, *The Political Economy of Colonialism in Ghana: A Collection of Documents and Statistics, 1900–1960* (Cambridge: Cambridge University Press, 1972)
Kaye, Barrington, *Bringing up Children in Ghana: An Impressionistic Survey* (London: George Allen & Unwin, 1962)
Keen, David, *The Benefits of Famine: A Political Economy of Famine and Relief in Southwestern Sudan, 1983–1989* (Oxford: James Currey, 1994)
Keys, A., J. Brozek, A. Henschel, O. Michelsen, and H.L. Taylor, *The Biology of Human Starvation* (Minneapolis, MN: University of Minnesota Press, 1950)
Killick, Tony, *Development Economics in Action: A Study of Economic Policies in Ghana* (London: Heinemann, 1978)
Komlos, John (ed.), *Stature, Living Standards, and Economic Development: Essays in Anthropometric History* (Chicago, IL: University of Chicago Press, 1994)
Konings, Piet, *The State and Rural Class Formation in Ghana: A Comparative Analysis* (London: KPI, 1986)
Kpedekpo, G.M.K., *Studies on Vital Registration Data from the Compulsory Registration Areas of Ghana, 1962–1967* (Legon, Accra: University of Ghana, 1970)
Kponkpogori, C.S., C.J. Natomah, and O. Rytz, *Gonja Proverbs* (Legon, Accra: University of Ghana, 1966)
Kuhanen, Jan, *Poverty, Health, and Reproduction in Early Colonial Uganda* (Joensuu, Finland: University of Joensuu, 2005)
Kunfaa, Ernest Y., *Consultations with the Poor: Ghana Country Synthesis Report* (Kumasi: CEDEP on behalf of the World Bank, 1999)
La Fleur, James D., *Fusion Foodways of Africa's Gold Coast in the Atlantic Era* (Leiden: Brill, 2012)
Ladouceur, Paul André, *Chiefs and Politicians: The Politics of Regionalism in Northern Ghana* (London: Longman, 1979)
Latour, Bruno, *Science in Action: How to Follow Scientists and Engineers through Society* (Milton Keynes: Open University Press, 1987)
Latour, Bruno, and Steve Woolgar, *Laboratory Life: The Construction of Scientific Facts* (London: Sage Publications, 1979)
Lavy, Victor, John Strauss, Duncan Thomas, and Philippe De Vreyer, *The Impact of the Quality of Health Care on Children's Nutrition and Survival in Ghana*, Living Standards Measurement Study (Washington, D.C.: World Bank, 1995)
Lentz, Carola, *Ethnicity and the Making of History in Northern Ghana* (Edinburgh: Edinburgh University Press, 2006)
Lewis, M. Paul, Charles D. Fennig, and Gary F. Simons, *Ethnologue: Languages of the World* (Dallas, TX: SIL International, 2016)

Liebig, Justus von, *Animal Chemistry, or Organic Chemistry in Its Applications to Physiology and Pathology* (London: Taylor and Walton, 1842)
Lock, Margaret, and Vinh-Kim Nguyen, *An Anthropology of Biomedicine* (Oxford: Wiley-Blackwell, 2010)
Logan, Amanda L., *The Scarcity Slot: Excavating Histories of Food Security in Ghana* (Berkeley, CA: University of California Press, 2020)
Lupton, Deborah, *Fat* (New York: Routledge, 2013)
Macdonald, George, *The Gold Coast, Past and Present: A Short Description of the Country and Its People* (London: Longmans, Green & Co., 1898)
MacGregor, D.R., *Non-Traditional Food Sources for Feeding Increasing Populations: An Inaugural Lecture Delivered on Thursday, 26th October 1972, at the University of Ghana, Legon* (Accra: University of Ghana, 1972)
Mamdani, Mahmood, *Citizen and Subject: Contemporary Africa and the Legacy of Late Colonialism* (Princeton, NJ: Princeton University Press, 1996)
Mamdani, Mahmood, *Politics and Class Formation in Uganda* (London: Heinemann, 1976)
Mandala, Elias C., *The End of Chidyerano: A History of Food and Everyday Life in Malawi, 1860–2004* (Portsmouth, NH: Heinemann, 2005)
Marshall, Alfred, *Principles of Economics* (London: Macmillan & Co., 1920)
Mavhunga, Clapperton Chakanetsa, *The Mobile Workshop: The Tsetse Fly and African Knowledge Production* (Cambridge, MA: MIT Press, 2018)
Maxwell, Daniel G., Carol E. Levin, Margaret Armar-Klemesu, Marie T. Ruel, Saul Sutkover Morris, and Clement Ahiadeke, *Urban Livelihoods and Food and Nutrition Security in Greater Accra, Ghana* (Washington, D.C.: International Food Policy Research Institute (IFPRI), 2000)
McCann, James C., *Stirring the Pot: A History of African Cuisine* (Athens, OH: Ohio University Press, 2009)
McCaskie, T.C., *Asante Identities: History and Modernity in an African Village, 1850–1950* (Edinburgh: Edinburgh University Press, 2001)
McCaskie, T.C., *State and Society in Pre-Colonial Asante* (Cambridge: Cambridge University Press, 1995)
Meillassoux, Claude, *Maidens, Meal and Money: Capitalism and the Domestic Community* (Cambridge: Cambridge University Press, 1981)
Metcalfe, G.E., *Great Britain and Ghana: Documents of Ghana History, 1807–1957* (London: Thomas Nelson & Sons for the University of Ghana, 1964)
Miescher, Stephan, *Making Men in Ghana* (Bloomington, IN: Indiana University Press, 2005)
Mikell, Gwendolyn, *Cocoa and Chaos in Ghana* (New York: Paragon House, 1989)
Mill, James, *An Essay on Government*, ed. by Currin V. Shields (Indianapolis, IN: Bobbs-Merrill, 1955)
Mintz, Sidney W., *Sweetness and Power: The Place of Sugar in Modern History* (New York: Penguin, 1986)
Mitchell, Timothy, *Rule of Experts: Egypt, Techno-Politics, Modernity* (Berkeley, CA: University of California Press, 2002)
Moore, Henrietta L., and Megan Vaughan, *Cutting down Trees: Gender, Nutrition, and Agricultural Change in the Northern Province of Zambia, 1890–1990*, Social History of Africa (London: James Currey, 1994)
Moradi, Alexander, Gareth Austin, and Joerg Baten, *Heights and Development in a Cash-Crop Colony: Living Standards in Ghana, 1870–1980* (Cape Town: ERSA, 2013)
Moran-Thomas, Amy, *Traveling with Sugar: Chronicles of a Global Epidemic* (Oakland, CA: University of California Press, 2019)
Muller, Mike, *The Baby Killer: A War on Want Investigation into the Promotion and Sale of Powdered Milks in the Third World* (London: War on Want, 1974)
Murphy, Michelle, *The Economization of Life* (Durham, NC: Duke University Press, 2017)
Nkrumah, Kwame, *Axioms of Kwame Nkrumah* (London: Panaf, 1969)
Nkrumah, Kwame, *Neo-Colonialism: The Last Stage of Imperialism* (London: Panaf, 1965)
North, J., *Women in National Development in Ghana* (Washington, D.C.: USAID, 1975)
Norton, Andy, Ellen Bortei-Doku Aryeetey, David Korboe, and D.K. Tony Dogbe, *Poverty Assessment in Ghana – Using Qualitative and Participatory Research Methods*, PSP Discussion Paper (Washington, D.C.: World Bank, 1995)
Nyanteng, V. K., and G. J. Van Apeldoorn, *The Farmer and the Marketing of Foodstuffs* (Legon, Accra: University of Ghana, 1971)

Ó Gráda, Cormac, *Black '47 and Beyond: The Great Irish Famine in History, Economy, and Memory* (Princeton, NJ: Princeton University Press, 1998)
Ó Gráda, Cormac, *Eating People Is Wrong, and Other Essays on Famine, Its Past, and Its Future* (Princeton, NJ: Princeton University Press, 2015)
Ó Gráda, Cormac, *Famine: A Short History* (Princeton, NJ: Princeton University Press, 2009)
Oelbaum, Jay, *Spatial Poverty Traps and Ethnic Conflict Traps: Lessons from Northern Ghana's 'Blood Yams'* (London: Overseas Development Institute, 2010)
Ofori-Sarpong, E., *Impact of Drought in Ghana and Upper Volta, 1970–1977* (Legon, Accra: University of Ghana, 1980)
Okali, C., and R.A. Kotey, *Akokoaso: A Resurvey* (Legon, Accra: University of Ghana, 1971)
Omari, T. Peter, *Kwame Nkrumah: The Anatomy of an African Dictatorship* (London: C. Hurst & Co., 1970)
Oppong, Christine, *Middle Class African Marriage: A Family Study of Ghanaian Senior Civil Servants* (London: George Allen & Unwin, 1981)
Osseo-Asare, Fran, *Food Culture in Sub-Saharan Africa* (Westport, CT: Greenwood Press, 2005)
Oti-Boateng, E., Kodwo Ewusi, Ravi Kanbur, and Andrew McKay, *A Poverty Profile for Ghana, 1987–88*, Social Dimensions of Adjustment in Sub-Saharan Africa Working Paper, 5 (Washington, D.C.: World Bank, 1990)
Palmer, Gabrielle, *The Politics of Breastfeeding: When Breasts Are Bad for Business* (London: Pinter & Martin, 2009)
Patterson, K. David, *Health in Colonial Ghana: Disease, Medicine, and Socio-Economic Change, 1900–1955* (Waltham, MA: Crossroads Press, 1981)
Perkins, John H., *Geopolitics and the Green Revolution: Wheat, Genes, and the Cold War* (Oxford: Oxford University Press, 1997)
Platt, B.S., and Jean Mayer, *Report of a Joint FAO/WHO Mission to Ghana* (Rome: WHO/FAO, 1959)
Poleman, Thomas T., *The Food Economies of Urban Middle Africa: The Case of Ghana* (Stanford, CA: Food Research Institute, Stanford University, 1961)
Price, Weston A., *Nutrition and Physical Degeneration: A Comparison of Primitive and Modern Diets and Their Effects* (London: P.B. Hoeber, 1939)
Purcell, F.M., *Diet and Ill-Health in the Forest Country of the Gold Coast* (London: Lewis, 1939)
Rathbone, Richard, *Nkrumah and the Chiefs: The Politics of Chieftaincy in Ghana, 1951–1960* (Oxford: James Currey, 1999)
Rattray, R.S., *Ashanti* (Oxford: Clarendon Press, 1923)
Rattray, R.S., *Ashanti Law and Constitution* (Oxford: Oxford University Press, 1929)
Rattray, R.S., *Ashanti Proverbs: The Primitive Ethics of a Savage People* (Oxford: Clarendon Press, 1916)
Rattray, R.S., *Religion and Art in Ashanti* (Oxford: Clarendon Press, 1927)
Rattray, R.S., *The Tribes of the Ashanti Hinterland* (Oxford: Clarendon Press, 1932)
Richards, A.I., *Land, Labour and Diet in Northern Rhodesia: An Economic Study of the Bemba Tribe* (London: Oxford University Press, 1939)
Riedmann, Agnes Czerwinski, *Science That Colonizes: A Critique of Fertility Studies in Africa* (Philadelphia, PA: Temple University Press, 1993)
Rijpma, Sjoerd, *David Livingstone and the Myth of African Poverty and Disease: A Close Examination of His Writing on the Pre-Colonial Era* (Leiden: Brill, 2015)
Rimmer, Douglas, *Staying Poor: Ghana's Political Economy, 1950–1990* (Oxford: Pergamon Press, 1992)
Robertson, Claire, *Sharing the Same Bowl?: A Socioeconomic History of Women and Class in Accra, Ghana* (Bloomington, IN: Indiana University Press, 1984)
Rock, Joeva Sean, *We Are Not Starving: The Struggle for Food Sovereignty in Ghana* (East Lansing, MI: Michigan State University Press, 2022)
Rodney, Walter, *How Europe Underdeveloped Africa* (Washington, D.C.: Howard University Press, 1974)
Ruel, Marie T., James L. Garrett, Saul S. Morris, Daniel Maxwell, Arne Oshaug, Patrice Engle, and others, *Urban Challenges to Food and Nutrition Security: A Review of Food Security, Health, and Caregiving in the Cities* (Washington, D.C.: IFPRI FCND Discussion Paper No. 51, 1998)
Sai, Fred T., *Dr Fred Sai Speaks Out* (London: International Planned Parenthood Federation, 1994)
Said, Edward W., *Orientalism* (London: Routledge & Kegan Paul, 1978)

Sarris, Alexander, and Hadi Shams, *Ghana under Structural Adjustment: The Impact on Agriculture and the Rural Poor* (New York: New York University Press for IFAD, 1991)
Schildkrout, Enid, *People of the Zongo: The Transformation of Ethnic Identities in Ghana* (Cambridge: Cambridge University Press, 1978)
Scott, David, *Epidemic Disease in Ghana 1901–1960* (London: Oxford University Press, 1965)
Scrinis, Gyorgy, *Nutritionism: The Science and Politics of Dietary Advice* (New York: Columbia University Press, 2013)
Searle, G.R., *The Quest for National Efficiency: A Study in British Politics and Political Thought, 1899–1914* (Oxford: Blackwell, 1971)
Seers, Dudley, *The Political Economy of Nationalism* (Oxford: Oxford University Press, 1983)
Sen, Amartya, *Poverty and Famines: An Essay on Entitlement and Deprivation* (Oxford: Oxford University Press, 1981)
Sen, Amartya, *Development as Freedom* (Oxford: Oxford University Press, 1999)
Shenton, Robert W., *The Development of Capitalism in Northern Nigeria* (Toronto: University of Toronto Press, 1986)
Silberschmidt, Margrethe, *'Women Forget That Men Are the Masters': Gender Antagonism and Socio-Economic Change in Kisii District, Kenya* (Uppsala: Nordiska Afrikainstitutet, 1999)
Simpson Miller, Brandi, *Food and Identity in Nineteenth and Twentieth Century Ghana: Food, Fights, and Regionalism* (Cham: Springer International Publishing, 2021)
Smith, Eustace, *On the Wasting Diseases of Infants and Children* (London: J. & A. Churchill, 1868)
Smith, Hugh, *Letters to Married Women* (London: C. and G. Kearsly, 1767)
Smith, Lisa C., and Lawrence J. Haddad, *Explaining Child Malnutrition in Developing Countries: A Cross-Country Analysis*, FCND Discussion Paper (Washington, D.C.: International Food Policy Research Institute, 1999)
Solomon, Harris, *Metabolic Living: Food, Fat and the Absorption of Illness in India* (Durham, NC: Duke University Press, 2016)
Songsore, Jacob, *Regional Development in Ghana: The Theory and the Reality* (Accra: Woeli, 2003)
Spary, E.C., *Feeding France: New Sciences of Food, 1760–1815* (Cambridge: Cambridge University Press, 2014).
Stein, Zena, *Famine and Human Development: The Dutch Hunger Winter of 1944–1945* (Oxford: Oxford University Press, 1975)
Strings, Sabrina, *Fearing the Black Body: The Racial Origins of Fat Phobia* (New York: NYU Press, 2019)
de Swaan, Abram, *In Care of the State: Health Care, Education and Welfare in Europe and the USA in the Modern Era* (Cambridge: Polity, 1988)
Tappan, Jennifer, *The Riddle of Malnutrition: The Long Arc of Biomedical and Public Health Interventions in Uganda* (Athens, OH: Ohio University Press, 2017)
Tauxier, Louis, *Le Noir Du Soudan: Pays Mossi et Gourounsi, Documents et Analyses* (Paris: Emile Larose, 1912)
Tiffen, Mary, Michael Mortimore, and Francis Gichuki, *More People, Less Erosion: Environmental Recovery in Kenya* (Chichester: Wiley, 1994)
Tilley, Helen, *Africa as a Living Laboratory: Empire, Development, and the Problem of Scientific Knowledge, 1870–1950* (Chicago, IL: University of Chicago Press, 2011)
Townsend, Peter, *Poverty in the United Kingdom: A Survey of Household Resources and Standards of Living* (Berkeley, CA: University of California Press, 1979)
Trowell, H.C., and D.P. Burkitt (eds), *Western Diseases: Their Emergence and Prevention* (Cambridge, MA: Harvard University Press, 1981)
Trowell, H.C., J.N.P. Davies, and R.F.A. Dean, *Kwashiorkor* (London: Edward Arnold, 1954)
UNICEF and Ghana Government, *Children and Women of Ghana: A Situation Analysis 1989–90* (Accra: UNICEF, 1990)
United Nations, *Report of the World Food Conference, Rome, 5–16th November 1974* (New York: United Nations Press, 1975)
Valenze, Deborah M., *Milk: A Local and Global History* (New Haven, CT: Yale University Press, 2011)
Vaughan, Megan, *Curing Their Ills: Colonial Power and African Illness* (Stanford, CA: Stanford University Press, 1991)
Vaughan, Megan, *The Story of an African Famine: Gender and Famine in Twentieth-Century Malawi* (Cambridge: Cambridge University Press, 1987)

Vernon, James, *Hunger: A Modern History* (Cambridge, MA: Harvard University Press, 2007)
Warren, Dennis M., *The Techiman-Bono of Ghana: An Ethnography of an Akan Society* (Dubuque, IA: Kendall/Hunt Pub. Co., 1975)
Waterlow, J.C. (ed.), *Protein Malnutrition: Proceedings of a Conference in Jamaica, 1953* (Cambridge: Cambridge University Press for the FAO, WHO and Josiah Macy Jr Foundation, 1955)
Watts, Michael, *Silent Violence: Food, Famine & Peasantry in Northern Nigeria* (Berkeley, CA: University of California Press, 1983)
Wilks, Ivor, *Asante in the Nineteenth Century: The Structure and Evolution of a Political Order* (Cambridge: Cambridge University Press, 1975)
Wilks, Ivor, Nehemia Levtzion, and Bruce M. Haight, *Chronicles from Gonja: A Tradition of West African Muslim Historiography* (Cambridge: Cambridge University Press, 1986)
Williams, Cicely D., *'Milk and Murder': Reprint of a Speech given to the Singapore Rotary Club, 1939* (Penang, Malaysia: International Organization of Consumers Unions, 1986)
Winterbottom, T.M., *An Account of the Native Africans in the Neighbourhood of Sierra Leone; to which is added an account of the present state of medicine among them* (London: C. Whittingham, 1803)
World Bank, *Ghana: Population, Health and Nutrition* (Washington, D.C.: World Bank, 1989)
World Bank, *Poverty and Hunger: Issues and Options for Food Security in Developing Countries.* (Washington, D.C.: World Bank, 1986)
World Bank, *The Social Dimensions of Adjustment in Africa: A Policy Agenda* (Washington, D.C.: World Bank, 31 March 1990)
World Health Organization, *Management of Severe Malnutrition: A Manual for Physicians and Other Senior Health Workers* (Geneva: World Health Organization, 1999)
World Health Organization, *WHO Child Growth Standards: Methods and Development* (Geneva: World Health Organization, 2006)
Wrigley, C.C., *Crops and Wealth in Uganda: A Short Agrarian History* (Kampala: East African Institute of Social Research, 1959)
Wylie, Diana, *Starving on a Full Stomach: Hunger and the Triumph of Cultural Racism in Modern South Africa*, Reconsiderations in Southern African History (Charlottesville, VI: University Press of Virginia, 2001)

Articles and book chapters

Abdul-Korah, Gariba B., '"Ka Biɛ Ba Yor": Labor Migration among the Dagaaba of the Upper West Region of Ghana, 1936–1957', *Nordic Journal of African Studies*, 17.1 (2008), 1–19
Abdul-Korah, Gariba B., '"Now If You Have Only Sons You Are Dead": Migration, Gender, and Family Economy in Twentieth Century Northwestern Ghana', *Journal of Asian and African Studies*, 46.4 (2011), 390–403
Abt, I.A., 'Injuries Produced by Starch', *Journal of the American Medical Association*, 61.14 (1913), 1275–7
Abu, Katherine, 'The Separateness of Spouses: Conjugal Resources in an Ashanti Town', in *Female and Male in West Africa*, ed. by Christine Oppong (London: George Allen & Unwin, 1983), pp. 156–68
Adams, Vincanne, 'Introduction', in *Metrics: What Counts in Global Health*, ed. by Vincanne Adams (Durham, NC: Duke University Press, 2016), pp. 1–18
Addai, Isaac, 'Determinants of Use of Maternal-Child Health Services in Rural Ghana', *Journal of Biosocial Science*, 32.1 (2000), 1–15
Agyei-Mensah, Samuel, and Ama de-Graft Aikins, 'Epidemiological Transition and the Double Burden of Disease in Accra, Ghana', *Journal of Urban Health*, 87 (2010), 879–97
Akurang-Parry, Kwabena O., '"The Loads Are Heavier than Usual": Forced Labor by Women and Children in the Central Province, Gold Coast (Colonial Ghana), c.1900–1940', *African Economic History*, 30 (2002), 31–51
Akyeampong, Emmanuel, 'Sexuality and Prostitution among the Akan of the Gold Coast c. 1650–1950', *Past & Present*, 156 (1997), 144–73
Akyeampong, Emmanuel, '"Wo Pe Tam Won Pe Ba" ("You like Cloth but You Don't Want Children"): Urbanization, Individualism & Gender Relations in Colonial Ghana, c.1900–39', in *Africa's Urban Past*, ed. by David M. Anderson and Richard Rathbone (Oxford: James Currey, 2000), pp. 222–34
Akyeampong, Emmanuel, and Samuel Agyei-Mensah, 'Itinerant Gold Mines? Mobility, Sexuality and the Spread of Gonorrhoea and Syphilis in Twentieth Century Ghana', in *Sex and Gender*

in an Era of AIDS: Ghana at the Turn of the Millennium, ed. by Christine Oppong, M. Yaa P.A. Oppong, and Irene K. Odotei (Legon, Accra: Sub-Saharan Publishers, 2006), pp. 41–58

Akyeampong, Emmanuel, and Pashington Obeng, 'Spirituality, Gender, and Power in Asante History', *The International Journal of African Historical Studies*, 28.3 (1995), 481–508

Alence, Rod, 'The 1937–1938 Gold Coast Cocoa Crisis: The Political Economy of Commercial Stalemate', *African Economic History*, 19 (1990), 77–104

Allman, Jean, 'Fathering, Mothering and Making Sense of Ntamoba: Reflections on the Economy of Child-Rearing in Colonial Asante', *Africa*, 67.2 (1997), 296–321

Allman, Jean, 'Making Mothers: Missionaries, Medical Officers and Women's Work in Colonial Asante, 1924–1945', *History Workshop*, 38.1 (1994), 23–47

Allman, Jean, 'Of "Spinsters", "Concubines" and "Wicked Women": Reflections on Gender and Social Change in Colonial Asante', *Gender & History*, 3.2 (1991), 176–89

Allman, Jean, 'Rounding up Spinsters: Gender Chaos and Unmarried Women in Colonial Asante', *Journal of African History*, 37.2 (1996), 195–214

Allman, Jean, Susan Geiger, and Nakanyike Musisi, 'Women in African Colonial Histories: An Introduction', in *Women in African Colonial Histories*, ed. by Jean Marie Allman, Susan Geiger, and Nakanyike Musisi (Bloomington, IN: Indiana University Press, 2002), pp. 1–18

Allotey, P., and D. Reidpath, 'Establishing the Causes of Childhood Mortality in Ghana: The "Spirit Child"', *Social Science & Medicine*, 52.7 (2001), 1007–12

Amin, Samir, 'Introduction', in *Modern Migrations in Western Africa*, ed. by Samir Amin (Oxford: Oxford University Press, 1974), pp. 65–151

Amin, Samir, 'Underdevelopment and Dependence in Black Africa – Origins and Contemporary Forms', *The Journal of Modern African Studies*, 10.4 (1972), 503–24

Amoah, Albert G.B., Samuel K. Owusu, and Samuel Adjei, 'Diabetes in Ghana: A Community Based Prevalence Study in Greater Accra', *Diabetes Research and Clinical Practice*, 56.3 (2002), 197–205

Amugsi, Dickson A., Maurice B. Mittelmark, and Anna Lartey, 'An Analysis of Socio-Demographic Patterns in Child Malnutrition Trends Using Ghana Demographic and Health Survey Data in the Period 1993–2008', *BMC Public Health*, 13 (2013), 960

Annim, Samuel Kobina, Kofi Awusabo-Asare, and Joshua Amo-Adjei, 'Household Nucleation, Dependency and Child Health Outcomes in Ghana', *Journal of Biosocial Science*, 47.5 (2015), 565–92

Anyinam, C.A., 'Spatial Implications of Structural Adjustment Programmes in Ghana', *Tijdschrift Voor Economische En Sociale Geografie*, 85.5 (1994), 446–60

Ardayfio-Schandorf, Elizabeth, 'Household Headship and Women's Earning in Ghana', in *Family and Development in Ghana*, ed. by Elizabeth Ardayfio-Schandorf (Legon, Accra: Ghana Universities Press, 1994), pp. 30–47

Arhin, Kwame, 'Monetisation and the Asante State', in *Money Matters: Instability, Values and Social Payments in the Modern History of West Africa Communities*, ed. by Jane I. Guyer (Portsmouth, NH: Heinemann, 1995), pp. 188–201

Arhin, Kwame, 'Succession and Gold Mining at Mansu Nkwanta', *Research Review, University of Ghana*, 6.3 (1970), 101–9

Arhin, Kwame, 'The Financing of the Ashanti Expansion (1700–1820)', *Africa*, 37.3 (1967), 283–91

Arhin, Kwame, 'The Structure of Greater Ashanti (1700–1824)', *Journal of African History*, 8.1 (1967), 65–85

Armah, Frederick A., Justice O. Odoi, Genesis T. Yengoh, Samuel Obiri, David O. Yawson, and Ernest K. A. Afrifa, 'Food Security and Climate Change in Drought-Sensitive Savanna Zones of Ghana', *Mitigation and Adaptation Strategies for Global Change*, 16.3 (2010), 291–306

Arnold, David, 'The "Discovery" of Malnutrition and Diet in Colonial India', *The Indian Economic & Social History Review*, 31.1 (1994), 1–26

Aryeetey, Ernest, and Andrew McKay, 'Growth with Poverty Reduction, but Increased Spatial Inequality: Ghana over the 1990s', in *Determinants of Pro Poor Growth: Analytical Issues and Findings from Country Cases*, ed. by Michael Grimm, Stephen Klasen, and Andrew McKay (Basingstoke: Palgrave Macmillan, 2007), pp. 57–80

Ashworth, Ann, 'Efficacy and Effectiveness of Community-Based Treatment of Severe Malnutrition', *Food and Nutrition Bulletin*, 27.3 (2006), S24–S48

Asibey, E.O.A., 'Utilisation of Wildlife in Ghana', *The Ghana Farmer*, 9.3 (1965), 91–3

Asiedu, Alex B., and Samuel Agyei-Mensah, 'Traders on the Run: Activities of Street Vendors in the Accra Metropolitan Area, Ghana', *Norwegian Journal of Geography*, 62.3 (2008), 191–202

Atkinson, A.B., 'Bringing Income Distribution in From the Cold', *The Economic Journal*, 107.441 (1997), 297–321

Austin, Gareth, 'Africa and the Anthropocene', in *Economic Development and Environmental History in the Anthropocene: Perspectives on Asia and Africa*, ed. by Gareth Austin (London: Bloomsbury Publishing, 2017), pp. 95–118

Austin, Gareth, 'African Economic Development and Colonial Legacies', *International Development Policy*, 1 (2010), 11–32

Austin, Gareth, 'Between Abolition and Jihad: The Asante Response to the Ending of the Atlantic Slave Trade, 1807–1896', in *From Slave Trade to 'Legitimate' Commerce: The Commercial Transition in Nineteenth-Century West Africa*, ed. by R. Law (Cambridge: Cambridge University Press, 1995), pp. 93–118

Austin, Gareth, 'Human Pawning in Asante 1800–1950: Markets and Coercion, Gender and Cocoa', in *Pawnship, Slavery and Colonialism in Africa*, ed. by Paul E. Lovejoy and Toyin Falola (Trenton, NJ: Africa World Press, 2003), pp. 187–224

Austin, Gareth, 'National Poverty and the "Vampire State" in Ghana: A Review Article', *Journal of International Development*, 8.4 (1996), 553–73

Austin, Gareth, '"No Elders Were Present": Commoners and Private Ownership in Asante, 1807–96', *The Journal of African History*, 37.1 (1996), 1–30

Austin, Gareth, 'Vent for Surplus or Productivity Breakthrough? The Ghanaian Cocoa Take-Off, c. 1890–1936', *The Economic History Review*, 67.4 (2014), 1035–64

Austin, Gareth, Joerg Baten, and Bas Van Leeuwen, 'The Biological Standard of Living in Early Nineteenth-Century West Africa: New Anthropometric Evidence for Northern Ghana and Burkina Faso', *The Economic History Review*, 65 (2012), 1280–302

Autret, M., 'Protein Malnutrition and the FAO Viewpoint', in *Progress in Meeting Protein Needs of Infants and Pre-School Children: Proceedings of an International Conference Held in Washington, D.C., August 21–24, 1960. Under the Auspices of the Committee on Protein Malnutrition, Food and Nutrition Board, and the Nutrition Study Section, National Institutes of Health*, ed. by National Academy of Sciences (Washington, D.C.: National Academy of Sciences, 1961), pp. 537–43

Ayee, Joseph R.A., 'Civil Service Reform in Ghana: A Case Study of Contemporary Reform Problems in Africa', *African Journal of Political Science*, 6.1 (2004), 1–41

Ball, Helen L., and Catherine M. Hill, 'Reevaluating "Twin Infanticide"', *Current Anthropology*, 37.5 (1996), 856–63

Bannister, David, 'The Sorcerer's Apprentice: Sleeping Sickness, Onchocerciasis, and Unintended Consequences in Ghana, 1930–60', *The Journal of African History*, 62.1 (2021), 29–57

Baten, Joerg, and Matthias Blum, 'Growing Tall but Unequal: New Findings and New Background Evidence on Anthropometric Welfare in 156 Countries, 1810–1989', *Economic History of Developing Regions*, 27.S1 (2012), S66–S85

Behrends, Andrea, '"Pogminga": The "Proper Dagara Woman": An Encounter between Christian Thought and Dagara Concepts', *Journal of Religion in Africa*, 32.2 (2002), 231–53

Beinart, William, 'Soil Erosion, Conservationism and Ideas about Development: A Southern African Exploration, 1900–1960', *Journal of Southern African Studies*, 11.1 (1984), 52–83

Benería, Lourdes, 'Toward a Greater Integration of Gender in Economics', *World Development*, 23.11 (1995), 1839–50

Bennett, F.J., and J.P. Stanfield, 'The Clinical Conditions and Aetiology of Malnutrition in Uganda', in *Nutrition and Food in an African Economy*, ed. by V.F. Amann, D.G.R. Belshaw, and J.P. Stanfield (Kampala: Department of Rural Economy, Makerere Library, 1972), pp. 1–9

Bennett, F.J., and J.P. Stanfield, 'The Pattern of Malnutrition in Uganda', *Journal of Tropical Pediatrics*, 17.1 (1971), S5–S10

Berg, A., 'Sliding toward Nutrition Malpractice: Time to Reconsider and Redeploy', *The American Journal of Clinical Nutrition*, 57.1 (1993), 3–7

Bernasko, F.G., 'Opening Address: Ghana's Operation Feed Yourself Programme', in *Food and Population: Ghana's Operation Feed Yourself Programme – A Case Study. Report of the 26th Annual New Year School of the Institute of Adult Education, 30 December 1974–8 January 1975*, ed. by Kwa O. Hagan (Legon, Accra: University of Ghana, 1975)

Bierlich, B., 'Injections and the Fear of Death: An Essay on the Limits of Biomedicine among the Dagomba of Northern Ghana', *Social Science & Medicine*, 50.5 (2000), 703–13

Bigland, A.D., 'Oedema as a Symptom in So-Called Food Deficiency Diseases', *The Lancet*, 195.5031 (1920), 243–7

Birdsall, Nancy, and Juan Luis Londoño, 'Asset Inequality Matters: An Assessment of the World Bank's Approach to Poverty Reduction', *The American Economic Review*, 87.2 (1997), 32–7

Black, Robert E., Cesar G. Victora, Susan P. Walker, Zulfiqar A. Bhutta, Parul Christian, Mercedes de Onis, et al., 'Maternal and Child Undernutrition and Overweight in Low-Income and Middle-Income Countries', *The Lancet*, 382.9890 (2013), 427–51

Bleek, Wolf, 'Did the Akan Resort to Abortion in Pre-Colonial Ghana? Some Conjectures', *Africa*, 60 (1990), 121–31

Bloch, C.E., 'Diseases of Infants Due to Prolonged Feeding With Excess of Carbohydrates', *British Medical Journal*, 1.3139 (1921), 293–5

Boadi, Kwasi Owusu, and Markku Kuitunen, 'Environment, Wealth, Inequality and the Burden of Disease in the Accra Metropolitan Area, Ghana', *International Journal of Environmental Health Research*, 15.3 (2005), 193–206

Bongaarts, John, 'The KAP-Gap and the Unmet Need for Contraception', *Population and Development Review*, 17.2 (1991), 293–313

Brantley, Cynthia, 'Kikuyu-Maasai Nutrition and Colonial Science: The Orr and Gilks Study in Late 1920s Kenya Revisited', *The International Journal of African Historical Studies*, 30.1 (1997), 49–86

Breschi, Marco, and Massimo Livi Bacci, 'Month of Birth as a Factor in Children's Survival', in *Infant and Child Mortality in the Past*, ed. by Alain Bideau, Bertrand Desjardins, and Héctor Pérez Brignoli (Oxford: Oxford University Press, 1997), pp. 157–73

Brewster, D.R., and B.M. Greenwood, 'Seasonal Variation of Paediatric Diseases in The Gambia, West Africa', *Annals of Tropical Paediatrics*, 13.2 (1993), 133–46

Briend, André, Radandi Lacsala, Claudine Prudhon, Béatrice Mounier, Yvonne Grellety, and Michael H.N. Golden, 'Ready-to-Use Therapeutic Food for Treatment of Marasmus', *The Lancet*, 353.9166 (1999), 1767–8

Brown, James W., 'Increased Intercommunication and Epidemic Disease in Early Colonial Ashanti', in *Disease in African History: An Introductory Survey and Case Studies*, ed. by K. David Patterson and Gerald W. Hartwig (Durham, NC: Duke University Press, 1978), pp. 180–207

Brown, Marjorie, 'Nutrition in the Gold Coast: A Summary of Information Relating to the Present Position of Nutrition in the Gold Coast', in *Conférence interafricaine sur l'alimentation et la nutrition. Dschang, Cameroun, 3–9 Octobre 1949* (Paris: La Documentation Française, 1949), pp. 96–103

Brydon, Lynne, 'Ghanaian Responses to the Nigerian Expulsions of 1983', *African Affairs*, 84.337 (1985), 561–85

Brydon, Lynne, 'Rice, Yams and Chiefs in Avatime: Speculations on the Development of a Social Order', *Africa*, 51.2 (1981), 659–77

Burnet, E., and W.R. Aykroyd, 'Nutrition and Public Health', *League of Nations: Quarterly Bulletin of the Health Organisation*, 4.2 (1935), 323–474

Caldwell, John C., 'Education as a Factor in Mortality Decline An Examination of Nigerian Data', *Population Studies*, 33.3 (1979), 395–413

Caldwell, John C., 'Fertility Attitudes in Three Economically Contrasting Rural Regions of Ghana', *Economic Development and Cultural Change*, 15.2 (1967), 217–38

Caldwell, John C., 'Routes to Low Mortality in Poor Countries', *Population and Development Review*, 12.2 (1986), 171–220

Cammack, Paul, 'Making the Poor Work for Globalisation?', *New Political Economy*, 6.3 (2001), 397–408

Cammack, Paul, 'What the World Bank Means by Poverty Reduction, and Why It Matters', *New Political Economy*, 9.2 (2004), 189–211

Carpenter, Kenneth J., 'A Short History of Nutritional Science: Part 1 (1785–1885)', *The Journal of Nutrition*, 133.3 (2003), 638–45

Carpenter, Kenneth J., 'A Short History of Nutritional Science: Part 2 (1885–1912)', *The Journal of Nutrition*, 133.4 (2003), 975–84

Carpenter, Kenneth J., 'A Short History of Nutritional Science: Part 4 (1945–1985)', *The Journal of Nutrition*, 133.11 (2003), 3331–42

Ceesay, S.M., A.M. Prentice, T.J. Cole, F. Foord, L.T. Weaver, E.M. Poskitt, et al., 'Effects on Birth Weight and Perinatal Mortality of Maternal Dietary Supplements in Rural Gambia: 5 Year Randomised Controlled Trial', *BMJ*, 315.7111 (1997), 786–90

Chalfin, Brenda, 'Risky Business: Economic Uncertainty, Market Reforms and Female Livelihoods in Northeast Ghana', *Development and Change*, 31.5 (2000), 987–1008

Christaller, J.G., 'Recent Explorations in the Basin of the Volta (Gold Coast) by Missionaries of the Basel Missionary Society', *Proceedings of the Royal Geographical Society and Monthly Record of Geography*, 8.4 (1886), 246–56

Ciliberto, Heather, Michael Ciliberto, André Briend, Per Ashorn, Dennis Bier, and Mark Manary, 'Antioxidant Supplementation for the Prevention of Kwashiorkor in Malawian Children: Randomised, Double Blind, Placebo Controlled Trial', *BMJ*, 330.7500 (2005), 1109–11

Clark, Gracia, 'Food Traders and Food Security in Ghana', in *The Political Economy of African Famine*, ed. by Richard Erskine Downs, Donna O. Kerner, and Stephen P. Reyna (London: Gordon and Breach, 1991), pp. 227–56

Clark, Gracia, 'From Fasting to Fast Food in Kumasi, Ghana', in *Food Consumption in Global Perspective: Essays in the Anthropology of Food in Honour of Jack Goody*, ed. by Jakob Klein and Anne Murcott (Basingstoke: Palgrave Macmillan, 2014), pp. 45–64

Clark, Gracia, 'Mothering, Work, and Gender in Urban Asante Ideology and Practice', *American Anthropologist*, 101.4 (1999), 717–29

Clarke, Edwin, 'Whistler and Glisson on Rickets', *Bulletin of the History of Medicine*, 36.1 (1962), 45–61

Cleveland, David A., 'Migration in West Africa: A Savanna Village Perspective', *Africa*, 61.2 (1991), 222–46

Codjoe, Samuel Nii Ardey, and Fred M. Dzanku, 'Long-Term Determinants of Deforestation in Ghana: The Role of Structural Adjustment Policies', *African Development Review*, 21.3 (2009), 558–88

Coghe, Samuël, 'Between Colonial Medicine and Global Health: Protein Malnutrition and UNICEF Milk in the Belgian Congo', *Medical History*, 65.4 (2021), 384–402

Colbourne, M.J., G.M. Edington, M.H. Hughes, and A. Ward-Brew, 'A Medical Survey in a Gold Coast Village', *Transactions of the Royal Society of Tropical Medicine and Hygiene*, 44.3 (1950), 271–90

Colecraft, Esi K., Grace S. Marquis, Alfred A. Bartolucci, LeaVonne Pulley, W. Bruce Owusu, and H. Michael Maetz, 'A Longitudinal Assessment of the Diet and Growth of Malnourished Children Participating in Nutrition Rehabilitation Centres in Accra, Ghana', *Public Health Nutrition*, 7.4 (2004), 487–94

Collins, Steve, Nicky Dent, Paul Binns, Paluku Bahwere, Kate Sadler, and Alistair Hallam, 'Management of Severe Acute Malnutrition in Children', *The Lancet*, 368.9551 (2006), 1992–2000

Collis, W.R.F., J. Dema, and A. Omololu, 'On the Ecology of Child Health and Nutrition in Nigerian Villages, Parts I and II', *Tropical and Geographical Medicine*, 14 (1962), 140–63, 201–29

Comaroff, Jean, 'The Diseased Heart of Africa: Medicine, Colonialism and the Black Body', in *Knowledge, Power, and Practice: The Anthropology of Medicine and Everyday Life*, ed. by Shirley Lindenbaum and Margaret M. Lock (Berkeley, CA: University of California Press, 1993)

Comaroff, Jean, and John L. Comaroff, 'Home-Made Hegemony: Modernity, Domesticity, and Colonialism in South Africa', in *African Encounters with Domesticity*, ed. by Karen Hansen (New Brunswick, NJ: Rutgers University Press, 1992), pp. 37–74

Comaroff, Jean, and John L. Comaroff, 'Millennial Capitalism: First Thoughts on a Second Coming', *Public Culture*, 12.2 (2000), 291–343

Comaroff, Jean, and John L. Comaroff, 'Second Comings: Neo-Protestant Ethics and Millennial Capitalism in Africa, and Elsewhere', in *2000 Years and Beyond: Faith, Identity, and the 'Common Era'*, ed. by Paul Gifford (London: Routledge, 2003), pp. 291–343

Côté, Anne-Marie, François Sobela, Agnes Dzokoto, Khonde Nzambi, Comfort Asamoah-Adu, Annie-Claude Labbé, et al., 'Transactional Sex Is the Driving Force in the Dynamics of HIV in Accra, Ghana', *AIDS*, 18.6 (2004), 917–25

Coulombe, Harold, and Andrew McKay, 'Growth with Selective Poverty Reduction – Ghana in the 1990s', in *Growth and Poverty Reduction: Case Studies from West Africa*, ed. by Quentin Wodon (Washington, D.C.: World Bank Publications, 2007), pp. 9–94

Curtin, Philip D., 'Nutrition in African History', in *Hunger and History: The Impact of Changing Food Production and Consumption Patterns on Society*, ed. by Robert I. Rotberg and Theodore K. Rabb (Cambridge: Cambridge University Press, 1985), pp. 173–84

Daloz, Jean-Pascal, '"Big Men" in Sub-Saharan Africa: How Elites Accumulate Positions and Resources', *Comparative Sociology*, 2.1 (2003), 271–85

Davey, P.L.H., 'Some Puzzling Spending Habits in Ghana', *Economic Bulletin of Ghana*, 7.1 (1963), 17–28

Davin, Anna, 'Imperialism and Motherhood', *History Workshop Journal*, 5 (1978), 9–65

de Waal, Alex, 'Famine Mortality: A Case Study of Darfur, Sudan 1984–5', *Population Studies*, 43 (1989), 5–24

Dei, George J.S., 'A Forest beyond the Trees: Tree Cutting in Rural Ghana', *Human Ecology*, 20.1 (1992), 57–88

Dei, George J.S., 'A Ghanaian Town Revisited: Changes and Continuities in Local Adaptive Strategies', *African Affairs*, 91.362 (1992), 95–120

Dei, George J.S., 'The Renewal of a Ghanaian Rural Economy', *Canadian Journal of African Studies*, 26.1 (1992), 24–53

Denham, Aaron R., Philip B. Adongo, Nicole Freydberg, and Abraham Hodgson, 'Chasing Spirits: Clarifying the Spirit Child Phenomenon and Infanticide in Northern Ghana', *Social Science & Medicine*, 71.3 (2010), 608–15

Destombes, Jerôme, 'From Long-Term Patterns of Seasonal Hunger to Changing Experiences of Everyday Poverty: Northeastern Ghana, c. 1930–2000', *Journal of African History*, 47.2 (2006), 181–205

Dodu, Silas R.A., 'Diabetes In The Tropics', *The British Medical Journal*, 2.5554 (1967), 747–50

Dodu, Silas R.A., 'The Incidence of Diabetes Mellitus in Accra (Ghana); A Study of 4,000 Patients', *The West African Medical Journal*, 7.3 (1958), 129–34

Dodu, Silas R.A., and N. De Heer, 'A Diabetes Case-Finding Survey in Ho, Ghana', *Ghana Medical Journal*, 3 (1964), 75–80

Doyle, Shane, 'Population Decline and Delayed Recovery in Bunyoro, 1860–1960', *Journal of African History*, 41.3 (2000), 429–58

Drewnowski, A., 'Taste Preferences and Food Intake', *Annual Review of Nutrition*, 17.1 (1997), 237–53

Drucker-Brown, Susan, 'Mamprusi Witchcraft, Subversion and Changing Gender Relations', *Africa*, 63.4 (1993), 531–49

Du, Shufa, Tom A Mroz, Fengying Zhai, and Barry M Popkin, 'Rapid Income Growth Adversely Affects Diet Quality in China – Particularly for the Poor!', *Social Science & Medicine*, 59.7 (2004), 1505–15

Dumett, Raymond, 'Disease and Mortality among Gold Miners of Ghana: Colonial Government and Mining Company Attitudes and Policies, 1900–1938', *Social Science & Medicine*, 37.2 (1993), 213–32

Editorial, 'Kwashiorkor', *The Lancet*, 253 (1949), 188–9 (p. 188)

England, Paula, 'The Separative Self: Androcentric Bias in Neoclassical Assumptions', in *Beyond Economic Man: Feminist Theory and Economics*, ed. by Marianne A. Ferber and Julie A. Nelson (Chicago, IL: University of Chicago Press, 1993), pp. 37–53

Engle, Patricia L., 'The Effect of Maternal Employment on Children's Welfare in Rural Guatemala', *New Directions for Child and Adolescent Development*, 20 (1983), 57–75

Esrey, S.A., J.P. Habicht, M.C. Latham, D.G. Sisler, and G. Casella, 'Drinking Water Source, Diarrheal Morbidity, and Child Growth in Villages with Both Traditional and Improved Water Supplies in Rural Lesotho, Southern Africa', *American Journal of Public Health*, 78.11 (1988), 1451–5

Evenson, R.E., and D. Gollin, 'Assessing the Impact of the Green Revolution, 1960 to 2000', *Science*, 300.5620 (2003), 758–62

Fee, Margery, 'Racializing Narratives: Obesity, Diabetes and the "Aboriginal" Thrifty Genotype', *Social Science & Medicine*, 62.12 (2006), 2988–97

Feierman, Steven, 'Struggles for Control: The Social Roots of Health and Healing in Modern Africa', *African Studies Review*, 28.2/3 (1985), 73–147

Fenn, Bridget, Saul S. Morris, and Chris Frost, 'Do Childhood Growth Indicators in Developing Countries Cluster? Implications for Intervention Strategies', *Public Health Nutrition*, 7.7 (2004), 829–34

Fiawoo, D.K., 'Physical Growth and the School Environment: A West African Example', in *Physiological and Morphological Adaptation and Evolution*, ed. by William A. Stini (The Hague: Mouton, 1979), pp. 301–14

Field, M.J., 'Gold Coast Food', *Petit Propos Culinaires*, 42 (1931), 7–21

Fine, Ben, and Kwabia Boateng, 'Labour and Employment under Structural Adjustment', in *Economic Reforms in Ghana: The Miracle and the Mirage*, ed. by Ernest Aryeetey, Jane Harrigan, and Machiko Nissanke (Oxford: James Currey, 2000), pp. 227–45

Finlay, Mark R., 'Early Marketing of the Theory of Nutrition: The Science and Culture of Liebig's Extract of Meat', in *The Science and Culture of Nutrition, 1840–1940*, ed. by Harmke Kamminga and Andrew Cunningham (Amsterdam: Brill Rodopi, 1995), pp. 48–74

Fortes, Meyer, 'A Demographic Field Study in Ashanti', in *Culture and Human Fertility: A Study of the Relation of Cultural Conditions to Fertility in Non-Industrial and Transitional Societies*, ed. by Lorimer Frank (Paris: UNESCO, 1954), pp. 253–340

Fortes, Meyer, 'Kinship and Marriage among the Ashanti', in *African Systems of Kinship and Marriage*, ed. by A.R. Radcliffe-Brown and D. Forde (Oxford: Oxford University Press, 1952), pp. 252–84

Fortes, Meyer, 'The Political System of the Tallensi of the Northern Territories of the Gold Coast', in *African Political Systems*, ed. by Meyer Fortes and Edward Evan Evans-Pritchard (Oxford: Oxford University Press, 1940), pp. 239–71

Fortes, Meyer, and S.L. Fortes, 'Food in the Domestic Economy of the Tallensi', *Africa*, 9.2 (1936), 237–76

Frisch, R. A., Lafayette B. Mendel, and John P. Peters, 'The Production of Edema and Serum Protein Deficiency in White Rats by Low Protein Diets', *Journal of Biological Chemistry*, 84.1 (1929), 167–77

Frongillo, E.A., M. de Onis, and K.M. Hanson, 'Socioeconomic and Demographic Factors Are Associated with Worldwide Patterns of Stunting and Wasting of Children', *The Journal of Nutrition*, 127.12 (1997), 2302–9

Gaisie, S.K., 'Levels and Patterns of Infant and Child Mortality in Ghana', *Demography*, 12.1 (1975), 21–34

Gary, Ian, 'Confrontation, Co-operation or Co-optation: NGOs and the Ghanaian State during Structural Adjustment', *Review of African Political Economy*, 23.68 (1996), 149–68

Gayi, Samuel K., 'Adjusting to the Social Costs of Adjustment in Ghana: Problems and Prospects', *The European Journal of Development Research*, 7.1 (1995), 77–100

van der Geest, Kees, 'North-South Migration in Ghana: What Role for the Environment?', *International Migration*, 49.S1 (2011), 69–94

Gifford, Paul, 'Ghana's Charismatic Churches', *Journal of Religion in Africa*, 24.3 (1994), 241–65

Gillespie, Tom, 'Accumulation by Urban Dispossession: Struggles over Urban Space in Accra, Ghana', *Transactions of the Institute of British Geographers*, 41.1 (2016), 66–77

Girdner, Janet, Victor Olorunsola, Myrna Froning, and Emmanuel Hansen, 'Ghana's Agricultural Food Policy: Operation Feed Yourself', *Food Policy*, 5.1 (1980), 14–25

Glasgow, Sara, and Ted Schrecker, 'The Double Burden of Neoliberalism? Noncommunicable Disease Policies and the Global Political Economy of Risk', *Health & Place*, 34 (2015), 279–86

Glewwe, Paul, and Jacques van der Gaag, 'Identifying the Poor in Developing Countries: Do Different Definitions Matter?', *World Development*, 18.6 (1990), 803–14

Gluckman, Max, 'The Lozi of Barotseland in North-Western Rhodesia', in *Seven Tribes of British Central Africa*, ed. by Elizabeth Colson and Max Gluckman (Manchester: Manchester University Press, 1951), pp. 1–93

Golden, M.H., 'Oedematous Malnutrition', *British Medical Bulletin*, 54.2 (1998), 433–44

Golden, M.H., 'Protein Deficiency, Energy Deficiency, and the Oedema of Malnutrition', *The Lancet*, 1.8284 (1982), 1261–5

Golden, M.H., 'The Development of Concepts of Malnutrition', *The Journal of Nutrition*, 132.7 (2002), 2117S–2122S

Goldsworthy, David, 'Ghana's Second Republic: A Post-Mortem', *African Affairs*, 72.286 (1973), 8–25

Goody, Esther, 'Legitimate and Illegitimate Aggression in a West African State', in *Witchcraft Confessions and Accusations*, ed. by Mary Douglas (London: Routledge, 2004)

Goody, Jack, 'Rice-Burning and the Green Revolution in Northern Ghana', *The Journal of Development Studies*, 16.2 (1980), 136–55

Grant, Faye Woodard, 'Nutrition and Health of Gold Coast Children. II. Care and Physical Status of Children', *Journal of the American Dietetic Association*, 31.7 (1955), 694–702

Granzberg, Gary, 'Twin Infanticide – A Cross-Cultural Test of a Materialistic Explanation', *Ethos*, 1.4 (1973), 405–12

Grier, Beverly, 'Pawns, Porters, and Petty Traders: Women in the Transition to Cash Crop Agriculture in Colonial Ghana', *Signs*, 17.2 (1992), 304–28

Grischow, Jeff D., 'Corruptions of Development in the Countryside of the Northern Territories of the Gold Coast, 1927–57', *The Journal of Peasant Studies*, 26.1 (1998), 139–58

Grischow, Jeff D., and Holger Weiss, 'Colonial Famine Relief and Development Policies: Towards an Environmental History of Northern Ghana', *Global Environment*, 7/8 (2012), 50–97

Guo, Guang, and Laurence M. Grummer-Strawn, 'Child Mortality Among Twins in Less Developed Countries', *Population Studies*, 47.3 (1993), 495–510

Guzmán, Juan Carlos, Andrew R. Morrison, and Mirja Sjöblom, 'The Impact of Remittances and Gender on Household Expenditure Patterns: Evidence from Ghana', in *The International Migration of Women*, ed. by Andrew R. Morrison, Maurice Schiff, and Mirja Sjöblom (Washington, D.C.: World Bank, 2008), pp. 125–52

Hardin, Garrett, 'The Tragedy of the Commons', *Science*, 162.3859 (1968), 1243–8

Hart, Keith, 'Informal Income Opportunities and Urban Employment in Ghana', *The Journal of Modern African Studies*, 11.1 (1973), 61–89

Hart, Keith, 'Migrations and the Opportunity Structure: A Ghanaian Case Study', in *Modern Migrations in Western Africa*, ed. by Samir Amin (Oxford: Oxford University Press, 1974), pp. 321–39

Hart, Keith, 'The Economic Basis of Tallensi Social History in the Early Twentieth Century', in *Research in Economic Anthropology: An Annual Compilation of Research*, ed. by George Dalton (London: JAI Press, 1978), pp. 185–216

Harvey, David, 'The "New" Imperialism: Accumulation by Dispossession', *Socialist Register*, 40.40 (2009), 63–87

Haukioja, Erkki, Risto Lemmetyinen, and Mirja Pikkola, 'Why Are Twins So Rare in Homo Sapiens?', *The American Naturalist*, 133.4 (1989), 572–7

Hawkins, Sean, '"The Woman in Question": Marriage and Identity in the Colonial Courts of Northern Ghana, 1907–1954', in *Women in African Colonial Histories*, ed. by Jean Allman, Susan Geiger, and Nakanyike Musisi (Bloomington, IN: Indiana University Press, 2002), pp. 116–43

Hawkins, Sean, 'To Pray or Not To Pray: Politics, Medicine, and Conversion among the LoDagaa of Northern Ghana, 1929–1939', *Canadian Journal of African Studies*, 31.1 (1997), 50–85

Hearn, Julie, 'The "Uses and Abuses" of Civil Society in Africa', *Review of African Political Economy*, 28.87 (2001), 43–53

Henry, C.J.K., P.A. Donachie, and J.P.W. Rivers, 'The Winged Bean: Will the Wonder Crop Be Another Flop?', *Ecology of Food and Nutrition*, 16.4 (1985), 331–8

Hill, Polly, 'Some Puzzling Spending Habits in Ghana', *Economic Bulletin of Ghana*, 1.10 (1957), 3–11

Hill, Polly, 'Women Cocoa Farmers', *Economic Bulletin of Ghana*, 2 (1958), 70–76

Hilson, Gavin, 'Child Labour in African Artisanal Mining Communities: Experiences from Northern Ghana', *Development and Change*, 41.3 (2010), 445–73

Hilson, Gavin, and Clive Potter, 'Structural Adjustment and Subsistence Industry: Artisanal Gold Mining in Ghana', *Development and Change*, 36.1 (2005), 103–31

Hong, Rathavuth, 'Effect of Economic Inequality on Chronic Childhood Undernutrition in Ghana', *Public Health Nutrition*, 10.4 (2007), 371–8

Howe, Paul, and Stephen Devereux, 'Famine Intensity and Magnitude Scales: A Proposal for an Instrumental Definition of Famine', *Disasters*, 28.4 (2004), 353–72

Hughes, M.H., and P.F. Daly, 'Onchocerciasis in the Southern Gold Coast', *Transactions of The Royal Society of Tropical Medicine and Hygiene*, 45.2 (1951), 243–52

Hunt, Nancy Rose, '"Le Bebe En Brousse": European Women, African Birth Spacing and Colonial Intervention in Breast Feeding in the Belgian Congo', *The International Journal of African Historical Studies*, 21.3 (1988), 401–32

Hunter, John M., 'River Blindness in Nangodi, Northern Ghana: A Hypothesis of Cyclical Advance and Retreat', *Geographical Review*, 56.3 (1966), 398–416

Hunter, John M., 'Seasonal Hunger in a Part of the West African Savanna: A Survey of Bodyweights in Nangodi, North-East Ghana', *Transactions of the Institute of British Geographers*, 41 (1967), 167–85

Hutchful, Eboe, '"Smoke and Mirrors": The World Bank's Social Dimensions of Adjustment (SDA) Programme', *Review of African Political Economy*, 21.62 (1994), 569–84

Hutchful, Eboe, 'Why Regimes Adjust: The World Bank Ponders Its "Star Pupil"', *Canadian Journal of African Studies*, 29.2 (1995), 303–17

Ittmann, Karl, '"Where Nature Dominates Man": Demographic Ideas and Policy in British Colonial Africa, 1890–1970', in *The Demographics of Empire*, ed. by Karl Ittmann, Dennis D. Cordell, and Gregory H. Maddox (Athens, OH: Ohio University Press, 2010), pp. 59–88

Jelliffe, D.B., 'Commerciogenic Malnutrition?', *Nutrition Reviews*, 30.9 (1972), 199–205

Jelliffe, D.B., 'Pediatrics in Uganda', *Clinical Pediatrics*, 4.1 (1965), 55–61

Jelliffe, D.B., 'Protein-Calorie Malnutrition in Tropical Preschool Children: A Review of Recent Knowledge', *The Journal of Pediatrics*, 54.2 (1959), 227–56

Jelliffe, D.B., 'Social Culture and Nutrition: Cultural Blocks and Protein Malnutrition in Early Childhood in Rural West Bengal', *Pediatrics*, 20.1 (1957), 128–38

Jelliffe, D.B., and F.J. Bennett, 'Cultural and Anthropological Factors in Infant and Maternal Nutrition', *Federation Proceedings*, 20 (1961), S185–7

Jelliffe, D.B., and J.P. Stanfield, 'Protein Deficiencies and Calorie Deficiencies', *The Lancet*, 288.7469 (1966), 207–8

Jellinek, E.H., 'The Russells of Edinburgh: A Medical Dynasty', *Proceedings of the Royal College of Physicians of Edinburgh*, 31.4 (2001), 342–51

Jerven, Morten, 'A Clash of Disciplines? Economists and Historians Approaching the African Past', *Economic History of Developing Regions*, 26.2 (2011), 111–24

Kasei, Raymond, Bernd Diekkrüger, and Constanze Leemhuis, 'Drought Frequency in the Volta Basin of West Africa', *Sustainability Science*, 5.1 (2009), 89–97

Katz, Cindi, 'Vagabond Capitalism and the Necessity of Social Reproduction', *Antipode*, 33 (2001), 709–28

Katz, Joanne, 'Sample-Size Implications for Population-Based Cluster Surveys of Nutritional Status', *The American Journal of Clinical Nutrition*, 61.1 (1995), 155–60

Katz, Joanne, Vincent J. Carey, Scott L. Zeger, and Alfred Sommer, 'Estimation of Design Effects and Diarrhea Clustering within Households and Villages', *American Journal of Epidemiology*, 138.11 (1993), 994–1006

Klausen, Susanne, 'The Race Welfare Society: Eugenics and Birth Control in Johannesburg, 1930–40', in *Science and Society in Southern Africa*, ed. by Saul Dubow (Manchester: Manchester University Press, 2000), pp. 164–87

Knapp, Vincent J., 'The Democratization of Meat and Protein in Late Eighteenth- and Nineteenth-Century Europe', *Historian*, 59.3 (1997), 541–51

Knight, J.B., 'Rural-Urban Income Comparisons and Migration in Ghana', *Bulletin of the Oxford University Institute of Economics & Statistics*, 34.2 (1972), 199–228

Komlos, John, 'Shrinking in a Growing Economy? The Mystery of Physical Stature during the Industrial Revolution', *The Journal of Economic History*, 58.3 (1998), 779–802

Konadu-Agyemang, Kwadwo, 'The Best of Times and the Worst of Times: Structural Adjustment Programs and Uneven Development in Africa: The Case Of Ghana', *The Professional Geographer*, 52.3 (2000), 469–83

Konotey-Ahulu, F.I.D., 'Issues in Kwashiorkor', *The Lancet*, 343.8896 (1994), 548

Kraus, Jon, 'The Political Economy of Agrarian Regression in Ghana', in *Africa's Agrarian Crisis: The Roots of Famine*, ed. by Stephen K. Commins, Michael F. Lofchie, and Rhys Payne (Boulder, CO: Lynne Rienner, 1986), pp. 103–32

Kwapong, A.A., 'Vice-Chancellor's Welcome Address', in *Food and Population: Ghana's Operation Feed Yourself Programme – A Case Study. Report of the 26th Annual New Year School of the Institute of Adult Education, 30 December 1974–8 January 1975*, ed. by Kwa O. Hagan (Legon, Accra: University of Ghana, 1975), pp. 15–19

La-Anyane, S., 'Research in Agriculture in Relation to National Economic Development', in *Scientific Research in Ghana: Proceedings of the Workshop on Research Priorities and Problems in the Execution of Research in Ghana* (Washington, D.C.: National Academy of Sciences, 1971)

Landecker, Hannah, 'Food as Exposure: Nutritional Epigenetics and the New Metabolism', *BioSocieties*, 6.2 (2011), 167–94

Landecker, Hannah, 'Postindustrial Metabolism: Fat Knowledge', *Public Culture*, 25.3 (2013), 495–522

Landman, J., and A.A. Jackson, 'The Role of Protein Deficiency in the Aetiology of Kwashiorkor', *The West Indian Medical Journal*, 29.4 (1980), 229–38
Lawson, Rowena M., 'Engel's Law and Its Application to Ghana', *Economic Bulletin of Ghana*, 6.4 (1962), 334–46
Lawson, Rowena M., 'The Distributive System in Ghana: A Review Article', *The Journal of Development Studies*, 3.2 (1967), 195–205
Le Vine, Victor T., 'Autopsy on a Régime: Ghana's Civilian Interregnum 1969–72', *The Journal of Modern African Studies*, 25.1 (1987), 169–78
Lelijveld, Natasha, Andrew Seal, Jonathan C. Wells, Jane Kirkby, Charles Opondo, Emmanuel Chimwezi, et al., 'Chronic Disease Outcomes after Severe Acute Malnutrition in Malawian Children (ChroSAM): A Cohort Study', *The Lancet. Global Health*, 4.9 (2016), e654–e662
Lentz, Carola, '"The Time When Politics Came": Ghana's Decolonisation from the Perspective of a Rural Periphery', *Journal of Contemporary African Studies*, 20.2 (2002), 245–74
Leslie, Joanne, 'Women's Work and Child Nutrition in the Third World', *World Development*, 16.11 (1988), 1341–62
Lock, Margaret, 'Comprehending the Body in the Era of the Epigenome', *Current Anthropology*, 56.2 (2015), 151–77
Lord, Jack, 'Child Labor in the Gold Coast: The Economics of Work, Education, and the Family in Late-Colonial African Childhoods, c. 1940–57', *The Journal of the History of Childhood and Youth*, 4.1 (2011), 88–115
Manesh, Alireza Olyaee, Trevor A. Sheldon, Kate E. Pickett, and Roy Carr-Hill, 'Accuracy of Child Morbidity Data in Demographic and Health Surveys', *International Journal of Epidemiology*, 37.1 (2008), 194–200
Manji, Firoze, and Carl O'Coill, 'The Missionary Position: NGOs and Development in Africa', *International Affairs*, 78.3 (2002), 567–83
Masih, I., S. Maskey, F.E.P. Mussá, and P. Trambauer, 'A Review of Droughts on the African Continent: A Geospatial and Long-Term Perspective', *Hydrol. Earth Syst. Sci.*, 18.9 (2014), 3635–49
McCaskie, T.C., 'Accumulation: Wealth and Belief in Asante History: II the Twentieth Century', *Africa*, 56.1 (1986), 3–23
McCaskie, T.C., 'State and Society, Marriage and Adultery: Some Considerations Towards a Social History of Pre-Colonial Asante', *Journal of African History*, 22.4 (1981), 477–94
McLaren, D.S., 'A Fresh Look at Protein-Calorie Malnutrition', *The Lancet*, 288.7461 (1966), 485–8
McLaren, D.S., 'Issues in Kwashiorkor', *The Lancet*, 343 (1994), 548–9
McLaren, D.S., 'The Great Protein Fiasco', *The Lancet*, 304.7872 (1974), 93–6
McMichael, Philip, 'Reframing Development: Global Peasant Movements and the New Agrarian Question', *Canadian Journal of Development Studies*, 27.4 (2006), 471–83
Meach, Rachel, 'From John Yudkin to Jamie Oliver: A Short but Sweet History on the War against Sugar', in *Proteins, Pathologies and Politics: Dietary Innovation and Disease from the Nineteenth Century*, ed. by David C. Gentilcore and Matthew Smith (London: Bloomsbury Academic, 2018), pp. 95–108
Messer, Ellen, 'Anthropological Perspectives on Diet', *Annual Review of Anthropology*, 13.1 (1984), 205–49
Meyer, Birgit, 'Commodities and the Power of Prayer: Pentecostalist Attitudes Towards Consumption in Contemporary Ghana', *Development and Change*, 29.4 (1998), 751–76
Meyer, Birgit, 'Visions of Blood, Sex and Money: Fantasy Spaces in Popular Ghanaian Cinema', *Visual Anthropology*, 16.1 (2003), 15–41
Mkhwanazi, Nolwazi, 'Medical Anthropology in Africa: The Trouble with a Single Story', *Medical Anthropology*, 35.2 (2016), 193–202
Moody, C.O., 'Malnutrition in Children under Five Years of Age in the Dagomba Villages of Northern Ghana', *The Journal of the Royal Institute of Public Health and Hygiene*, 26 (1963), 224–41
Moradi, Alexander, 'Confronting Colonial Legacies – Lessons from Human Development in Ghana and Kenya, 1880–2000', *Journal of International Development*, 20 (2008), 1107–21
Moradi, Alexander, and Joerg Baten, 'Inequality in Sub-Saharan Africa: New Data and New Insights from Anthropometric Estimates', *World Development*, 33.8 (2005), 1233–65
Moran-Thomas, Amy, 'The Para-Communicable: Living between Infectious and Non-Communicable Conditions', in *Epidemiological Change and Chronic Disease in Sub-Saharan Africa: Historical*

and Anthropological Perspectives, ed. by Megan Vaughan, Kafui Adjaye-Gbewonyo, and Marissa Mika (London: UCL Press, 2021), pp. 233–51

Morgan, W.B., 'Food Imports of West Africa', *Economic Geography*, 39.4 (1963), 351–62

Morris, Saul S., Carol E. Levin, Margaret Armar-Klemesu, Daniel Maxwell, and Marie T. Ruel, 'Does Geographic Targeting of Nutrition Interventions Make Sense in Cities? Evidence from Abidjan and Accra', *World Development*, 27.11 (1999), 2011–19

Murton, John, 'Population Growth and Poverty in Machakos District, Kenya', *The Geographical Journal*, 165.1 (1999), 37–46

Musoke, Latimer K., 'An Analysis of Admissions to the Paediatric Division, Mulago Hospital in 1959', *Archives of Disease in Childhood*, 36.187 (1961), 305–15

Neel, James V., 'Diabetes Mellitus: A "Thrifty" Genotype Rendered Detrimental by "Progress"?', *American Journal of Human Genetics*, 14.4 (1962), 353–62

Nicholas, Stephen, and Deborah Oxley, 'The Living Standards of Women during the Industrial Revolution, 1795–1820', *The Economic History Review*, 46.4 (1993), 723–49

Niewöhner, Jörg, 'Epigenetics: Embedded Bodies and the Molecularisation of Biography and Milieu', *BioSocieties*, 6.3 (2011), 279–98

Niewöhner, Jörg, and Margaret Lock, 'Situating Local Biologies: Anthropological Perspectives on Environment/Human Entanglements', *BioSocieties*, 13.4 (2018), 681–97

Nixon, J.A., 'Famine Dropsy as a Food-Deficiency Disease', *Bristol Medico-Chirurgical Journal*, 37.140 (1920), 137–48

Normet, L., 'La Bouffissure d'Annam', *Bulletin de La Société de Pathologie Exotique*, 3 (1926), 207–13

Nott, John, '"How Little Progress"? A Political Economy of Postcolonial Nutrition', *Population and Development Review*, 44.4 (2018), 771–91

Nott, John, 'Malnutrition in a Modernising Economy: The Changing Aetiology and Epidemiology of Malnutrition in an African Kingdom, Buganda c.1940–73', *Medical History*, 60.2 (2016), 229–49

Nott, John, 'Material History, Historied Materials and the Question of Epistemic Freedom in Ghana's Medical Schools', *Social History of Medicine*, 37.1 (2023), pp. 116–40

Nott, John, '"No One May Starve in the British Empire": Kwashiorkor, Protein and the Politics of Nutrition Between Britain and Africa', *Social History of Medicine*, 34.2 (2021), 553–76

Nugent, Paul, 'Educating Rawlings: The Evolution of Government Strategy Towards Smuggling', in *Ghana: The Political Economy of Recovery*, ed. by Donald S. Rothchild (Boulder, CO: Lynne Rienner, 1991), pp. 69–84

Nweke, Felix I., 'Direct Governmental Production in Agriculture in Ghana: Consequences for Food Production and Consumption, 1960–1966 and 1967–1975', *Food Policy*, 3.3 (1978), 202–8

Nweke, Felix I., 'The Organisation of Agricultural Research in Ghana: Priorities, Problems, Implications for Domestic Food Production and Policy Issues', *Agricultural Administration*, 6.1 (1979), 19–29

Nyanteng, V.K., and A. Wayo Seini, 'Agricultural Policy and the Impact on Growth and Productivity 1970–95', in *Economic Reforms in Ghana: The Miracle and the Mirage*, ed. by Ernest Aryeetey, Jane Harrigan, and Machiko Nissanke (Oxford: James Curry, 2000), pp. 267–83

Ó Gráda, Cormac, and Kevin H. O'Rourke, 'Migration as Disaster Relief: Lessons from the Great Irish Famine', *European Review of Economic History*, 1.1 (1997), 3–25

Obeng-Odoom, Franklin, 'Neoliberalism and the Urban Economy in Ghana: Urban Employment, Inequality, and Poverty', *Growth and Change*, 43.1 (2012), 85–109

Obeng-Odoom, Franklin, 'The Informal Sector in Ghana under Siege', *Journal of Developing Societies*, 27.3–4 (2011), 355–92

Ofori-Sarpong, E., 'The 1981–1983 Drought in Ghana', *Singapore Journal of Tropical Geography*, 7.2 (1986), 108–27

Ofosu-Amaah, S., 'The Maternal and Child Health Services in Ghana', *Ghana Medical Journal*, 6.2 (1967), 51–59

Omran, Abdel R., 'The Epidemiologic Transition: A Theory of the Epidemiology of Population Change', *The Milbank Memorial Fund Quarterly*, 49.4 (1971), 509–38

de Onis, M., 'Assessment of Differences in Linear Growth among Populations in the WHO Multicentre Growth Reference Study', *Acta Pædiatrica*, 95 (2006), 56–65

de Onis, M., and R. Yip, 'The WHO Growth Chart: Historical Considerations and Current Scientific Issues', *Bibliotheca Nutritio Et Dieta*, 53 (1996), 74–89

Opare, Mary, and Judy E. Mill, 'The Evolution of Nursing Education in a Postindependence Context: Ghana from 1957 to 1970', *Western Journal of Nursing Research*, 22.8 (2000), 936–44
Oppong, Christine, 'Some Roles of Women: What Do We Know?', in *Family and Development in Ghana*, ed. by Elizabeth Ardayfio-Schandorf (Legon, Accra: Ghana Universities Press, 1994), pp. 57–94
Orraca-Tetteh, R., 'Effects of Rapid Population Growth in Ghana on Nutritional Needs', in *Symposium on Implications of Population Trends for Policy Measures in West Africa*, ed. by N.O. Addo et al., Ghana Population Studies No. 3 (Legon, Accra: University of Ghana, 1971), pp. 57–68
Osei, Philip D., 'Political Liberalisation and the Implementation of Value Added Tax in Ghana', *The Journal of Modern African Studies*, 38.2 (2000), 255–78
Ostry, Jonathan D., Prakash Loungani, and Davide Furceri, 'Neoliberalism: Oversold?', *Finance & Development*, 53.2 (2016), 38–41
Otero, Gerardo, Gabriela Pechlaner, Giselle Liberman, and Efe Gürcan, 'The Neoliberal Diet and Inequality in the United States', *Social Science & Medicine*, 142 (2015), 47–55
Overå, Ragnhild, 'When Men Do Women's Work: Structural Adjustment, Unemployment and Changing Gender Relations in the Informal Economy of Accra, Ghana', *The Journal of Modern African Studies*, 45.4 (2007), 539–63
Owen, Christopher G., Richard M. Martin, Peter H. Whincup, George Davey Smith, and Derek G. Cook, 'Does Breastfeeding Influence Risk of Type 2 Diabetes in Later Life? A Quantitative Analysis of Published Evidence', *The American Journal of Clinical Nutrition*, 84.5 (2006), 1043–54
Owen, Christopher G., Richard M. Martin, Peter H. Whincup, George Davey Smith, and Derek G. Cook, 'Effect of Infant Feeding on the Risk of Obesity across the Life Course: A Quantitative Review of Published Evidence', *Pediatrics*, 115.5 (2005), 1367–77
Parker, John, 'Northern Gothic: Witches, Ghosts and Werewolves in the Savanna Hinterland of the Gold Coast, 1900s–1950s', *Africa*, 76.3 (2006), 352–80
Patterson, K. David, 'Health in Urban Ghana: The Case of Accra 1900–1940', *Social Science & Medicine. Medical Anthropology*, 13B.4 (1979), 251–68
Patterson, K. David, 'River Blindness in Northern Ghana', in *Disease in African History: An Introductory Survey and Case Studies*, ed. by K. David Patterson and Gerald W. Hartwig (Durham, NC: Duke University Press, 1978), pp. 88–117
Patterson, K. David, 'The Influenza Epidemic of 1918–19 in the Gold Coast', *Journal of African History*, 24.4 (1983), 485–502
Patterson, K. David, 'The Veterinary Department and the Animal Industry in the Gold Coast, 1909–1955', *The International Journal of African Historical Studies*, 13 (1980), 457–91
Petty, Celia, 'Primary Research and Public Health: The Prioritisation of Nutrition Research in Inter-War Britain', in *Historical Perspectives on the Role of the MRC: Essays in the History of the Medical Research Council of the United Kingdom and Its Predecessor, the Medical Research Committee, 1913–1953*, ed. by J. Austoker and L. Bryder (Oxford: Oxford University Press, 1989), pp. 83–108
Pfeiffer, James, and Rachel Chapman, 'Anthropological Perspectives on Structural Adjustment and Public Health', *Annual Review of Anthropology*, 39.1 (2010), 149–65
Piwoz, Ellen G., and Sandra L. Huffman, 'The Impact of Marketing of Breast-Milk Substitutes on WHO-Recommended Breastfeeding Practices', *Food and Nutrition Bulletin*, 36.4 (2015), 373–86
Plange, Nii-K., 'Underdevelopment in Northern Ghana: Natural Causes or Colonial Capitalism?', *Review of African Political Economy*, 6.15/16 (1979), 4–14
Platteau, Jean-Philippe, 'The Food Crisis in Africa: A Comparative Structural Analysis', in *The Political Economy of Hunger: Volume 2, Famine Prevention*, ed. by Jean Drèze and Amartya Sen (Oxford: Oxford University Press, 1991), pp. 279–388
Popkin, Barry M., 'The Nutrition Transition in Low-Income Countries: An Emerging Crisis', *Nutrition Reviews*, 52.9 (1994), 285–98
Procter, R.A.W., 'Medical Work in a Native Reserve', *Kenya Medical Journal*, 3 (1926), 284–9
Purcell, F.M., 'Beri-Beri or Epidemic Dropsy', *West African Medical Journal*, 7.4 (1934), 143–5
Randall, Sara, and Ernestina Coast, 'Poverty in African Households: The Limits of Survey and Census Representations', *The Journal of Development Studies*, 51.2 (2015), 162–77
Rangasami, Amrita, '"Failure of Exchange Entitlements" Theory of Famine: A Response', *Economic and Political Weekly*, 20 (1985), 1797–801

Rebrovick, Tripp, 'The Politics of Diet: "Eco-Dietetics," Neoliberalism, and the History of Dietetic Discourses', *Political Research Quarterly*, 68.4 (2015), 678–89
Redfield, Peter, 'Bioexpectations: Life Technologies as Humanitarian Goods', *Public Culture*, 24.1 66 (2012), 157–84
Rhodie, Sam, 'The Gold Coast Cocoa Hold-up of 1930–31', *Transactions of the Historical Society of Ghana*, 9 (1968), 105–18
Rijpma, Sjoerd, 'Malnutrition in the History of Tropical Africa', *Civilisations*, 43.2 (1996), 45–63
Robbins, Joel, 'The Globalization of Pentecostal and Charismatic Christianity', *Annual Review of Anthropology*, 33.1 (2004), 117–43
Roberts, Penelope, 'The State and the Regulation of Marriage: Sefwi Wiawso (Ghana), 1900–40', in *Women, State, and Ideology: Studies from Africa and Asia*, ed. by Haleh Afshar (Albany, NY: SUNY Press, 1987), pp. 48–69
Robertson, Claire, 'The Death of Makola and Other Tragedies', *Canadian Journal of African Studies*, 17.3 (1983), 469–95
Robins, Jonathan E., '"Food Comes First": The Development of Colonial Nutritional Policy in Ghana, 1900–1950', *Global Food History*, 4.2 (2018), 168–88
Robotham, Don, 'The Ghana Problem', *Labour, Capital and Society*, 21.1 (1988), 12–35
Roemer, Michael, 'Ghana 1950–80: Missed Opportunities', in *World Economic Growth: Case Studies of Developed and Developing Nations*, ed. by Arnold C. Harberger (San Francisco, CA: ICS Press, 1984), pp. 201–26
Rönnbäck, Klas, 'The Idle and the Industrious – European Ideas about the African Work Ethic in Precolonial West Africa', *History in Africa*, 41 (2014), 117–45
Ruel, Marie T., Carol E. Levin, Margaret Armar-Klemesu, Daniel Maxwell, and Saul S. Morris, 'Good Care Practices Can Mitigate the Negative Effects of Poverty and Low Maternal Schooling on Children's Nutritional Status: Evidence from Accra', *World Development*, 27.11 (1999), 1993–2009
Russell, Beatrice A.S., 'Malnutrition in Children under Three Years of Age in Ashanti, West Africa', *Archives of Disease in Childhood*, 21.106 (1946), 110–12
Ruttan, Vernon W., 'The Politics of U.S. Food Aid Policy: A Historical Review', in *Why Food Aid?*, ed. by Vernon W. Ruttan (Baltimore, MD: Johns Hopkins University Press, 1993), pp. 2–38
Saha, Jonathan, 'Milk to Mandalay: Dairy Consumption, Animal History and the Political Geography of Colonial Burma', *Journal of Historical Geography*, 54 (2016), 1–12
Sai, Fred T., 'Changing Perspectives of Population in Africa and International Responses', *African Affairs*, 87.347 (1988), 267–76
Sai, Fred T., 'Introducing New Foods Against Protein Deficiency', *Nutrition Reviews*, 18.12 (1960), 353–5
Sai, Fred T., 'Nutrition in Ghana', in *Nutrition and National Policy*, ed. by Beverly Winikoff (Cambridge, MA: MIT Press, 1978), pp. 81–107
Sai, Fred T., 'The Impact of Urban Life on the Diets of Rural Immigrants and Its Repercussions on the Nutritional Status of the Community', *Ghana Medical Journal*, 6.4 (1967), 134–9
Sai, F.T., P.L.H. Davey, and P. Whitby, 'A National Food and Nutrition Survey Project', *Postgraduate Medical Journal*, 38.436 (1962), 112–20
Sanuade, Olutobi, 'Estimating and Monitoring the Burden of Non-Communicable and Chronic Diseases in Ghana', in *Epidemiological Change and Chronic Disease in Sub-Saharan Africa: Historical and Anthropological Perspectives*, ed. by Megan Vaughan, Kafui Adjaye-Gbewonyo, and Marissa Mika (London: UCL Press, 2021), pp. 212–30
Sanjek, Roger, 'Maid Servants and Market Women's Apprentices in Adabraka', in *At Work in Homes: Household Workers in World Perspective*, ed. by Roger Sanjek and Shellee Cohen (Washington, D.C.: American Anthropological Association, 1990), pp. 35–62
Sarfo-Kantanka, Osei, F.S. Sarfo, E. Oparebea Ansah, B. Eghan, N.K. Ayisi-Boateng, and E. Acheamfour-Akowuah, 'Secular Trends in Admissions and Mortality Rates from Diabetes Mellitus in the Central Belt of Ghana: A 31-Year Review', *PLOS ONE*, 11.11 (2016), 1–14
Sasson, Tehila, 'Milking the Third World? Humanitarianism, Capitalism, and the Moral Economy of the Nestlé Boycott', *The American Historical Review*, 121.4 (2016), 1196–224
Sasson, Tehila, and James Vernon, 'Practising the British Way of Famine: Technologies of Relief, 1770–1985', *European Review of History: Revue Européenne d'histoire*, 22.6 (2015), 860–72
Schoenmaeckers, R., I.H. Shah, R. Lesthaeghe, and O. Tambashe, 'The Child-Spacing Tradition and the Postpartum Taboo in Tropical Africa: Anthropological Evidence', in *Child-Spacing in*

Tropical Africa: Traditions and Change, ed. by H.J. Page and R. Schoenmaeckers (New York: Academic Press, 1981), pp. 25–71
Schofield, C., and A. Ashworth, 'Why Have Mortality Rates for Severe Malnutrition Remained so High?', *Bulletin of the World Health Organization*, 74.2 (1996), 223–9
Scott-Smith, Tom, 'Beyond the "Raw" and the "Cooked": A History of Fortified Blended Foods', *Disasters*, 39.2 (2015), 244–60
Scott-Smith, Tom, 'Control and Biopower in Contemporary Humanitarian Aid: The Case of Supplementary Feeding', *Journal of Refugee Studies*, 28.1 (2014), 1–17
Scott-Smith, Tom, 'Humanitarian Neophilia: The "Innovation Turn" and Its Implications', *Third World Quarterly*, 37.12 (2016), 2229–51
Scott-Smith, Tom, 'The Fetishism of Humanitarian Objects and the Management of Malnutrition in Emergencies', *Third World Quarterly*, 34.5 (2013), 913–28
Shaffer, Paul, 'Seasonal Hunger in the Northern Territories of the Gold Coast, 1900–40', *Economic History of Developing Regions*, 32.3 (2017), 270–300
Shammas, Carole, 'The Eighteenth-Century English Diet and Economic Change', *Explorations in Economic History*, 21.3 (1984), 254–69
Shanahan, T.M., J.T. Overpeck, K.J. Anchukaitis, J.W. Beck, J.E. Cole, D.L. Dettman, et al., 'Atlantic Forcing of Persistent Drought in West Africa', *Science*, 324.5925 (2009), 377–80
Shapin, Steven, 'How to Eat Like a Gentleman: Dietetics and Ethics in Early Modern England', in *In Right Living: An Anglo-American Tradition of Self-Help Medicine and Hygiene*, ed. by C. Rosenberg (Baltimore, MD: Johns Hopkins University Press, 2003), pp. 21–58
Shee, George F., 'The Deterioration in the National Physique', *Nineteenth Century*, 52 (1903), 797–805
Shepherd, Andrew, 'Agrarian Change in Northern Ghana: Public Investment, Capitalist Farming and Famine', in *Rural Development in Tropical Africa*, ed. by Judith Heyer, Pepe Roberts, and Gavin Williams (London: Palgrave Macmillan, 1981), pp. 168–92
Shore, Cris, and Susan Wright, 'Governing by Numbers: Audit Culture, Rankings and the New World Order', *Social Anthropology*, 23.1 (2015), 22–8
Simpson Miller, Brandi, 'Food and Nationalism in an Independent Ghana', in *The Emergence of National Food: The Dynamics of Food and Nationalism*, ed. by Atsuko Ichijo, Venetia Johannes, and Ronald Ranta (London: Bloomsbury Publishing, 2019), pp. 61–70
Smith, Lisa C., Marie T. Ruel, and Aida Ndiaye, 'Why Is Child Malnutrition Lower in Urban Than in Rural Areas? Evidence from 36 Developing Countries', *World Development*, 33.8 (2005), 1285–305
Smith, Robyn, 'The Emergence of Vitamins as Bio-Political Objects during World War I', *Studies in History and Philosophy of Biological and Biomedical Sciences*, 40.3 (2009), 179–89
Soloway, Richard, 'Counting the Degenerates: The Statistics of Race Deterioration in Edwardian England', *Journal of Contemporary History*, 17.1 (1982), 137–64
Southall, Roger J., 'Farmers, Traders and Brokers in the Gold Coast Cocoa Economy', *Canadian Journal of African Studies*, 12.2 (1978), 185–211
Sparr, Pamela, 'Feminist Critiques of Structural Adjustment', in *Mortgaging Women's Lives: Feminist Critiques of Structural Adjustment*, ed. by Pamela Sparr (London: ZED Books, 1994), pp. 13–39
Stannus, Hugh S., 'Kwashiorkor', *The Lancet*, 226.5856 (1935), 1207–8
Stanton, J., 'Listening to the Ga: Cicely Williams' Discovery of Kwashiorkor on the Gold Coast', *Clio Medica*, 61 (2001), 149–71
Steckel, Richard H., 'Heights and Human Welfare: Recent Developments and New Directions', *Explorations in Economic History*, 46.1 (2009), 1–23
Steckel, Richard H., 'Stature and the Standard of Living', *Journal of Economic Literature*, 33.4 (1995), 1903–40
Steel, Robert W., 'Problems of Population Pressure in Tropical Africa', *Transactions of the Institute of British Geographers*, 49 (1970), 1–14
Stephens, Rhiannon, 'Poverty's Pasts: A Case for Longue Durée Studies', *The Journal of African History*, 59.3 (2018), 399–409
Stewart, Frances, 'The Many Faces of Adjustment', *World Development*, 19.12 (1991), 1847–64
Stoces, Ferdinand, 'Agricultural Production in Ghana, 1955–65', *The Economic Bulletin of Ghana*, 10.3 (1966), 3–32
Street, Alice, 'Food as Pharma: Marketing Nutraceuticals to India's Rural Poor', *Critical Public Health*, 25.3 (2015), 361–72

Sutton, Inez, 'Colonial Agricultural Policy: The Non-Development of the Northern Territories of the Gold Coast', *The International Journal of African Historical Studies*, 22.4 (1989), 637–69

de Swaan, Abram, 'Elite Perceptions of the Poor: Reflections on a Comparative Research Project', in *Elite Perceptions of Poverty and Inequality*, ed. by Elisa Pereira Reis and Mick Moore (London: ZED Books, 2005), pp. 182–94

Szreter, Simon, 'The Epidemiologic Transition Turned Upside down: Britain's Mortality History as an Imaginative Resource for Africa', in *Epidemiological Change and Chronic Disease in Sub-Saharan Africa: Historical and Anthropological Perspectives*, ed. by Megan Vaughan, Kafui Adjaye-Gbewonyo, and Marissa Mika (London: UCL Press, 2021), pp. 39–79

Szreter, Simon, 'The Idea of Demographic Transition and the Study of Fertility Change: A Critical Intellectual History', *Population and Development Review*, 19.4 (1993), 659–701

Tait, David, 'A Sorcery Hunt in Dagomba', *Africa*, 33.2 (1963), 136–47

Takyiwaa, Manu, 'Ghana: Women in the Public and Informal Sectors under the Economic Recovery Programme', in *Mortgaging Women's Lives: Feminist Critiques of Structural Adjustment*, ed. by Pamela Sparr (London: ZED Books, 1994), pp. 61–77

Tanko, Mohammed, Salifu Ismaila, and Saeed Abu Sadiq, 'Planting for Food and Jobs (PFJ): A Panacea for Productivity and Welfare of Rice Farmers in Northern Ghana', *Cogent Economics & Finance*, 7.1 (2019), 1693121

Tedlie, H., 'Materia Medica and Diseases', in *Mission from Cape Coast Castle to Ashantee: With a Statistical Account of That Kingdom and Geographical Notices of Other Parts of the Interior of Africa*, by T.E. Bowdich (London: John Murray, 1819), pp. 370–80

Tette, Edem M.A., Margaret Neizer, Maame Yaa Nyarko, Eric K. Sifah, Edmund T. Nartey, and Eric S. Donkor, 'Changing Patterns of Disease and Mortality at the Children's Hospital, Accra: Are Infections Rising?', *PLOS ONE*, 11.4 (2016), 1–12

Tette, Edem M.A., Eric K. Sifah, Edmund T. Nartey, Peter Nuro-Ameyaw, Pricilla Tete-Donkor, and Richard B. Biritwum, 'Maternal Profiles and Social Determinants of Malnutrition and the MDGs: What Have We Learnt?', *BMC Public Health*, 16 (2016), 214

Thang, Nguyen Minh, and Barry M. Popkin, 'In an Era of Economic Growth, Is Inequity Holding Back Reductions in Child Malnutrition in Vietnam?', *Asia Pacific Journal of Clinical Nutrition*, 12.4 (2003), 405–10

Thomas, Roger G., 'Forced Labour in British West Africa: The Case of the Northern Territories of the Gold Coast 1906–1927', *Journal of African History*, 14.1 (1973), 79–103

Tommaselli, Giovanni A., Maurizio Guida, Stefano Palomba, Michele Barbato, and Carmine Nappi, 'Using Complete Breastfeeding and Lactational Amenorrhoea as Birth Spacing Methods', *Contraception*, 61.4 (2000), 253–7

Townsend, Peter, 'Poverty as Relative Deprivation: Resources and Style of Living', in *Poverty, Inequality & Class Structure*, ed. by Dorothy Wedderburn (Cambridge: Cambridge University Press, 1975), pp. 15–42

Trowell, H.C., 'Infantile Pellagra', *Transactions of the Royal Society of Tropical Medicine and Hygiene*, 33 (1940), 389–404

Trowell, H.C., 'Malignant Malnutrition (Kwashiorkor)', *Transactions of the Royal Society of Tropical Medicine and Hygiene*, 42.5 (1949), 417–42

Trowell, H.C., 'The Beginning of the Kwashiorkor Story in Africa', *Central African Journal of Medicine*, 21.1 (1975), 1–5

Trowell, H.C., J.N.P. Davies, and R.F.A. Dean, 'Kwashiorkor – II. Clinical Picture, Pathology, and Diagnosis', *British Medical Journal*, 2.4788 (1952), 798–801

Truswell, A. Stewart, 'Protein-Energy Malnutrition', in *Essentials of Human Nutrition*, ed. by A. Stewart Truswell and Jim Mann (Oxford: Oxford University Press, 2012), pp. 301–9

Tsey, Komla, and Stephanie D. Short, 'From Headloading to the Iron Horse: The Unequal Health Consequences of Railway Construction and Expansion in the Gold Coast, 1898–1929', *Social Science & Medicine*, 40.5 (1995), 613–21

Twumasi, P.A., 'Colonialism and International Health: A Study in Social Change in Ghana', *Social Science & Medicine. Medical Anthropology*, 15B.2 (1981), 147–51

Uauy, Ricardo, Cecilia Albala, and Juliana Kain, 'Obesity Trends in Latin America: Transiting from Under- to Overweight', *The Journal of Nutrition*, 131.3 (2001), 893S–899S

UNICEF, 'Adjustment Policies and Programmes to Protect Children and Other Vulnerable Groups in Ghana', in *Adjustment with a Human Face: Country Case Studies*, ed. by Giovanni Andrea Cornia, Richard Jolly, and Frances Stewart, 2 vols (Oxford: Clarendon Press, 1987), ii, 93–125

Vail, Leroy, 'Ecology and History: The Example of Eastern Zambia', *Journal of Southern African Studies*, 3.2 (1977), 129–55
Van de Poel, Ellen, Ahmad Reza Hosseinpoor, Caroline Jehu-Appiah, Jeanette Vega, and Niko Speybroeck, 'Malnutrition and the Disproportional Burden on the Poor: The Case of Ghana', *International Journal for Equity in Health*, 6 (2007), 1–12
Vaughan, Megan, 'Conceptualising Metabolic Disorder in Southern Africa: Biology, History and Global Health', *BioSocieties*, 14.1 (2019), 123–42
Vella, Venanzio, Andrew Tomkins, John Nviku, and Tom Marshall, 'Determinants of Nutritional Status in South-West Uganda', *Journal of Tropical Pediatrics*, 41.2 (1995), 89–98
Vellenga, Dorothy Dee, 'Matriliny, Patriliny, and Class Formation Among Women Cocoa Farmers in Two Rural Areas of Ghana', in *Women and Class in Africa*, ed. by Claire Robertson and Iris Berger (New York: Africana Publishing Company, 1986), pp. 62–77
Vellenga, Dorothy Dee, 'Who Is a Wife? Legal Expressions of Heterosexual Conflicts in Ghana', in *Female and Male in West Africa*, ed. by Christine Oppong (London: George Allen & Unwin, 1983), pp. 144–55
Vernon, James, 'The Ethics of Hunger and the Assembly of Society: The Techno-Politics of the School Meal in Modern Britain', *The American Historical Review*, 110.3 (2005), 693–725
Volta, B., 'The Future of Ghana's Wildlife', *The Ghana Farmer*, 15.1 (1971), 30–5
Waddington, C.J., and K.A. Enyimayew, 'A Price to Pay: The Impact of User Charges in Ashanti-Akim District, Ghana', *The International Journal of Health Planning and Management*, 4.1 (1989), 17–47
Waddy, B.B., 'A District Medical Officer in North-West Ghana', in *Health in Tropical Africa During the Colonial Period*, ed. by E.E. Sabben-Clarke, D.J. Bradley, and K. Kirkwood (Oxford: Clarendon Press, 1980), pp. 159–65
Waddy, B.B., 'Heights and Weights of Children in the Northern Territories of the Gold Coast', *Journal of Tropical Medicine and Hygiene*, 59.1 (1956), 1–4
Waddy, B.B., 'Organization and Work of the Gold Coast Medical Field Units', *Transactions of The Royal Society of Tropical Medicine and Hygiene*, 50.4 (1956), 313–43
Wallace, Tina, 'NGO Dilemmas: Trojan Horses for Global Neoliberalism?', *Socialist Register*, 40 (2009), 202–19
Waterlow, J.C., and P.R. Payne, 'The Protein Gap', *Nature*, 258.5531 (1975), 113–17
Watts, Michael, 'Entitlements or Empowerment? Famine and Starvation in Africa', *Review of African Political Economy*, 51 (1991), 9–26
Webber, Paul, 'Agrarian Change in Kusasi, North-East Ghana', *Africa*, 66.3 (1996), 437–57
Weiss, Holger, 'Crop Failures, Food Shortages and Colonial Famine Relief Policies in the Northern Territories of the Gold Coast', *Ghana Studies*, 6 (2003), 5–58
Welbourn, H.F., 'Backgrounds and Follow-Up of Children with Kwashiorkor', *Journal of Tropical Pediatrics*, 5 (1959), 91
Welbourn, H.F., 'Bottle Feeding: A Problem of Modern Civilization', *Journal of Tropical Pediatrics*, 3.4 (1958), 157–66
Welbourn, H.F., 'The Danger Period During Weaning', *Journal of Tropical Pediatrics*, 1.1 (1955), 34–46
Werlin, Herbert H., 'The Consequences of Corruption: The Ghanaian Experience', *Political Science Quarterly*, 88.1 (1973), 71–85
Westoff, Charles F., 'Is the KAP-Gap Real?', *Population and Development Review*, 14.2 (1988), 225–32
White, Howard, 'Combining Quantitative and Qualitative Approaches in Poverty Analysis', *World Development*, 30.3 (2002), 511–22
White, Howard, and Edward Anderson, 'Growth versus Distribution: Does the Pattern of Growth Matter?', *Development Policy Review*, 19.3 (2001), 267–89
White, H.P., 'Internal Exchange of Staple Foods in the Gold Coast', *Economic Geography*, 32.2 (1956), 115–25
Whiting, J.W.M., 'Effects of Climate on Certain Cultural Practices', in *Explorations in Cultural Anthropology*, by W. Goodenough (New York: McGraw-Hill, 1964), pp. 511–44
Whyte, Susan Reynolds, 'Knowing Hypertension and Diabetes: Conditions of Treatability in Uganda', *Health & Place*, 39 (2016), 219–25
Wiemers, Alice, 'A "Time of Agric": Rethinking the "Failure" of Agricultural Programs in 1970s Ghana', *World Development*, 66 (2015), 104–17

Wilhelm, Lola, '"One of the Most Urgent Problems to Solve": Malnutrition, Trans-Imperial Nutrition Science, and Nestlé's Medical Pursuits in Late Colonial Africa', *The Journal of Imperial and Commonwealth History*, 48.5 (2020), 914–33

Wilkinson, Richard G., and Kate E. Pickett, 'Income Inequality and Social Dysfunction', *Annual Review of Sociology*, 35 (2009), 493–511

Williams, Cicely D., 'A Nutritional Disease of Childhood Associated with a Maize Diet', *Archives of Disease in Childhood*, 8 (1933), 423–33

Williams, Cicely D., 'Child Health in the Gold Coast', *The Lancet*, 231 (1938), 97–102

Williams, Cicely D., 'Council on Foods and Nutrition', *Journal of the American Medical Association*, 153.14 (1953), 1280–5

Williams, Cicely D., 'Kwashiorkor: A Nutritional Disease of Children Associated with a Maize Diet', *The Lancet*, 226 (1935), 1151

Williams, Cicely D., 'Maternal and Child Health in Kumasi in 1935', *Journal of Tropical Pediatrics*, 2.3 (1956), 141–6

Worboys, Michael, 'The Discovery of Colonial Malnutrition Between the Wars', in *Imperial Medicine and Indigenous Societies*, ed. by David Arnold (Manchester: Manchester University Press, 1988), pp. 208–25

Wrigley-Asante, Charlotte, Samuel Agyei-Mensah, and Faustina Adomaa Obeng, 'It's Not All about Wealth and Beauty: Changing Perceptions of Fatness among Makola Market Women of Accra, Ghana', *Singapore Journal of Tropical Geography*, 3.38 (2017), 414–28

Yaro, Joseph Awetori, 'Is Deagrarianisation Real? A Study of Livelihood Activities in Rural Northern Ghana', *The Journal of Modern African Studies*, 44.1 (2006), 125–56

Yarom, R., and J. McFie, 'Kwashiorkor in the Congo: A Clinical Survey of a Hundred Successive Cases in the Kasai Province', *The Journal of Tropical Pediatrics and Environmental Child Health*, 9 (1963), 56–63

Zeng, Ning, 'Drought in the Sahel', *Science*, 302.5647 (2003), 999–1000

Index

Page references in *italics* are to figures; references to notes are indicated by n.